OPCS Classification of Interventions and Procedures, Version 4.7

Volume I

Tabular List

London: TSO

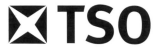

information & publishing solutions

Published by TSO (The Stationery Office) and available from:

Online
www.tsoshop.co.uk

Mail, Telephone, Fax & E-mail
TSO
PO Box 29, Norwich, NR3 1GN
Telephone orders/General enquiries: 0870 600 5522
Fax orders: 0870 600 5533
E-mail: customer.services@tso.co.uk
Textphone: 0870 240 3701

TSO@Blackwell and other Accredited Agents

An Alphabetical Index Tabular List (volume II) is available separately under ISBN 978 0 11 322991 8
Both volumes can be purchased together at a discounted price, if ordered under
ISBN 978 0 11 322992 5

First published 2014

ISBN 978 0 11 322990 1

Printed in the United Kingdom for The Stationery Office

TABLE OF CONTENTS

INTRODUCTION

Welcome to the OPCS Classification of Interventions and Procedures Version 4.7, to be used in the NHS from 1 April 2014.

The classification is an NHS Fundamental Information Standard developed and maintained by the Health and Social Care Information Centre, Clinical Classifications Service. The classification is used by health care providers and commissioners throughout the NHS.

The OPCS-4 is available as an eVersion and replicates the familiar style of the OPCS-4 Tabular List and Alphabetical Index, with the added benefits of a powerful search engine and annotation.

THE CLASSIFICATION

The OPCS-4 classification supports various forms of data collection, such as Central Returns and Commissioning Data Sets, as well as other secondary uses of information essential to planning and improving patient care. Among these secondary uses are:

- Operational and strategic planning,
- Resource use,
- National and local planning and performance management,
- Epidemiology,
- Department of Health initiatives, and
- Information grouped by Healthcare Resource Groups.

Developments in healthcare and the increasing diversity of interventions and procedures mean that any classification system can rapidly become out of date.

The enhancements provided in OPCS-4.7 continue to reflect changes to clinical care in recent years, and enable clinicians (in collaboration with clinical coders) to better describe interventions and procedures. As a result the enhanced classification will further improve the quality of coded clinical data. The ability to provide improved clinical information continues to ensure the classification also meets the needs of NHS funding via Payment by Results (PbR).

This version has been completed in collaboration with Consultant Specialists from the Craniofacial Unit at Oxford University Hospitals, Consultant Gynaecology Specialist at University College London Hospitals (UCLH), the Department of Health, and clinical Expert Working Groups representing the Royal Colleges. Their support in delivering the revised classification is gratefully acknowledged.

The Clinical Classifications Service is also indebted to all those who made time available to support the development. It would not have been achieved without the valuable input of all those that submitted requests for change, reviewed the proposed changes and tested the eVersion.

The Revision Process

The first major revision of OPCS-4 in 15 years was successfully implemented in the NHS in April 2006. The revision was not only a long overdue improvement in the ability to record clinical coding detail, but also met the needs of Government health policy at that time. OPCS-4.3 allowed the NHS to better record clinical interventions and procedures. This feature, which went beyond the recording of surgical procedures found in previous versions of the classification, was reflected in the change of name to OPCS Classification of Interventions and Procedures.

The following table lists OPCS-4 versions and the financial year in which they were mandated for use:

Financial Year	Version of OPCS-4
Up to 31 March 2006	OPCS-4.2
1 April 2006 – 31 March 2007	OPCS-4.3
1 April 2007 – 31 March 2009	OPCS-4.4
1 April 2009 – 31 March 2011	OPCS-4.5
1 April 2011 – 31 March 2014	OPCS-4.6
1 April 2014 until further notice	OPCS-4.7

Since September 2007, the Clinical Classifications Service has made it easier for stakeholders to provide requests for change and track their progress with the launch of the online OPCS-4 Requests Portal. This was designed so anyone could submit their suggestions whenever it suited them. The OPCS-4.5 release of the classification was the first which included requests for change received through the portal from all stakeholders of the NHS.

In addition, an up-to-date electronic platform was introduced which provides a more structured and controlled environment in which to produce and validate changes. This enables continual improvements to the content of both the Tabular List and Alphabetical Index for future releases.

Among the improvements to this current updated version of OPCS-4 are:

- More procedures and interventions are available in the Tabular List
- Refinement and addition of includes, excludes and notes in the tabular list
- Refinement and additional entries in the Alphabetical Index

The Structure of the Classification

The basic structure of OPCS-4 remains unchanged in the latest revision.

The Tabular List is mainly comprised of anatomically based chapters, most of which relate to the whole or part of a body system. Each chapter is also designated alphabetically, e.g. Chapter A covers the nervous system and Chapter K the heart. The alphabetic character for each chapter forms the prefix of the 3- and 4- character codes within it.

Capacity

The hierarchical body system structure is no longer as evident when using OPCS-4 and so strict use of the Alphabetical Index and Tabular List notes is imperative to ensure accuracy.

New 3-character categories are placed within chapter ranges, and 4-character codes are added to existing categories where space allows. Alternatively, new codes are placed at the end of the specific body system chapter. For example, categories H01 to H03 are operations on the appendix, whereas category H04 relates to operations on the colon and rectum. Therefore, if there is a requirement for a specific operation on the appendix to be included in OPCS-4, and no room exists within the categories (H01–H03), the code will be placed in the most suitable available space, typically at the end of the chapter.

There are also instances where an existing full category needs extension. In such cases, and dependent on the chapter capacity, an extended category has been added within the chapter.

These categories are referred to as principal category or extended category, and are identified by an accompanying note to ease navigation.

For example:

Principal Category

C46 Plastic operations on cornea
Note: Principal category, extended at C44

Extended Category

C44 Other plastic operations on cornea
Note: Principal C46

The extended categories amplify the capacity of the principal category, containing 4-character codes that have a relationship with the 3-character title of the principal category. The four-step coding process will direct the coder from the Alphabetical Index to both the principal and extended categories in the Tabular List.

When assigning a .8 or .9 code in the Tabular List, the coder should always select the .8 or .9 code from the principal category. The principal category can be distinguished from the extended category by reference to the note, as in the example above.

Once a chapter is full then alpha-numeric categories are assigned using the free alpha O. This has occurred within:

- Chapter L Arteries and Veins,

- Chapter W Other Bones and Joints, and

- Chapter Z Subsidiary Classification of Sites of Operation.

Codes created in this way still form part of an existing chapter, even though they have a different alpha prefix to the rest of that chapter. Such new codes will therefore logically sit at the end of the body system chapter. These codes can be identified by using the Alphabetical Index to determine alignment of the codes to the relevant chapter.

In line with previous practice, the Tabular List incorporates a number of inclusion terms, exclusion terms and notes which assist in the correct assignment of appropriate codes.

Scope of OPCS-4

The scope of OPCS-4 is regulated by the definition of an intervention (as expressed below) and by OPCS-4 Editorial Policy. An Editorial Committee oversee the content development of the OPCS-4 update.

Definition of an Intervention

Interventions are those aspects of clinical care carried out on patients undergoing treatment:

- for the prevention, diagnosis, care or relief of disease

- for the correction of deformity or deficit, including those performed for cosmetic reasons

- associated with pregnancy, childbirth or contraceptive or procreative management.

Typically this will be:

- surgical in nature; and/or

- carries a procedural risk; and/or

- carries an anaesthetic risk; and/or

- requires specialist training; and/or

- requires special facilities or equipment only available in an acute care setting.

Single Procedure Analysis and Multiple Coding

When a series of operations is recorded, it is traditional, as with diagnostic information, to select the first mentioned procedure or intervention for routine analysis.

Main intervention or procedure

When classifying diagnostic information the International Classification of Diseases (ICD) recommends criteria for the selection of the MAIN condition for single-cause analysis. OPCS-4 follows this precedent in that the intervention selected for single-procedure analysis from consultant episodes is the MAIN intervention or procedure carried out during the relevant episode.

Multiple interventions are often carried out simultaneously. OPCS-4 adopts the same rules that applied previously; which are that some combinations have been encompassed within a single category whilst others, with a seemingly similar relationship, are required to be coded separately.

NB: Users of the classification need to ensure that they apply the instruction notes within the Tabular List – Volume I. These are provided to ensure the selection of the correct codes.

Subsidiary Classification of Methods of Operations

Chapter Y provides 'Methods of Operation' codes which are intended for the incorporation of otherwise unclassifiable detail in a far wider range of procedures. For example, Y08 covers different types of laser procedure and identifies the use of this form of treatment when associated with a particular operation. It is not intended that the subsidiary codes derived from this chapter be used in a primary position. They will always be used in a secondary position following a main code from Chapters A–X.

Subsidiary Classification of Sites of Operation

Chapter Z provides a series of site codes which are not intended as primary codes.

Radical Operations

Radical operations are usually neither listed nor tabulated as such in the classification. The term 'radical' can imply an operation on more than one site, e.g. removal of an organ and its associated lymph nodes. Users of the classification must ensure that the classification instructional notes are applied in these cases to fully reflect the intervention performed.

Incomplete or Failed Operations or Procedures

These must be coded to the stage reached at the abandonment of the operation or procedure; the intention must not be coded.

Retirement of a code

Codes fall out of favour for various reasons and there is a mechanism, called retiring, for handling such codes. However, the retirement of a code is only ever considered as a very last option. If an extraordinary circumstance arises where a code/description is considered invalid or incorrect (usually following classification review) the code, the associated problem, an options appraisal to address it and recommendation(s) are provided to the Editorial Committee for a decision. The support of the relevant professional body would also be required in these circumstances to provide appropriate clinical input.

In practice, the code is retired in the classification with a note to that effect and excluded from the metadata file so that it is no longer perpetuated. Additionally, the successor code and the retired code are mapped in the Table of Coding Equivalence.

Instances of retirement are represented in the OPCS-4 Tabular Volume 1 and the Codes and Titles file as follows:

OPCS-4.7:

R03	**Category retired – refer to introduction**
X15.3	**Code retired – refer to introduction**

OPCS-4.5:

X63	**Category retired – refer to introduction**
X64	**Category retired – refer to introduction**

Abbreviations

Specific abbreviations are used in this volume. Their meanings are as follows:

HFQ	However Further Qualified
NEC	Not Elsewhere Classified
NFQ	Not Further Qualified
NOC	Not Otherwise Classifiable
>	Greater than
<	Less than

Prosthesis

For operations involving prosthesis, a special terminology is used to cover the various associated procedures:

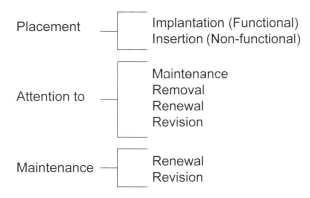

Prosthesis

Placement —— Implantation (Functional)
Insertion (Non-functional)

Attention to —— Maintenance
Removal
Renewal
Revision

Maintenance —— Renewal
Revision

Training and Advice

The Clinical Classifications Service provides a national service with the primary objective of supporting the NHS.

In addition to developing the OPCS-4 information standard, the Clinical Classifications Service provides expert clinical classifications knowledge on the coding standards in use in the NHS. This covers all aspects of guidance, advice, maintenance, implementation, cross-mapping, coding audit, data quality standards, training and accreditation.

The Classifications and Coding Standards Advisory Service promotes consistent application of the coding standards and use of classifications.

The Clinical Classifications Service is committed to ensuring the clinical coder has access to the highest quality clinical coding training. Our training and accreditation strategy sets a framework to support the NHS and to ensure consistent application of coding standards, giving confidence in the quality of coded clinical data.

For more information on our work:
http://systems.hscic.gov.uk/data/clinicalcoding

For all queries relating to clinical coding including the Classifications and Coding Standards Advisory Service (helpdesk):
Email: Information.standards@hscic.gov.uk   Tel: 08451300114

For more information on OPCS-4
http://systems.hscic.gov.uk/data/clinicalcoding/codingstandards/opcs4

To access the online web portal to offer requests for change:
http://systems.hscic.gov.uk/data/clinicalcoding/codingstandards/opcs4/44submissions

To download the eVersion of the OPCS-4 Tabular List and Index go to the Technology Reference Update Distribution Service (TRUD):
http://www.uktcregistration.nss.cfh.nhs.uk/trud3

Part 1

Tabular List
of
Three Digit Categories

A. NERVOUS SYSTEM

Tissue of brain (A01–A11)

A01	Major excision of tissue of brain
A02	Excision of lesion of tissue of brain
A03	Stereotactic ablation of tissue of brain
A04	Open biopsy of lesion of tissue of brain
A05	Drainage of lesion of tissue of brain
A06	Other excision of lesion of tissue of brain
A07	Other open operations on tissue of brain
A08	Other biopsy of lesion of tissue of brain
A09	Neurostimulation of brain
A10	Other operations on tissue of brain
A11	Operations on tissue of brain

Ventricle of brain and subarachnoid space (A12–A22)

A12	Creation of connection from ventricle of brain
A13	Attention to component of connection from ventricle of brain
A14	Other operations on connection from ventricle of brain
A16	Other open operations on ventricle of brain
A17	Therapeutic endoscopic operations on ventricle of brain
A18	Diagnostic endoscopic examination of ventricle of brain
A20	Other operations on ventricle of brain
A22	Operations on subarachnoid space of brain

Cranial nerves (A24–A36)

A24	Graft to cranial nerve
A25	Intracranial transection of cranial nerve
A26	Other intracranial destruction of cranial nerve
A27	Extracranial extirpation of vagus nerve (x)
A28	Extracranial extirpation of other cranial nerve
A29	Excision of lesion of cranial nerve
A30	Repair of cranial nerve
A31	Intracranial stereotactic release of cranial nerve
A32	Other decompression of cranial nerve
A33	Neurostimulation of cranial nerve
A34	Exploration of cranial nerve
A36	Other operations on cranial nerve

Meninges of brain (A38–A43)

A38	Extirpation of lesion of meninges of brain
A39	Repair of dura
A40	Drainage of extradural space
A41	Drainage of subdural space
A42	Other operations on meninges of brain
A43	Other extirpation of lesion of meninges of brain

Spinal cord and other contents of spinal canal (A44–A57)

A44	Partial extirpation of spinal cord
A45	Other open operations on spinal cord
A47	Other destruction of spinal cord
A48	Other operations on spinal cord
A49	Repair of spina bifida
A51	Other operations on meninges of spinal cord
A52	Therapeutic epidural injection
A53	Drainage of spinal canal
A54	Therapeutic spinal puncture
A55	Diagnostic spinal puncture
A57	Operations on spinal nerve root

Peripheral nerves (A59–A73)

A59	Excision of peripheral nerve
A60	Destruction of peripheral nerve
A61	Extirpation of lesion of peripheral nerve
A62	Microsurgical repair of peripheral nerve
A63	Other graft to peripheral nerve
A64	Other repair of peripheral nerve
A65	Release of entrapment of peripheral nerve at wrist
A66	Release of entrapment of peripheral nerve at ankle
A67	Release of entrapment of peripheral nerve at other site
A68	Other release of peripheral nerve
A69	Revision of release of peripheral nerve
A70	Neurostimulation of peripheral nerve
A73	Other operations on peripheral nerve

Other parts of nervous system (A75–A84)

A75	Excision of sympathetic nerve
A76	Chemical destruction of sympathetic nerve
A77	Cryotherapy to sympathetic nerve
A78	Radiofrequency controlled thermal destruction of sympathetic nerve
A79	Other destruction of sympathetic nerve
A81	Other operations on sympathetic nerve
A83	Electroconvulsive therapy
A84	Neurophysiological operations

B. ENDOCRINE SYSTEM AND BREAST

Pituitary and pineal glands (B01–B06)

B01	Excision of pituitary gland
B02	Destruction of pituitary gland
B04	Other operations on pituitary gland
B06	Operations on pineal gland

Thyroid and parathyroid glands (B08–B17)

B08	Excision of thyroid gland
B09	Operations on aberrant thyroid tissue
B10	Operations on thyroglossal tissue
B12	Other operations on thyroid gland
B14	Excision of parathyroid gland
B16	Other operations on parathyroid gland
B17	Transplantation of thymus gland

Other endocrine glands (B18–B25)

B18	Excision of thymus gland
B20	Other operations on thymus gland
B22	Excision of adrenal gland
B23	Operations on aberrant adrenal tissue
B25	Other operations on adrenal gland

Breast (B27–B40)

B27	Total excision of breast
B28	Other excision of breast
B29	Reconstruction of breast
B30	Prosthesis for breast
B31	Other plastic operations on breast
B32	Biopsy of breast
B33	Incision of breast
B34	Operations on duct of breast
B35	Operations on nipple
B36	Reconstruction of nipple and areola
B37	Other operations on breast
B38	Reconstruction of breast using flap of skin of buttock
B39	Reconstruction of breast using abdominal flap
B40	Destruction of lesion of breast

C. EYE

Orbit (C01–C08)

C01	Excision of eye
C02	Extirpation of lesion of orbit
C03	Insertion of prosthesis of eye
C04	Attention to prosthesis of eye
C05	Plastic repair of orbit
C06	Incision of orbit
C08	Other operations on orbit

Eyebrow and eyelid (C09–C23)

C09	Replacement of canthal tendon
C10	Operations on eyebrow
C11	Operations on canthus
C12	Extirpation of lesion of eyelid
C13	Excision of redundant skin of eyelid
C14	Reconstruction of eyelid
C15	Correction of deformity of eyelid
C16	Other plastic repair of eyelid
C17	Other repair of eyelid
C18	Correction of ptosis of eyelid
C19	Incision of eyelid
C20	Protective suture of eyelid
C22	Other operations on eyelid
C23	Operations on eyelid

Lacrimal apparatus (C24–C29)

C24	Operations on lacrimal gland
C25	Connection between lacrimal apparatus and nose
C26	Other operations on lacrimal sac
C27	Operations on nasolacrimal duct
C29	Other operations on lacrimal apparatus

Muscles of eye (C31–C37)

C31	Combined operations on muscles of eye
C32	Recession of muscle of eye
C33	Resection of muscle of eye
C34	Partial division of tendon of muscle of eye
C35	Other adjustment to muscle of eye
C37	Other operations on muscle of eye

Conjunctiva and cornea (C39–C51)

C39	Extirpation of lesion of conjunctiva
C40	Repair of conjunctiva
C41	Incision of conjunctiva
C43	Other operations on conjunctiva
C44	Other plastic operations on cornea
C45	Extirpation of lesion of cornea
C46	Plastic operations on cornea
C47	Closure of cornea
C48	Removal of foreign body from cornea
C49	Incision of cornea
C51	Other operations on cornea

Sclera and iris (C52–C65)

C52	Excision of sclera
C53	Extirpation of lesion of sclera
C54	Buckling operations for attachment of retina
C55	Incision of sclera
C57	Other operations on sclera
C59	Excision of iris
C60	Filtering operations on iris
C61	Other operations on trabecular meshwork of eye
C62	Incision of iris
C64	Other operations on iris
C65	Operations following glaucoma surgery

Anterior chamber of eye and lens (C66–C77)

C66	Extirpation of ciliary body
C67	Other operations on ciliary body
C69	Other operations on anterior chamber of eye
C71	Extracapsular extraction of lens
C72	Intracapsular extraction of lens
C73	Incision of capsule of lens
C74	Other extraction of lens
C75	Prosthesis of lens
C77	Other operations on lens

Retina, other parts of eye and anaesthetics (C79–C90)

C79	Operations on vitreous body
C80	Operations on retinal membrane
C81	Photocoagulation of retina for detachment
C82	Destruction of lesion of retina
C83	Translocation of retina
C84	Other operations on retina
C85	Fixation of retina
C86	Other operations on eye
C87	Evaluation of retina
C88	Destruction of subretinal lesion
C89	Operations on posterior segment of eye
C90	Local anaesthetics for ophthalmology procedures

D. EAR

External ear and external auditory canal (D01–D08)

D01	Excision of external ear
D02	Extirpation of lesion of external ear
D03	Plastic operations on external ear
D04	Drainage of external ear
D05	Attachment of auricular prosthesis
D06	Other operations on external ear
D07	Clearance of external auditory canal
D08	Other operations on external auditory canal

Mastoid and middle ear (D10–D20)

D10 Exenteration of mastoid air cells
D12 Other operations on mastoid
D13 Attachment of bone anchored hearing prosthesis
D14 Repair of eardrum
D15 Drainage of middle ear
D16 Reconstruction of ossicular chain
D17 Other operations on ossicle of ear
D19 Extirpation of lesion of middle ear
D20 Other operations on middle ear

Inner ear and eustachian canal (D22–D28)

D22 Operations on eustachian canal
D23 Operations on inner ear
D24 Operations on cochlea
D26 Operations on vestibular apparatus
D28 Other operations on ear

E. RESPIRATORY TRACT

Nose (E01–E11, E64–E65)

E01 Excision of nose
E02 Plastic operations on nose
E03 Operations on septum of nose
E04 Operations on turbinate of nose
E05 Surgical arrest of bleeding from internal nose
E06 Packing of cavity of nose
E07 Other plastic operations on nose
E08 Other operations on internal nose
E09 Operations on external nose
E10 Other operations on nose
E11 Operations on fixtures for nasal prosthesis
E64 Therapeutic endoscopic operations on nasal cavity
E65 Diagnostic endoscopic examination of nasal cavity

Nasal sinuses (E12–E17)

E12 Operations on maxillary antrum using sublabial approach
E13 Other operations on maxillary antrum
E14 Operations on frontal sinus
E15 Operations on sphenoid sinus
E16 Other operations on frontal sinus
E17 Operations on unspecified nasal sinus

Pharynx (E19–E28)

E19	Excision of pharynx
E20	Operations on adenoid
E21	Repair of pharynx
E23	Other open operations on pharynx
E24	Therapeutic endoscopic operations on pharynx
E25	Diagnostic endoscopic examination of pharynx
E27	Other operations on pharynx
E28	Operations on cricopharyngeus muscle

Larynx (E29–E38)

E29	Excision of larynx
E30	Open extirpation of lesion of larynx
E31	Reconstruction of larynx
E33	Other open operations on larynx
E34	Microtherapeutic endoscopic operations on larynx
E35	Other therapeutic endoscopic operations on larynx
E36	Diagnostic endoscopic examination of larynx
E37	Diagnostic microendoscopic examination of larynx
E38	Other operations on larynx

Trachea and bronchus (E39–E52)

E39	Partial excision of trachea
E40	Plastic operations on trachea
E41	Open placement of prosthesis in trachea
E42	Exteriorisation of trachea
E43	Other open operations on trachea
E44	Open operations on carina
E45	Code deleted
E46	Partial extirpation of bronchus
E47	Other open operations on bronchus
E48	Therapeutic fibreoptic endoscopic operations on lower respiratory tract
E49	Diagnostic fibreoptic endoscopic examination of lower respiratory tract
E50	Therapeutic endoscopic operations on lower respiratory tract using rigid bronchoscope
E51	Diagnostic endoscopic examination of lower respiratory tract using rigid bronchoscope
E52	Other operations on bronchus

Lung and mediastinum (E53–E63)

E53	Transplantation of lung
E54	Excision of lung
E55	Open extirpation of lesion of lung
E57	Other open operations on lung
E59	Other operations on lung
E61	Open operations on mediastinum
E62	Therapeutic endoscopic operations on mediastinum
E63	Diagnostic endoscopic examination of mediastinum

Non operations on lower respiratory tract (E85–E98)

E85	Ventilation support
E87	Oxygen therapy support
E89	Other respiratory support
E91	Oximetry testing
E92	Respiratory tests
E93	Respiratory measurements
E94	Bronchial reaction studies
E95	Tuberculosis support
E97	Respiratory education
E98	Smoking cessation therapy

F. MOUTH

Lip (F01–F06)

F01	Partial excision of lip
F02	Extirpation of lesion of lip
F03	Correction of deformity of lip
F04	Other reconstruction of lip
F05	Other repair of lip
F06	Other operations on lip

Tooth and gingiva (F08–F20)

F08	Implantation of tooth
F09	Surgical removal of tooth
F10	Simple extraction of tooth
F11	Preprosthetic oral surgery
F12	Surgery on apex of tooth
F13	Restoration of tooth
F14	Orthodontic operations
F15	Other orthodontic operations
F16	Other operations on tooth
F17	Operations on teeth using dental crown or bridge
F18	Excision of dental lesion of jaw
F20	Operations on gingiva

Tongue and palate (F22–F32)

F22	Excision of tongue
F23	Extirpation of lesion of tongue
F24	Incision of tongue
F26	Other operations on tongue
F28	Extirpation of lesion of palate
F29	Correction of deformity of palate
F30	Other repair of palate
F32	Other operations on palate

Tonsil and other parts of mouth (F34–F43)

F34	Excision of tonsil
F36	Other operations on tonsil
F38	Extirpation of lesion of other part of mouth
F39	Reconstruction of other part of mouth
F40	Other repair of other part of mouth
F42	Other operations on mouth
F43	Other examinations of mouth

Salivary apparatus (F44–F58)

F44	Excision of salivary gland
F45	Extirpation of lesion of salivary gland
F46	Incision of salivary gland
F48	Other operations on salivary gland
F50	Transposition of salivary duct
F51	Open extraction of calculus from salivary duct
F52	Ligation of salivary duct
F53	Other open operations on salivary duct
F55	Dilation of salivary duct
F56	Manipulative removal of calculus from salivary duct
F58	Other operations on salivary duct

Other dental (F63)

F63	Insertion of dental prosthesis

G. UPPER DIGESTIVE TRACT

Oesophagus including hiatus hernia (G01–G25)

G01	Excision of oesophagus and stomach
G02	Total excision of oesophagus
G03	Partial excision of oesophagus
G04	Open extirpation of lesion of oesophagus
G05	Bypass of oesophagus
G06	Attention to connection of oesophagus
G07	Repair of oesophagus
G08	Artificial opening into oesophagus
G09	Incision of oesophagus
G10	Open operations on varices of oesophagus
G11	Open placement of prosthesis in oesophagus
G13	Other open operations on oesophagus
G14	Fibreoptic endoscopic extirpation of lesion of oesophagus
G15	Other therapeutic fibreoptic endoscopic operations on oesophagus
G16	Diagnostic fibreoptic endoscopic examination of oesophagus
G17	Endoscopic extirpation of lesion of oesophagus using rigid oesophagoscope
G18	Other therapeutic endoscopic operations on oesophagus using rigid oesophagoscope
G19	Diagnostic endoscopic examination of oesophagus using rigid oesophagoscope
G21	Other operations on oesophagus
G23	Repair of diaphragmatic hernia
G24	Antireflux operations
G25	Revision of antireflux operations

Stomach pylorus and general upper gastrointestinal tract endoscopy (G26–G48)

G26	Transplantation of stomach
G27	Total excision of stomach
G28	Partial excision of stomach
G29	Open extirpation of lesion of stomach
G30	Plastic operations on stomach
G31	Connection of stomach to duodenum
G32	Connection of stomach to transposed jejunum
G33	Other connection of stomach to jejunum
G34	Artificial opening into stomach
G35	Operations on ulcer of stomach
G36	Other repair of stomach
G38	Other open operations on stomach
G40	Incision of pylorus
G41	Other operations on pylorus
G42	Other fibreoptic endoscopic extirpation of lesion of upper gastrointestinal tract
G43	Fibreoptic endoscopic extirpation of lesion of upper gastrointestinal tract
G44	Other therapeutic fibreoptic endoscopic operations on upper gastrointestinal tract
G45	Diagnostic fibreoptic endoscopic examination of upper gastrointestinal tract
G46	Therapeutic fibreoptic endoscopic operations on upper gastrointestinal tract
G47	Intubation of stomach
G48	Other operations on stomach

Duodenum (G49–G57)

G49	Excision of duodenum
G50	Open extirpation of lesion of duodenum
G51	Bypass of duodenum
G52	Operations on ulcer of duodenum
G53	Other open operations on duodenum
G54	Therapeutic endoscopic operations on duodenum
G55	Diagnostic endoscopic examination of duodenum
G57	Other operations on duodenum

Jejunum (G58–G67)

G58	Excision of jejunum
G59	Extirpation of lesion of jejunum
G60	Artificial opening into jejunum
G61	Bypass of jejunum
G62	Open endoscopic operations on jejunum
G63	Other open operations on jejunum
G64	Therapeutic endoscopic operations on jejunum
G65	Diagnostic endoscopic examination of jejunum
G67	Other operations on jejunum

Ileum (G68–G82)

G68	Transplantation of ileum
G69	Excision of ileum
G70	Open extirpation of lesion of ileum
G71	Bypass of ileum
G72	Other connection of ileum
G73	Attention to connection of ileum
G74	Creation of artificial opening into ileum
G75	Attention to artificial opening into ileum
G76	Intra-abdominal manipulation of ileum
G78	Other open operations on ileum
G79	Therapeutic endoscopic operations on ileum
G80	Diagnostic endoscopic examination of ileum
G82	Other operations on ileum

H. LOWER DIGESTIVE TRACT

Appendix (H01–H03)

H01	Emergency excision of appendix
H02	Other excision of appendix
H03	Other operations on appendix

Colon (H04–H32)

H04	Total excision of colon and rectum
H05	Total excision of colon
H06	Extended excision of right hemicolon
H07	Other excision of right hemicolon
H08	Excision of transverse colon
H09	Excision of left hemicolon
H10	Excision of sigmoid colon
H11	Other excision of colon
H12	Extirpation of lesion of colon
H13	Bypass of colon
H14	Exteriorisation of caecum
H15	Other exteriorisation of colon
H16	Incision of colon
H17	Intra-abdominal manipulation of colon
H18	Open endoscopic operations on colon
H19	Other open operations on colon
H20	Endoscopic extirpation of lesion of colon
H21	Other therapeutic endoscopic operations on colon
H22	Diagnostic endoscopic examination of colon
H23	Endoscopic extirpation of lesion of lower bowel using fibreoptic sigmoidoscope
H24	Other therapeutic endoscopic operations on lower bowel using fibreoptic sigmoidoscope
H25	Diagnostic endoscopic examination of lower bowel using fibreoptic sigmoidoscope
H26	Endoscopic extirpation of lesion of sigmoid colon using rigid sigmoidoscope
H27	Other therapeutic endoscopic operations on sigmoid colon using rigid sigmoidoscope
H28	Diagnostic endoscopic examination of sigmoid colon using rigid sigmoidoscope
H29	Subtotal excision of colon
H30	Other operations on colon
H31	Image guided colorectal therapeutic operations
H32	Exteriorisation of colon

Rectum (H33–H46)

H33	Excision of rectum
H34	Open extirpation of lesion of rectum
H35	Fixation of rectum for prolapse
H36	Other abdominal operations for prolapse of rectum
H40	Operations on rectum through anal sphincter
H41	Other operations on rectum through anus
H42	Perineal operations for prolapse of rectum
H44	Manipulation of rectum
H46	Other operations on rectum

Anus and perianal region (H47–H70)

H47	Excision of anus
H48	Excision of lesion of anus
H49	Destruction of lesion of anus
H50	Repair of anus
H51	Excision of haemorrhoid
H52	Destruction of haemorrhoid
H53	Other operations on haemorrhoid
H54	Dilation of anal sphincter
H55	Other operations on perianal region
H56	Other operations on anus
H57	Other operations on the anal sphincter to control continence
H58	Drainage through perineal region
H59	Excision of pilonidal sinus
H60	Other operations on pilonidal sinus
H62	Other operations on bowel
H66	Therapeutic operations on ileoanal pouch
H68	Diagnostic endoscopic examination of enteric pouch using colonoscope
H69	Diagnostic endoscopic examination of enteric pouch using fibreoptic sigmoidoscope
H70	Diagnostic endoscopic examination of enteric pouch using rigid sigmoidoscope

J. OTHER ABDOMINAL ORGANS – PRINCIPALLY DIGESTIVE

Liver (J01–J17)

J01	Transplantation of liver
J02	Partial excision of liver
J03	Extirpation of lesion of liver
J04	Repair of liver
J05	Incision of liver
J06	Other transjugular intrahepatic operations on blood vessel of liver
J07	Other open operations on liver
J08	Therapeutic endoscopic operations on liver using laparoscope
J09	Diagnostic endoscopic examination of liver using laparoscope
J10	Transluminal operations on blood vessel of liver
J11	Transjugular intrahepatic operations on blood vessel of liver
J12	Other therapeutic percutaneous operations on liver
J13	Diagnostic percutaneous operations on liver
J14	Other puncture of liver
J15	Transluminal insertion of prosthesis into blood vessel of liver
J16	Other operations on liver
J17	Endoscopic ultrasound examination of liver

Gall bladder (J18–J26)

J18	Excision of gall bladder
J19	Connection of gall bladder
J20	Repair of gall bladder
J21	Incision of gall bladder
J23	Other open operations on gall bladder
J24	Therapeutic percutaneous operations on gall bladder
J25	Diagnostic percutaneous operations on gall bladder
J26	Other operations on gall bladder

Bile duct (J27–J53)

J27	Excision of bile duct
J28	Extirpation of lesion of bile duct
J29	Connection of hepatic duct
J30	Connection of common bile duct
J31	Open introduction of prosthesis into bile duct
J32	Repair of bile duct
J33	Incision of bile duct
J34	Plastic repair of sphincter of Oddi using duodenal approach
J35	Incision of sphincter of Oddi using duodenal approach
J36	Other operations on ampulla of Vater using duodenal approach
J37	Other open operations on bile duct
J38	Endoscopic incision of sphincter of Oddi
J39	Other therapeutic endoscopic operations on ampulla of Vater
J40	Endoscopic retrograde placement of prosthesis in bile duct
J41	Other therapeutic endoscopic retrograde operations on bile duct
J42	Therapeutic endoscopic retrograde operations on pancreatic duct
J43	Diagnostic endoscopic retrograde examination of bile duct and pancreatic duct
J44	Diagnostic endoscopic retrograde examination of bile duct
J45	Diagnostic endoscopic retrograde examination of pancreatic duct
J46	Therapeutic percutaneous attention to connection of bile duct
J47	Therapeutic percutaneous insertion of prosthesis into bile duct
J48	Other therapeutic percutaneous operations on bile duct
J49	Therapeutic operations on bile duct along T tube track
J50	Percutaneous examination of bile duct
J51	Laparoscopic ultrasound examination of bile duct
J52	Other operations on bile duct
J53	Endoscopic ultrasound examination of bile duct

Pancreas (J54–J68)

J54	Transplantation of pancreas
J55	Total excision of pancreas
J56	Excision of head of pancreas
J57	Other partial excision of pancreas
J58	Extirpation of lesion of pancreas
J59	Connection of pancreatic duct
J60	Other open operations on pancreatic duct
J61	Open drainage of lesion of pancreas
J62	Incision of pancreas
J63	Open examination of pancreas
J65	Other open operations on pancreas
J66	Therapeutic percutaneous operations on pancreas
J67	Diagnostic percutaneous operations on pancreas
J68	Other operations on pancreas

Spleen (J69–J72)

J69	Total excision of spleen
J70	Other excision of spleen
J72	Other operations on spleen

Pancreas (J73–J77)

J73	Laparoscopic ultrasound examination of pancreas
J74	Endoscopic ultrasound examination of pancreas
J76	Therapeutic percutaneous operations on bile duct
J77	Other transluminal operations on blood vessel of liver

K. HEART

Wall septum and chambers of heart (K01–K24)

K01	Transplantation of heart and lung
K02	Other transplantation of heart
K04	Repair of tetralogy of Fallot
K05	Atrial inversion operations for transposition of great arteries
K06	Other repair of transposition of great arteries
K07	Correction of total anomalous pulmonary venous connection
K08	Repair of double outlet ventricle
K09	Repair of defect of atrioventricular septum
K10	Repair of defect of interatrial septum
K11	Repair of defect of interventricular septum
K12	Repair of defect of unspecified septum of heart
K13	Transluminal repair of defect of septum
K14	Other open operations on septum of heart
K15	Closed operations on septum of heart
K16	Other therapeutic transluminal operations on septum of heart
K17	Repair of univentricular heart
K18	Creation of valved cardiac conduit
K19	Creation of other cardiac conduit
K20	Refashioning of atrium
K22	Other operations on wall of atrium
K23	Other operations of wall of heart
K24	Other operations on ventricles of heart

Valves of heart and adjacent structures (K25–K38)

K25	Plastic repair of mitral valve
K26	Plastic repair of aortic valve
K27	Plastic repair of tricuspid valve
K28	Plastic repair of pulmonary valve
K29	Plastic repair of unspecified valve of heart
K30	Revision of plastic repair of valve of heart
K31	Open incision of valve of heart
K32	Closed incision of valve of heart
K33	Operations on aortic root
K34	Other open operations on valve of heart
K35	Therapeutic transluminal operations on valve of heart
K36	Excision of valve of heart
K37	Removal of obstruction from structure adjacent to valve of heart
K38	Other operations on structure adjacent to valve of heart

Coronary artery (K40–K51)

K40	Saphenous vein graft replacement of coronary artery
K41	Other autograft replacement of coronary artery
K42	Allograft replacement of coronary artery
K43	Prosthetic replacement of coronary artery
K44	Other replacement of coronary artery
K45	Connection of thoracic artery to coronary artery
K46	Other bypass of coronary artery
K47	Repair of coronary artery
K48	Other open operations on coronary artery
K49	Transluminal balloon angioplasty of coronary artery
K50	Other therapeutic transluminal operations on coronary artery
K51	Diagnostic transluminal operations on coronary artery

Other parts of heart and pericardium (K52–K78)

K52	Open operations on conducting system of heart
K53	Other incision of heart
K54	Open heart assist operations
K55	Other open operations on heart
K56	Transluminal heart assist operations
K57	Other therapeutic transluminal operations on heart
K58	Diagnostic transluminal operations on heart
K59	Cardioverter defibrillator introduced through the vein
K60	Cardiac pacemaker system introduced through vein
K61	Other cardiac pacemaker system
K62	Therapeutic transluminal operations on heart
K63	Contrast radiology of heart
K64	Percutaneous operations on heart
K65	Catheterisation of heart
K66	Other operations on heart
K67	Excision of pericardium
K68	Drainage of pericardium
K69	Incision of pericardium
K71	Other operations on pericardium
K72	Other cardioverter defibrillator
K75	Percutaneous transluminal balloon angioplasty and insertion of stent into coronary artery
K76	Transluminal operations on cardiac conduit
K77	Transluminal drainage of pericardium
K78	Transluminal operations on internal mammary artery side branch

L. ARTERIES AND VEINS

Great vessels and pulmonary artery (L01–L13)

L01	Open operations for combined abnormality of great vessels
L02	Open correction of patent ductus arteriosus
L03	Transluminal operations on abnormality of great vessel
L04	Open operations on pulmonary arterial tree
L05	Creation of shunt to pulmonary artery from aorta using interposition tube prosthesis
L06	Other connection to pulmonary artery from aorta
L07	Creation of shunt to pulmonary artery from subclavian artery using interposition tube prosthesis
L08	Other connection to pulmonary artery from subclavian artery
L09	Other connection to pulmonary artery
L10	Repair of pulmonary artery
L12	Other open operations on pulmonary artery
L13	Transluminal operations on pulmonary artery

Aorta (L16–L28)

L16	Extra-anatomic bypass of aorta
L18	Emergency replacement of aneurysmal segment of aorta
L19	Other replacement of aneurysmal segment of aorta
L20	Other emergency bypass of segment of aorta
L21	Other bypass of segment of aorta
L22	Attention to prosthesis of aorta
L23	Plastic repair of aorta
L25	Other open operations on aorta
L26	Transluminal operations on aorta
L27	Transluminal insertion of stent graft for aneurysmal segment of aorta
L28	Transluminal operations on aneurysmal segment of aorta

Carotid cerebral and subclavian arteries (L29–L39)

L29	Reconstruction of carotid artery
L30	Other open operations on carotid artery
L31	Transluminal operations on carotid artery
L33	Operations on aneurysm of cerebral artery
L34	Other open operations on cerebral artery
L35	Transluminal operations on cerebral artery
L37	Reconstruction of subclavian artery
L38	Other open operations on subclavian artery
L39	Transluminal operations on subclavian artery

Abdominal branches of aorta (L41–L47)

L41	Reconstruction of renal artery
L42	Other open operations on renal artery
L43	Transluminal operations on renal artery
L45	Reconstruction of other visceral branch of abdominal aorta
L46	Other open operations on other visceral branch of abdominal aorta
L47	Transluminal operations on other visceral branch of abdominal aorta

Iliac and femoral arteries (L48–L63)

L48   Emergency replacement of aneurysmal iliac artery
L49   Other replacement of aneurysmal iliac artery
L50   Other emergency bypass of iliac artery
L51   Other bypass of iliac artery
L52   Reconstruction of iliac artery
L53   Other open operations on iliac artery
L54   Transluminal operations on iliac artery
L56   Emergency replacement of aneurysmal femoral artery
L57   Other replacement of aneurysmal femoral artery
L58   Other emergency bypass of femoral artery
L59   Other bypass of femoral artery
L60   Reconstruction of femoral artery
L62   Other open operations on femoral artery
L63   Transluminal operations on femoral artery

Other arteries (L65–L72)

L65   Revision of reconstruction of artery
L66   Other therapeutic transluminal operations on artery
L67   Excision of other artery
L68   Repair of other artery
L69   Operations on major systemic to pulmonary collateral arteries
L70   Other open operations on other artery
L71   Therapeutic transluminal operations on other artery
L72   Diagnostic transluminal operations on other artery

Veins and other blood vessels (L73–L99)

L73	Mechanical embolic protection of blood vessel
L74	Arteriovenous shunt
L75	Other arteriovenous operations
L76	Endovascular placement of stent
L77	Connection of vena cava or branch of vena cava
L79	Other operations on vena cava
L80	Operations on individual pulmonary veins
L81	Other bypass operations on vein
L82	Repair of valve of vein
L83	Other operations for venous insufficiency
L84	Combined operations on varicose vein of leg
L85	Ligation of varicose vein of leg
L86	Injection into varicose vein of leg
L87	Other operations on varicose vein of leg
L88	Transluminal operations on varicose vein of leg
L89	Other endovascular placement of stent
L90	Open removal of thrombus from vein
L91	Other vein related operations
L92	Unblocking of access catheter
L93	Other open operations on vein
L94	Therapeutic transluminal operations on vein
L95	Diagnostic transluminal operations on vein
L96	Percutaneous removal of thrombus from vein
L97	Other operations on blood vessel
L98	Operations on microvascular vessel
L99	Other therapeutic transluminal operations on vein

Overflow arteries and veins (O01–O05, O15, O20)

O01	Transluminal coil embolisation of aneurysm of artery
O02	Transluminal balloon assisted coil embolisation of aneurysm of artery
O03	Transluminal stent assisted coil embolisation of aneurysm of artery
O04	Other transluminal embolisation of aneurysm of artery
O05	Operations on dural arteriovenous fistula
O15	Operations on blood vessel
O20	Endovascular placement of stent graft

M. URINARY

Kidney (M01–M17)

M01	Transplantation of kidney
M02	Total excision of kidney
M03	Partial excision of kidney
M04	Open extirpation of lesion of kidney
M05	Open repair of kidney
M06	Incision of kidney
M08	Other open operations on kidney
M09	Therapeutic endoscopic operations on calculus of kidney
M10	Other therapeutic endoscopic operations on kidney
M11	Diagnostic endoscopic examination of kidney
M12	Percutaneous studies of upper urinary tract
M13	Percutaneous puncture of kidney
M14	Extracorporeal fragmentation of calculus of kidney
M15	Operations on kidney along nephrostomy tube track
M16	Other operations on kidney
M17	Interventions associated with transplantation of kidney

Ureter (M18–M33)

M18	Excision of ureter
M19	Urinary diversion
M20	Replantation of ureter
M21	Other connection of ureter
M22	Repair of ureter
M23	Incision of ureter
M25	Other open operations on ureter
M26	Therapeutic nephroscopic operations on ureter
M27	Therapeutic ureteroscopic operations on ureter
M28	Other endoscopic removal of calculus from ureter
M29	Other therapeutic endoscopic operations on ureter
M30	Diagnostic endoscopic examination of ureter
M31	Extracorporeal fragmentation of calculus of ureter
M32	Operations on ureteric orifice
M33	Percutaneous ureteric stent procedures

Bladder (M34–M49)

M34	Total excision of bladder
M35	Partial excision of bladder
M36	Enlargement of bladder
M37	Other repair of bladder
M38	Open drainage of bladder
M39	Other open operations on contents of bladder
M41	Other open operations on bladder
M42	Endoscopic extirpation of lesion of bladder
M43	Endoscopic operations to increase capacity of bladder
M44	Other therapeutic endoscopic operations on bladder
M45	Diagnostic endoscopic examination of bladder
M47	Urethral catheterisation of bladder
M48	Operations on bladder
M49	Other operations on bladder

Outlet of bladder and prostate (M51–M71)

M51	Combined abdominal and vaginal operations to support outlet of female bladder
M52	Abdominal operations to support outlet of female bladder
M53	Vaginal operations to support outlet of female bladder
M54	Open operations on outlet of female bladder
M55	Other open operations on outlet of female bladder
M56	Therapeutic endoscopic operations on outlet of female bladder
M58	Other operations on outlet of female bladder
M60	Open operations on outlet of male bladder
M61	Open excision of prostate
M62	Other open operations on prostate
M64	Other open operations on outlet of male bladder
M65	Endoscopic resection of outlet of male bladder
M66	Other therapeutic endoscopic operations on outlet of male bladder
M67	Other therapeutic endoscopic operations on prostate
M68	Endoscopic insertion of prosthesis into prostate
M70	Other operations on outlet of male bladder
M71	Other operations on prostate

Urethra and other parts of urinary tract (M72–M86)

M72	Excision of urethra
M73	Repair of urethra
M75	Other open operations on urethra
M76	Therapeutic endoscopic operations on urethra
M77	Diagnostic endoscopic examination of urethra
M79	Other operations on urethra
M81	Operations on urethral orifice
M83	Other operations on urinary tract
M85	Diagnostic endoscopic examination of urinary diversion
M86	Therapeutic endoscopic operations on urinary diversion

N. MALE GENITAL ORGANS

Scrotum and testis (N01–N13)

N01	Extirpation of scrotum
N03	Other operations on scrotum
N05	Bilateral excision of testes
N06	Other excision of testis
N07	Extirpation of lesion of testis
N08	Bilateral placement of testes in scrotum
N09	Other placement of testis in scrotum
N10	Prosthesis of testis
N11	Operations on hydrocele sac
N13	Other operations on testis

Spermatic cord and male perineum (N15–N24)

N15	Operations on epididymis
N17	Excision of vas deferens
N18	Repair of spermatic cord
N19	Operations on varicocele
N20	Other operations on spermatic cord
N22	Operations on seminal vesicle
N24	Operations on male perineum

Penis and other male genital organs (N26–N35)

N26	Amputation of penis
N27	Extirpation of lesion of penis
N28	Plastic operations on penis
N29	Prosthesis of penis
N30	Operations on prepuce
N32	Other operations on penis
N34	Other operations on male genital tract
N35	Non-operative interventions to male genitalia

P. LOWER FEMALE GENITAL TRACT

Vulva and female perineum (P01–P13)

P01	Operations on clitoris
P03	Operations on Bartholin gland
P05	Excision of vulva
P06	Extirpation of lesion of vulva
P07	Repair of vulva
P09	Other operations on vulva
P11	Extirpation of lesion of female perineum
P13	Other operations on female perineum

Vagina (P14–P32)

P14   Incision of introitus of vagina
P15   Other operations on introitus of vagina
P17   Excision of vagina
P18   Other obliteration of vagina
P19   Excision of band of vagina
P20   Extirpation of lesion of vagina
P21   Plastic operations on vagina
P22   Repair of prolapse of vagina and amputation of cervix uteri
P23   Other repair of prolapse of vagina
P24   Repair of vault of vagina
P25   Other repair of vagina
P26   Introduction of supporting pessary into vagina
P27   Exploration of vagina
P29   Other operations on vagina
P31   Operations on pouch of Douglas
P32   Other plastic operations on vagina

Q. UPPER FEMALE GENITAL TRACT

Uterus (Q01–Q21)

Q01   Excision of cervix uteri
Q02   Destruction of lesion of cervix uteri
Q03   Biopsy of cervix uteri
Q05   Other operations on cervix uteri
Q07   Abdominal excision of uterus
Q08   Vaginal excision of uterus
Q09   Other open operations on uterus
Q10   Curettage of uterus
Q11   Other evacuation of contents of uterus
Q12   Intrauterine contraceptive device
Q13   Introduction of gametes into uterine cavity
Q14   Introduction of abortifacient into uterine cavity
Q15   Introduction of other substance into uterine cavity
Q16   Other vaginal operations on uterus
Q17   Therapeutic endoscopic operations on uterus
Q18   Diagnostic endoscopic examination of uterus
Q19   Plastic operations on uterus
Q20   Other operations on uterus
Q21   Other introduction of gametes into uterine cavity

Fallopian tube (Q22–Q41)

Q22	Bilateral excision of adnexa of uterus
Q23	Unilateral excision of adnexa of uterus
Q24	Other excision of adnexa of uterus
Q25	Partial excision of fallopian tube
Q26	Placement of prosthesis in fallopian tube
Q27	Open bilateral occlusion of fallopian tubes
Q28	Other open occlusion of fallopian tube
Q29	Open reversal of female sterilisation
Q30	Other repair of fallopian tube
Q31	Incision of fallopian tube
Q32	Operations on fimbria
Q34	Other open operations on fallopian tube
Q35	Endoscopic bilateral occlusion of fallopian tubes
Q36	Other endoscopic occlusion of fallopian tube
Q37	Endoscopic reversal of female sterilisation
Q38	Other therapeutic endoscopic operations on fallopian tube
Q39	Diagnostic endoscopic examination of fallopian tube
Q41	Other operations on fallopian tube

Ovary and broad ligament (Q43–Q56)

Q43	Partial excision of ovary
Q44	Open destruction of lesion of ovary
Q45	Repair of ovary
Q47	Other open operations on ovary
Q48	Oocyte recovery
Q49	Therapeutic endoscopic operations on ovary
Q50	Diagnostic endoscopic examination of ovary
Q51	Other operations on ovary
Q52	Operations on broad ligament of uterus
Q54	Operations on other ligament of uterus
Q55	Other examination of female genital tract
Q56	Other operations on female genital tract

R. FEMALE GENITAL TRACT ASSOCIATED WITH PREGNANCY, CHILDBIRTH AND PUERPERIUM

Fetus and gravid uterus (R01–R12)

R01	Therapeutic endoscopic operations on fetus
R02	Diagnostic endoscopic examination of fetus
R03	Category retired – refer to introduction
R04	Therapeutic percutaneous operations on fetus
R05	Diagnostic percutaneous examination of fetus
R06	Destruction of fetus
R07	Therapeutic endoscopic operations for twin to twin transfusion syndrome
R08	Therapeutic percutaneous operations for twin to twin transfusion syndrome
R10	Other operations on amniotic cavity
R12	Operations on gravid uterus

Induction and delivery (R14–R27)

R14	Surgical induction of labour
R15	Other induction of labour
R17	Elective caesarean delivery
R18	Other caesarean delivery
R19	Breech extraction delivery
R20	Other breech delivery
R21	Forceps cephalic delivery
R22	Vacuum delivery
R23	Cephalic vaginal delivery with abnormal presentation of head at delivery without instrument
R24	Normal delivery
R25	Other methods of delivery
R27	Other operations to facilitate delivery

Other obstetric (R28–R34)

R28	Instrumental removal of products of conception from delivered uterus
R29	Manual removal of products of conception from delivered uterus
R30	Other operations on delivered uterus
R32	Repair of obstetric laceration
R34	Other obstetric operations

Obstetric scans and studies (R36–R43)

R36	Routine obstetric scan
R37	Non-routine obstetric scan for fetal observations
R38	Other non-routine obstetric scan
R40	Other maternal physiological assessments
R42	Obstetric doppler ultrasound
R43	Ultrasound monitoring

S. SKIN

Skin or subcutaneous tissue (S01–S63)

S01	Plastic excision of skin of head or neck
S02	Plastic excision of skin of abdominal wall
S03	Plastic excision of skin of other site
S04	Other excision of skin
S05	Microscopically controlled excision of lesion of skin
S06	Other excision of lesion of skin
S07	Photodynamic therapy of skin
S08	Curettage of lesion of skin
S09	Photodestruction of lesion of skin
S10	Other destruction of lesion of skin of head or neck
S11	Other destruction of lesion of skin of other site
S12	Phototherapy to skin
S13	Punch biopsy of skin
S14	Shave biopsy of skin
S15	Other biopsy of skin
S17	Distant flap of skin and muscle
S18	Distant flap of skin and fascia

S19	Distant pedicle flap of skin
S20	Other distant flap of skin
S21	Hair bearing flap of skin
S22	Sensory flap of skin
S23	Flap operations to relax contracture of skin
S24	Local flap of skin and muscle
S25	Local flap of skin and fascia
S26	Local subcutaneous pedicle flap of skin
S27	Other local flap of skin
S28	Flap of mucosa
S30	Other operations on flap of skin to head or neck
S31	Other operations on flap of skin to other site
S33	Hair bearing graft of skin to scalp
S34	Hair bearing graft of skin to other site
S35	Split autograft of skin
S36	Other autograft of skin
S37	Other graft of skin
S38	Graft of mucosa
S39	Graft of other tissue to skin
S40	Other closure of skin
S41	Suture of skin of head or neck
S42	Suture of skin of other site
S43	Removal of repair material from skin
S44	Removal of other inorganic substance from skin
S45	Removal of other substance from skin
S47	Opening of skin
S48	Insertion of skin expander into subcutaneous tissue
S49	Attention to skin expander in subcutaneous tissue
S50	Introduction of other inert substance into subcutaneous tissue
S51	Introduction of destructive substance into subcutaneous tissue
S52	Introduction of therapeutic substance into subcutaneous tissue
S53	Introduction of substance into skin
S54	Exploration of burnt skin of head or neck
S55	Exploration of burnt skin of other site
S56	Exploration of other skin of head or neck
S57	Exploration of other skin of other site
S58	Larvae therapy of skin
S59	Leech therapy of skin
S60	Other operations on skin
S62	Other operations on subcutaneous tissue
S63	Operations on subcutaneous tissue

Nail (S64–S70)

S64	Extirpation of nail bed
S66	Other operations on nail bed
S68	Excision of nail
S70	Other operations on nail

T. SOFT TISSUE

Chest wall pleura and diaphragm (T01–T17)

T01	Partial excision of chest wall
T02	Reconstruction of chest wall
T03	Opening of chest
T05	Other operations on chest wall
T07	Open excision of pleura
T08	Open drainage of pleural cavity
T09	Other open operations on pleura
T10	Therapeutic endoscopic operations on pleura
T11	Diagnostic endoscopic examination of pleura
T12	Puncture of pleura
T13	Introduction of substance into pleural cavity
T14	Other operations on pleura
T15	Repair of rupture of diaphragm
T16	Other repair of diaphragm
T17	Other operations on diaphragm

Abdominal wall (T19–T31, T97–T98)

T19	Simple excision of inguinal hernial sac
T20	Primary repair of inguinal hernia
T21	Repair of recurrent inguinal hernia
T22	Primary repair of femoral hernia
T23	Repair of recurrent femoral hernia
T24	Primary repair of umbilical hernia
T25	Primary repair of incisional hernia
T26	Repair of recurrent incisional hernia
T27	Repair of other hernia of abdominal wall
T28	Other repair of anterior abdominal wall
T29	Operations on umbilicus
T30	Opening of abdomen
T31	Other operations on anterior abdominal wall
T97	Repair of recurrent umbilical hernia
T98	Repair of recurrent other hernia of abdominal wall

Peritoneum (T33–T48)

T33	Open extirpation of lesion of peritoneum
T34	Open drainage of peritoneum
T36	Operations on omentum
T37	Operations on mesentery of small intestine
T38	Operations on mesentery of colon
T39	Operations on posterior peritoneum
T41	Other open operations on peritoneum
T42	Therapeutic endoscopic operations on peritoneum
T43	Diagnostic endoscopic examination of peritoneum
T45	Image controlled operations on abdominal cavity
T46	Other drainage of peritoneal cavity
T48	Other operations on peritoneum

Fascia ganglion and bursa (T50–T62)

T50	Transplantation of fascia
T51	Excision of fascia of abdomen
T52	Excision of other fascia
T53	Extirpation of lesion of fascia
T54	Division of fascia
T55	Release of fascia
T56	Other excision of other fascia
T57	Other operations on fascia
T59	Excision of ganglion
T60	Re–excision of ganglion
T61	Other operations on ganglion
T62	Operations on bursa

Tendon (T64–T74)

T64	Transposition of tendon
T65	Excision of tendon
T67	Primary repair of tendon
T68	Secondary repair of tendon
T69	Freeing of tendon
T70	Adjustment to length of tendon
T71	Excision of sheath of tendon
T72	Other operations on sheath of tendon
T74	Other operations on tendon

Muscle (T76–T83)

T76	Transplantation of muscle
T77	Excision of muscle
T79	Repair of muscle
T80	Release of contracture of muscle
T81	Biopsy of muscle
T83	Other operations on muscle

Lymphatic tissue (T85–T96)

T85	Block dissection of lymph nodes
T86	Sampling of lymph nodes
T87	Excision or biopsy of lymph node
T88	Drainage of lesion of lymph node
T89	Operations on lymphatic duct
T90	Contrast radiology of lymphatic tissue
T91	Operations on sentinel lymph node
T92	Other operations on lymphatic tissue
T94	Operations on branchial cleft
T96	Other operations on soft tissue

U. DIAGNOSTIC IMAGING, TESTING AND REHABILITATION

Diagnostic Imaging (U01–U21)

U01	Diagnostic imaging of whole body
U04	Diagnostic imaging of mouth
U05	Diagnostic imaging of central nervous system
U06	Diagnostic imaging of face and neck
U07	Diagnostic imaging of chest
U08	Diagnostic imaging of abdomen
U09	Diagnostic imaging of pelvis
U10	Diagnostic imaging of heart
U11	Diagnostic imaging of vascular system
U12	Diagnostic imaging of genitourinary system
U13	Diagnostic imaging of musculoskeletal system
U14	Nuclear bone scan
U15	Diagnostic imaging of respiratory system
U16	Diagnostic imaging of hepatobiliary system
U17	Diagnostic imaging of digestive tract
U18	Diagnostic imaging of breast
U19	Diagnostic electrocardiography
U20	Diagnostic echocardiography
U21	Diagnostic imaging procedures

Diagnostic tests (U22–U40)

U22	Neuropsychology tests
U23	Nuclear medicine haematological tests
U24	Diagnostic audiology
U25	Breath tests
U26	Diagnostic testing of genitourinary system
U27	Diagnostic application tests on skin
U28	Other diagnostic tests on skin
U29	Diagnostic endocrinology
U30	Autonomic cardiovascular testing
U31	Pacemaker testing
U32	Diagnostic blood tests
U33	Other diagnostic tests
U34	Other diagnostic electrocardiography
U35	Other diagnostic imaging of vascular system
U36	Other diagnostic imaging procedures
U37	Other diagnostic imaging of genitourinary system
U40	Diagnostic tests on skin

Rehabilitation (U50–U54)

U50	Rehabilitation for musculoskeletal disorders
U51	Rehabilitation for neurological disorders
U52	Rehabilitation for psychiatric disorders
U53	Rehabilitation for trauma and reconstructive surgery
U54	Rehabilitation for other disorders

V. BONES AND JOINTS OF SKULL AND SPINE

Bones and joints of cranium, face and jaw (V01–V21)

V01	Plastic repair of cranium
V02	Other plastic repair of cranium
V03	Opening of cranium
V04	Reshaping of cranium
V05	Other operations on cranium
V06	Excision of maxilla
V07	Excision of bone of face
V08	Reduction of fracture of maxilla
V09	Reduction of fracture of other bone of face
V10	Division of bone of face
V11	Fixation of bone of face
V12	Operations on bones of skull
V13	Other operations on bone of face
V14	Excision of mandible
V15	Reduction of fracture of mandible
V16	Division of mandible
V17	Fixation of mandible
V18	Distraction osteogenesis of bones of skull
V19	Other operations on mandible
V20	Reconstruction of temporomandibular joint
V21	Other operations on temporomandibular joint

Bones and joints of spine (V22–V68)

V22	Primary decompression operations on cervical spine
V23	Revisional decompression operations on cervical spine
V24	Decompression operations on thoracic spine
V25	Primary decompression operations on lumbar spine
V26	Revisional decompression operations on lumbar spine
V27	Decompression operations on unspecified spine
V28	Insertion of lumbar interspinous process spacer
V29	Primary excision of cervical intervertebral disc
V30	Revisional excision of cervical intervertebral disc
V31	Primary excision of thoracic intervertebral disc
V32	Revisional excision of thoracic intervertebral disc
V33	Primary excision of lumbar intervertebral disc
V34	Revisional excision of lumbar intervertebral disc
V35	Excision of unspecified intervertebral disc
V36	Prosthetic replacement of intervertebral disc
V37	Primary fusion of joint of cervical spine
V38	Primary fusion of other joint of spine
V39	Revisional fusion of joint of spine
V40	Stabilisation of spine
V41	Instrumental correction of deformity of spine
V42	Other correction of deformity of spine
V43	Extirpation of lesion of spine
V44	Decompression of fracture of spine
V45	Other reduction of fracture of spine
V46	Fixation of fracture of spine
V47	Biopsy of spine
V48	Denervation of spinal facet joint of vertebra
V49	Exploration of spine
V50	Manipulation of spine
V52	Other operations on intervertebral disc
V54	Other operations on spine
V55	Levels of spine
V56	Primary foraminoplasty of spine
V57	Revisional formaminoplasty of spine
V58	Primary automated percutaneous mechanical excision of intervertebral disc
V59	Revisional automated percutaneous mechanical excision of intervertebral disc
V60	Primary percutaneous decompression using coblation to intervertebral disc
V61	Revisional percutaneous decompression using coblation to intervertebral disc
V62	Primary percutaneous intradiscal radiofrequency thermocoagulation to intervertebral disc
V63	Revisional percutaneous intradiscal radiofrequency thermocoagulation to intervertebral disc
V66	Other revisional fusion of joint of spine
V67	Other primary decompression operations on lumbar spine
V68	Other revisional decompression operations on lumbar spine

W. OTHER BONES AND JOINTS

Complex reconstruction of hand and foot (W01–W04)

W01	Complex reconstruction of thumb
W02	Other complex reconstruction of hand
W03	Complex reconstruction of forefoot
W04	Complex reconstruction of hindfoot

Bone (W05–W36)

W05	Prosthetic replacement of bone
W06	Total excision of bone
W07	Excision of ectopic bone
W08	Other excision of bone
W09	Extirpation of lesion of bone
W10	Open surgical fracture of bone
W11	Other surgical fracture of bone
W12	Angulation periarticular division of bone
W13	Other periarticular division of bone
W14	Diaphyseal division of bone
W15	Division of bone of foot
W16	Other division of bone
W17	Other reconstruction of bone
W18	Drainage of bone
W19	Primary open reduction of fracture of bone and intramedullary fixation
W20	Primary open reduction of fracture of bone and extramedullary fixation
W21	Primary open reduction of intra-articular fracture of bone
W22	Other primary open reduction of fracture of bone
W23	Secondary open reduction of fracture of bone
W24	Closed reduction of fracture of bone and internal fixation
W25	Closed reduction of fracture of bone and external fixation
W26	Other closed reduction of fracture of bone
W27	Fixation of epiphysis
W28	Other internal fixation of bone
W29	Skeletal traction of bone
W30	Other external fixation of bone
W31	Other autograft of bone
W32	Other graft of bone
W33	Other open operations on bone
W34	Graft of bone marrow
W35	Therapeutic puncture of bone
W36	Diagnostic puncture of bone

Joint (W37–W99)

W37	Total prosthetic replacement of hip joint using cement
W38	Total prosthetic replacement of hip joint not using cement
W39	Other total prosthetic replacement of hip joint
W40	Total prosthetic replacement of knee joint using cement
W41	Total prosthetic replacement of knee joint not using cement
W42	Other total prosthetic replacement of knee joint
W43	Total prosthetic replacement of other joint using cement

W44	Total prosthetic replacement of other joint not using cement
W45	Other total prosthetic replacement of other joint
W46	Prosthetic replacement of head of femur using cement
W47	Prosthetic replacement of head of femur not using cement
W48	Other prosthetic replacement of head of femur
W49	Prosthetic replacement of head of humerus using cement
W50	Prosthetic replacement of head of humerus not using cement
W51	Other prosthetic replacement of head of humerus
W52	Prosthetic replacement of articulation of other bone using cement
W53	Prosthetic replacement of articulation of other bone not using cement
W54	Other prosthetic replacement of articulation of other bone
W55	Prosthetic interposition reconstruction of joint
W56	Other interposition reconstruction of joint
W57	Excision reconstruction of joint
W58	Other reconstruction of joint
W59	Fusion of joint of toe
W60	Fusion of other joint and extra-articular bone graft
W61	Fusion of other joint and other articular bone graft
W62	Other primary fusion of other joint
W63	Revisional fusion of other joint
W64	Conversion to fusion of other joint
W65	Primary open reduction of traumatic dislocation of joint
W66	Primary closed reduction of traumatic dislocation of joint
W67	Secondary reduction of traumatic dislocation of joint
W68	Primary reduction of injury to growth plate
W69	Open operations on synovial membrane of joint
W70	Open operations on semilunar cartilage
W71	Other open operations on intra-articular structure
W72	Prosthetic replacement of ligament
W73	Prosthetic reinforcement of ligament
W74	Other reconstruction of ligament
W75	Other open repair of ligament
W76	Other operations on ligament
W77	Stabilising operations on joint
W78	Release of contracture of joint
W79	Soft tissue operations on joint of toe
W80	Debridement and irrigation of joint
W81	Other open operations on joint
W82	Therapeutic endoscopic operations on semilunar cartilage
W83	Therapeutic endoscopic operations on other articular cartilage
W84	Therapeutic endoscopic operations on other joint structure
W85	Therapeutic endoscopic operations on cavity of knee joint
W86	Therapeutic endoscopic operations on cavity of other joint
W87	Diagnostic endoscopic examination of knee joint
W88	Diagnostic endoscopic examination of other joint
W89	Other therapeutic endoscopic operations on other articular cartilage
W90	Puncture of joint
W91	Other manipulation of joint
W92	Other operations on joint
W93	Hybrid prosthetic replacement of hip joint using cemented acetabular component
W94	Hybrid prosthetic replacement of hip joint using cemented femoral component

W95	Hybrid prosthetic replacement of hip joint using cement
W96	Total prosthetic replacement of shoulder joint using cement
W97	Total prosthetic replacement of shoulder joint not using cement
W98	Total prosthetic replacement of shoulder joint
W99	Graft of cord blood stem cells to bone marrow

Overflow other bones and joints (O06–O10, O17–O19, O21–O27, O29, O32)

O06	Hybrid prosthetic replacement of shoulder joint using cemented humeral component
O07	Hybrid prosthetic replacement of shoulder joint using cemented glenoid component
O08	Hybrid prosthetic replacement of shoulder joint using cement
O09	Placement of bone prosthesis
O10	Complex reconstruction of shoulder
O17	Secondary closed reduction of fracture of bone and internal fixation
O18	Hybrid prosthetic replacement of knee joint using cement
O19	Other therapeutic endoscopic operations on other joint structure
O21	Total prosthetic replacement of elbow joint using cement
O22	Total prosthetic replacement of elbow joint not using cement
O23	Total prosthetic replacement of elbow joint
O24	Prosthetic replacement of head of radius using cement
O25	Prosthetic replacement of head of radius not using cement
O26	Other prosthetic replacement of head of radius
O27	Other stabilising operations on joint
O29	Excision of bone
O32	Total prosthetic replacement of ankle joint

X. MISCELLANEOUS OPERATIONS

Operations covering multiple systems (X01–X27)

X01	Replantation of upper limb
X02	Replantation of lower limb
X03	Replantation of other organ
X04	Transplantation between systems
X05	Implantation of prosthesis for limb
X07	Amputation of arm
X08	Amputation of hand
X09	Amputation of leg
X10	Amputation of foot
X11	Amputation of toe
X12	Operations on amputation stump
X14	Clearance of pelvis
X15	Operations for sexual transformation
X16	Operations for disorders of sex development
X17	Separation of conjoined twins
X19	Correction of congenital deformity of shoulder or upper arm
X20	Correction of congenital deformity of forearm
X21	Correction of congenital deformity of hand
X22	Correction of congenital deformity of hip
X23	Correction of congenital deformity of leg
X24	Primary correction of congenital deformity of foot
X25	Other correction of congenital deformity of foot
X27	Correction of minor congenital deformity of foot

Miscellaneous operations (X28–X68)

X28	Intermittent infusion of therapeutic substance
X29	Continuous infusion of therapeutic substance
X30	Injection of therapeutic substance
X31	Injection of radiocontrast material
X32	Exchange blood transfusion
X33	Other blood transfusion
X34	Other intravenous transfusion
X35	Other intravenous injection
X36	Blood withdrawal
X37	Intramuscular injection
X38	Subcutaneous injection
X39	Other route of administration of therapeutic substance
X40	Compensation for renal failure
X41	Placement of ambulatory apparatus for compensation for renal failure
X42	Placement of other apparatus for compensation for renal failure
X43	Compensation for liver failure
X44	Administration of vaccine
X45	Donation of organ
X46	Donation of other tissue
X47	Other exchange blood transfusion
X48	Immobilisation using plaster cast
X49	Other external support of limb
X50	External resuscitation
X51	Change of body temperature
X52	Oxygen therapy
X53	Extirpation of unspecified organ
X55	Other operations on unspecified organ
X56	Intubation of trachea
X58	Artificial support for body system
X59	Anaesthetic without surgery
X60	Rehabilitation assessment
X61	Complementary therapy
X62	Assessment
X63	Category retired – refer to introduction
X64	Category retired – refer to introduction
X65	Radiotherapy delivery
X66	Cognitive behavioural therapy
X67	Preparation for external beam radiotherapy
X68	Preparation for brachytherapy

Specified Drug therapy (X70–X98)

X70	Procurement of drugs for chemotherapy for neoplasm in Bands 1–5
X71	Procurement of drugs for chemotherapy for neoplasm in Bands 6–10
X72	Delivery of chemotherapy for neoplasm
X73	Delivery of oral chemotherapy for neoplasm
X74	Other chemotherapy drugs
X81	High cost gastrointestinal drugs
X82	High cost hypertension drugs
X83	High cost other cardiovascular drugs
X84	High cost respiratory drugs
X85	High cost neurology drugs
X86	High cost anti-infective drugs
X87	High cost endocrinology drugs
X88	High cost reproductive and urinary tract drugs
X89	High cost immunosuppressant drugs
X90	High cost haematology and nutrition drugs
X91	High cost metabolic drugs
X92	High cost musculoskeletal drugs
X93	High cost ophthalmology drugs
X94	High cost ear, nose and throat drugs
X95	High cost dermatology drugs
X96	High cost immunology drugs
X97	High cost anaesthesia drugs
X98	Other high cost drugs

Y. SUBSIDIARY CLASSIFICATION OF METHODS OF OPERATION

Methods of operation not otherwise classifiable (Y01–Y44)

Y01	Replacement of organ NOC
Y02	Placement of prosthesis in organ NOC
Y03	Attention to prosthesis in organ NOC
Y04	Replantation of organ NOC
Y05	Excision of organ NOC
Y06	Excision of lesion of organ NOC
Y07	Obliteration of cavity of organ NOC
Y08	Laser therapy to organ NOC
Y09	Chemical destruction of organ NOC
Y10	Destruction of organ NOC
Y11	Other destruction of organ NOC
Y12	Chemical destruction of lesion of organ NOC
Y13	Other destruction of lesion of organ NOC
Y14	Placement of stent in organ NOC
Y15	Attention to stent in organ NOC
Y16	Connection of organ NOC
Y17	Destruction of lesion of organ NOC
Y18	Release of organ NOC
Y20	Biopsy of organ NOC
Y21	Cytology of organ NOC
Y22	Drainage of organ NOC
Y24	Microvascular repair of organ NOC
Y25	Suture of organ NOC
Y26	Other repair of organ NOC
Y27	Graft to organ NOC
Y29	Removal of foreign body from organ NOC
Y30	Incision of organ NOC
Y31	Exploration of organ NOC
Y32	Re-exploration of organ NOC
Y33	Puncture of organ NOC
Y35	Introduction of removable radioactive material into organ NOC
Y36	Introduction of non-removable material into organ NOC
Y37	Introduction of other substance into organ NOC
Y38	Injection of therapeutic substance into organ NOC
Y39	Injection of other substance into organ NOC
Y40	Dilation of organ NOC
Y41	Examination of organ NOC
Y42	Manipulation of organ NOC
Y44	Other methods of operation on organ NOC

Approach to organ (Y46–Y53)

Y46	Open approach to contents of cranium
Y47	Burrhole approach to contents of cranium
Y48	Approach to spine through back
Y49	Approach through thoracic cavity
Y50	Approach through abdominal cavity
Y51	Approach to organ through artificial opening into gastrointestinal tract
Y52	Approach to organ through other opening
Y53	Approach to organ under image control

Harvest of organ (Y54–Y69)

Y54	Harvest of nerve
Y55	Harvest of random pattern flap of skin from limb
Y56	Harvest of random pattern flap of skin from other site
Y57	Harvest of axial pattern flap of skin
Y58	Harvest of skin for graft
Y59	Harvest of flap of skin and fascia
Y60	Other harvest of fascia
Y61	Harvest of flap of skin and muscle of trunk
Y62	Harvest of flap of skin and muscle of other site
Y63	Harvest of flap of muscle of trunk
Y64	Harvest of flap of muscle of other site
Y65	Harvest of tendon
Y66	Harvest of bone
Y67	Harvest of other multiple tissue
Y69	Harvest of other tissue

Staged procedures etc and minimal access approaches (Y70–Y79)

Y70	Early operations NOC
Y71	Late operations NOC
Y73	Facilitating operations NOC
Y74	Minimal access to thoracic cavity
Y75	Minimal access to abdominal cavity
Y76	Minimal access to other body cavity
Y78	Arteriotomy approach to organ under image control
Y79	Approach to organ through artery

Anaesthetic etc (Y80–Y89, Y91–Y94)

Y80	General anaesthetic
Y81	Spinal anaesthetic
Y82	Local anaesthetic
Y84	Other anaesthetic
Y89	Brachytherapy
Y91	External beam radiotherapy
Y92	Support for preparation for radiotherapy
Y93	Gallium-67 imaging
Y94	Radiopharmaceutical imaging

Non-operations relating to fetus or embryo (Y95–Y96)

Y95   Gestational age
Y96   In vitro fertilisation

Radiology (Y97–Y98)

Y97   Radiology with contrast
Y98   Radiology procedures

Non-operations relating to status (Y99)

Y99   Donor status

Non-operations (Y90)

Y90   Other non-operations

Z. SUBSIDIARY CLASSIFICATION OF SITES OF OPERATION

Nervous system (Z01–Z12)

Z01   Tissue of brain
Z02   Ventricle of brain
Z03   Upper cranial nerve
Z04   Other cranial nerve
Z05   Meninges of brain
Z06   Spinal cord
Z07   Spinal nerve root
Z08   Brachial plexus
Z09   Peripheral nerve of arm
Z10   Lumbar plexus
Z11   Sacral plexus
Z12   Other nerve

Endocrine breast and special senses (Z13–Z21)

Z13   Endocrine gland of neck
Z14   Other endocrine gland
Z15   Breast
Z16   External structure of eye
Z17   Muscle of eye
Z18   Anterior chamber of eye
Z19   Other part of eye
Z20   Outer ear
Z21   Other part of ear

Respiratory tract and mouth (Z22–Z26)

Z22   Nose
Z23   Nasal sinus
Z24   Other respiratory tract
Z25   Mouth
Z26   Salivary apparatus

Digestive tract and abdominal organs (Z27–Z31)

Z27	Upper digestive tract
Z28	Large intestine
Z29	Other part of bowel
Z30	Biliary tract
Z31	Other abdominal organ

Heart arteries and veins (Z32–Z40)

Z32	Valve of heart
Z33	Other part of heart
Z34	Aorta
Z35	Cerebral artery
Z36	Branch of thoracic aorta
Z37	Lateral branch of abdominal aorta
Z38	Terminal branch of aorta
Z39	Vein
Z40	Other vascular tissue

Urinary tract and male genital organs (Z41–Z43)

Z41	Upper urinary tract
Z42	Lower urinary tract
Z43	Male genital organ

Female genital tract (Z44–Z46)

Z44	Vagina
Z45	Uterus
Z46	Other female genital tract

Skin (Z47–Z51)

Z47	Skin of face
Z48	Skin of other part of head or neck
Z49	Skin of trunk
Z50	Skin of other site
Z51	Nail

Soft tissue (Z52–Z62)

Z52	Chest wall
Z53	Abdominal wall
Z54	Muscle of shoulder or upper arm
Z55	Muscle of forearm
Z56	Muscle of hand
Z57	Muscle of hip or thigh
Z58	Muscle of lower leg
Z59	Muscle of foot
Z60	Other muscle
Z61	Lymph node
Z62	Other soft tissue

Bones and joints of skull and spine (Z63–Z67)

Z63	Bone of cranium
Z64	Bone of face
Z65	Jaw
Z66	Vertebra
Z67	Intervertebral joint

Other bones and joints (Z68–Z87)

Z68	Bone of shoulder girdle
Z69	Humerus
Z70	Radius
Z71	Ulna
Z72	Other bone of arm or wrist
Z73	Other bone of hand
Z74	Rib cage
Z75	Bone of pelvis
Z76	Femur
Z77	Tibia
Z78	Other bone of lower leg
Z79	Bone of tarsus
Z80	Other bone of foot
Z81	Joint of shoulder girdle or arm
Z82	Joint of wrist or hand
Z83	Joint of finger
Z84	Joint of pelvis or upper leg
Z85	Joint of lower leg or tarsus
Z86	Other joint of foot
Z87	Other part of musculoskeletal system

Other sites (Z89–Z99)

Z89	Arm region
Z90	Leg region
Z91	Other vein of upper body
Z92	Other region of body
Z93	Other veins of pelvis
Z94	Laterality of operation
Z95	Other branch of thoracic aorta
Z96	Other lateral branch of abdominal aorta
Z97	Other terminal branch of aorta
Z98	Other veins of lower limb
Z99	Intervertebral disc

Overflow sites of operation (O11–O14, O16, O28, O30–O31, O33)

O11	Other upper digestive tract
O12	Branch of external carotid artery
O13	Other leg region
O14	Other lymph node
O16	Body region
O28	Other cerebral artery
O30	Other large intestine
O31	Other arm region
O33	Bone of skull

Part 2

Tabular List
of
Four Digit Subcategories

CHAPTER A
NERVOUS SYSTEM
(CODES A01–A84)

Excludes:	ANAESTHETIC PROCEDURES	*(Chapter Y)*
Note:	*Use a subsidiary code for minimal access approach (Y74–Y76)*	
	Use a subsidiary code to identify method of image control (Y53)	

A01   **Major excision of tissue of brain**

A01.1   Hemispherectomy
A01.2   Total lobectomy of brain
A01.3   Partial lobectomy of brain
A01.8   Other specified
A01.9   Unspecified

A02   **Excision of lesion of tissue of brain**
         Note: *Principal category, extended at A06*

A02.1   Excision of lesion of tissue of frontal lobe of brain
A02.2   Excision of lesion of tissue of temporal lobe of brain
A02.3   Excision of lesion of tissue of parietal lobe of brain
A02.4   Excision of lesion of tissue of occipital lobe of brain
A02.5   Excision of lesion of tissue of cerebellum
A02.6   Excision of lesion of tissue of brain stem
A02.7   Excision of transcranial dermoid cyst
         Note: *Use additional codes for concurrent procedures on the skull (V01–V13)*
A02.8   Other specified
A02.9   Unspecified

A03   **Stereotactic ablation of tissue of brain**

A03.1   Stereotactic leucotomy
A03.2   Stereotactic ablation of tissue of thalamus
A03.3   Stereotactic ablation of tissue of globus pallidus
A03.4   Stereotactic ablation of tissue of brain stem
A03.8   Other specified
A03.9   Unspecified

A04   **Open biopsy of lesion of tissue of brain**
         Includes: *Tissue of brain*

A04.1   Open biopsy of lesion of tissue of frontal lobe of brain
A04.2   Open biopsy of lesion of tissue of temporal lobe of brain
A04.3   Open biopsy of lesion of tissue of parietal lobe of brain
A04.4   Open biopsy of lesion of tissue of occipital lobe of brain
A04.5   Open biopsy of lesion of tissue of cerebellum
A04.6   Open biopsy of lesion of tissue of brain stem
A04.8   Other specified
A04.9   Unspecified

A05   **Drainage of lesion of tissue of brain**
         Excludes: *Drainage of subarachnoid space of brain (A22.1)*
                     Drainage of extradural space (A40)

A05.1   Drainage of abscess of tissue of brain
A05.2   Evacuation of haematoma from temporal lobe of brain
A05.3   Evacuation of haematoma from cerebellum
A05.4   Evacuation of intracerebral haematoma NEC
A05.8   Other specified
A05.9   Unspecified

A06   **Other excision of lesion of tissue of brain**
         Note: *Principal A02*

A06.1   Excision of basal encephalocele
         Note: ***Use additional codes for concurrent procedures on the skull (V01–V13)***

A06.2   Excision of occipital encephalocele
         Includes: *Excision of parietal encephalocele*
         Note: ***Use additional codes for concurrent procedures on the skull (V01–V13)***

A06.3   Excision of syncipital encephalocele
         Includes: *Excision of interfrontal encephalocele*
                     Excision of frontoethmoidal encephalocele
         Note: ***Use additional codes for concurrent procedures on the skull (V01–V13)***

A06.4   Repair of post-traumatic meningoencephalocele
         Includes: *Repair of growing fracture of cranium*
         Excludes: *Repair of meningoencephalocele (A39.1)*
         Note: ***Use an additional code for associated repair of cranium (V02.3)***

A06.8   Other specified
A06.9   Unspecified

A07   **Other open operations on tissue of brain**

A07.1   Open division of tissue of brain
A07.2   Removal of foreign body from tissue of brain
A07.3   Exploration of tissue of brain
A07.4   Excision of abscess of tissue of brain
A07.5   Multiple subpial transections
A07.6   Complete callosotomy
A07.7   Partial callosotomy
A07.8   Other specified
A07.9   Unspecified

A08   **Other biopsy of lesion of tissue of brain**
         Includes: *Tissue of brain*

A08.1   Biopsy of lesion of tissue of frontal lobe of brain NEC
A08.2   Biopsy of lesion of tissue of temporal lobe of brain NEC
A08.3   Biopsy of lesion of tissue of parietal lobe of brain NEC
A08.4   Biopsy of lesion of tissue of occipital lobe of brain NEC
A08.5   Biopsy of lesion of tissue of cerebellum NEC
A08.6   Biopsy of lesion of tissue of brain stem NEC
A08.8   Other specified
A08.9   Unspecified

A09   **Neurostimulation of brain**
         Includes: *Neurostimulation of brainstem*

A09.1   Implantation of neurostimulator into brain
A09.2   Maintenance of neurostimulator in brain
A09.3   Removal of neurostimulator from brain
A09.4   Operation on neurostimulator in brain NEC
A09.5   Insertion of neurostimulator electrodes into the brain
A09.8   Other specified
A09.9   Unspecified

A10   **Other operations on tissue of brain**
         Note: *Principal category, extended at A11*

A10.1   Leucotomy NEC
A10.2   Aspiration of abscess of tissue of brain
A10.3   Aspiration of haematoma of tissue of brain
A10.4   Aspiration of lesion of tissue of brain NEC
A10.5   Puncture of tissue of brain NEC
A10.6   Insertion of carmustine wafers in neoplasm of tissue of brain
A10.7   Stereotactic radiosurgery on tissue of brain
         Note: *Use an additional code to specify radiotherapy delivery (X65)*
A10.8   Other specified
A10.9   Unspecified

A11   **Operations on tissue of brain**
         Note: *Principal A10*

A11.1   Placement of depth electrodes for electroencephalography
A11.2   Placement of surface electrodes for electroencephalography
A11.3   Monitoring of pressure in tissue of brain
         Excludes: Monitoring of pressure in ventricle of brain (A20.3)
A11.4   Cortical mapping
         Includes: *Cortical stimulation mapping*
A11.8   Other specified
A11.9   Unspecified

A12   **Creation of connection from ventricle of brain**

A12.1   Ventriculocisternostomy
A12.2   Creation of ventriculovascular shunt
         Includes: *Creation of ventriculoatrial shunt*
A12.3   Creation of ventriculopleural shunt
A12.4   Creation of ventriculoperitoneal shunt
A12.5   Creation of subcutaneous cerebrospinal fluid reservoir
A12.8   Other specified
A12.9   Unspecified

A13   **Attention to component of connection from ventricle of brain**

A13.1   Maintenance of proximal catheter of cerebroventricular shunt
A13.2   Maintenance of distal catheter of cerebroventricular shunt
A13.3   Insertion of antisyphon device into cerebroventricular shunt
A13.4   Renewal of valve of cerebroventricular shunt
A13.8   Other specified
A13.9   Unspecified

A14   **Other operations on connection from ventricle of brain**

A14.1   Renewal of cerebroventricular shunt
A14.2   Revision of cerebroventricular shunt NEC
         Includes: *Conversion of cerebroventricular shunt NEC*
A14.3   Removal of cerebroventricular shunt
A14.4   Irrigation of cerebroventricular shunt
A14.5   Attention to cerebroventricular shunt NEC
A14.8   Other specified
A14.9   Unspecified

A16   **Other open operations on ventricle of brain**

A16.1   Open drainage of ventricle of brain NEC
A16.8   Other specified
A16.9   Unspecified

A17   **Therapeutic endoscopic operations on ventricle of brain**
              Note: It is not necessary to code additionally any mention of diagnostic endoscopic
              examination of ventricle of brain (A18.9)

A17.1   Endoscopic extirpation of lesion of ventricle of brain
A17.2   Endoscopic third ventriculostomy
A17.8   Other specified
A17.9   Unspecified

A18   **Diagnostic endoscopic examination of ventricle of brain**

A18.1   Diagnostic endoscopic examination of ventricle of brain and biopsy of lesion of ventricle
              of brain
              Includes: Diagnostic endoscopic examination of ventricle of brain and biopsy of
              ventricle of brain
              Endoscopic biopsy of lesion of brain
              Endoscopic biopsy of brain
A18.8   Other specified
A18.9   Unspecified
              Includes: Ventriculoscopy of brain NEC

A20   **Other operations on ventricle of brain**

A20.1   Drainage of ventricle of brain NEC
A20.2   Ventriculography of brain
A20.3   Monitoring of pressure in ventricle of brain
A20.8   Other specified
A20.9   Unspecified

A22   **Operations on subarachnoid space of brain**

A22.1   Drainage of subarachnoid space of brain
A22.2   Puncture of cistern of brain
A22.3   Isotopic cisternography
A22.8   Other specified
A22.9   Unspecified

A24   **Graft to cranial nerve**

A24.1   Primary microsurgical graft to facial nerve (vii)
A24.2   Secondary microsurgical graft to facial nerve (vii)
A24.3   Microsurgical graft to facial nerve (vii) NEC
A24.4   Primary microsurgical graft to cranial nerve NEC
A24.5   Secondary microsurgical graft to cranial nerve NEC
A24.6   Microsurgical graft to cranial nerve NEC
A24.8   Other specified
A24.9   Unspecified

A25   **Intracranial transection of cranial nerve**

A25.1   Intracranial transection of optic nerve (ii)
A25.2   Intracranial transection of oculomotor nerve (iii)
          Includes: *Intracranial transection of trochlear nerve (iv)*
                         Intracranial transection of abducens nerve (vi)
A25.3   Intracranial transection of trigeminal nerve (v)
A25.4   Intracranial transection of facial nerve (vii)
A25.5   Intracranial transection of acoustic nerve (viii)
A25.6   Intracranial transection of glossopharyngeal nerve (ix)
A25.7   Intracranial transection of vagus nerve (x)
A25.8   Intracranial transection of specified cranial nerve NEC
          Includes: *Intracranial transection of accessory nerve (xi)*
                         Intracranial transection of hypoglossal nerve (xii)
A25.9   Unspecified

A26   **Other intracranial destruction of cranial nerve**

A26.1   Intracranial destruction of optic nerve (ii)
A26.2   Intracranial destruction of oculomotor nerve (iii)
          Includes: *Intracranial destruction of trochlear nerve (iv)*
                         Intracranial destruction of abducens nerve (vi)
A26.3   Intracranial destruction of trigeminal nerve (v)
          Includes: *Intracranial destruction of trigeminal ganglion*
A26.4   Intracranial destruction of facial nerve (vii)
A26.5   Intracranial destruction of acoustic nerve (viii)
A26.6   Intracranial destruction of glossopharyngeal nerve (ix)
A26.7   Intracranial destruction of vagus nerve (x)
A26.8   Intracranial destruction of specified cranial nerve NEC
          Includes: *Intracranial destruction of accessory nerve (xi)*
                         Intracranial destruction of hypoglossal nerve (xii)
A26.9   Unspecified

A27   **Extracranial extirpation of vagus nerve (x)**
          Note: ***Use a supplementary code for concurrent pyloroplasty (G40.3)***

A27.1   Extracranial truncal vagotomy
          Includes: *Truncal vagotomy*
A27.2   Proximal gastric vagotomy
          Includes: *Highly selective vagotomy*
                         Parietal cell vagotomy
A27.3   Selective extracranial vagotomy NEC
          Includes: *Selective vagotomy NEC*
A27.8   Other specified
A27.9   Unspecified
          Includes: *Extracranial vagotomy NEC*
                         Vagotomy NEC

A28   **Extracranial extirpation of other cranial nerve**

A28.1   Extracranial transection of trigeminal nerve (v) NEC
         Includes: Transection of trigeminal nerve (v) NEC
         Excludes: Neurectomy of vidian nerve NEC (E13.7)
                    Transantral neurectomy of vidian nerve using sublabial approach (E12.4)
A28.2   Extracranial transection of accessory nerve (xi) NEC
         Includes: Transection of accessory nerve (xi) NEC
A28.8   Other specified
A28.9   Unspecified

A29   **Excision of lesion of cranial nerve**

A29.1   Excision of lesion of optic nerve (ii)
A29.2   Excision of lesion of oculomotor nerve (iii)
         Includes: Excision of lesion of trochlear nerve (iv)
                    Excision of lesion of abducens nerve (vi)
A29.3   Excision of lesion of trigeminal nerve (v)
A29.4   Excision of lesion of facial nerve (vii)
A29.5   Excision of lesion of acoustic nerve (viii)
A29.6   Excision of lesion of glossopharyngeal nerve (ix)
A29.7   Excision of lesion of vagus nerve (x)
A29.8   Excision of lesion of specified cranial nerve NEC
         Includes: Excision of lesion of accessory nerve (xi)
                    Excision of lesion of hypoglossal nerve (xii)
A29.9   Unspecified

A30   **Repair of cranial nerve**

A30.1   Repair of optic nerve (ii)
A30.2   Repair of oculomotor nerve (iii)
         Includes: Repair of trochlear nerve (iv)
                    Repair of abducens nerve (vi)
A30.3   Repair of trigeminal nerve (v)
A30.4   Repair of facial nerve (vii)
A30.5   Repair of acoustic nerve (viii)
A30.6   Repair of glossopharyngeal nerve (ix)
A30.7   Repair of vagus nerve (x)
A30.8   Repair of specified cranial nerve NEC
         Includes: Repair of accessory nerve (xi)
                    Repair of hypoglossal nerve (xii)
A30.9   Unspecified

A31   **Intracranial stereotactic release of cranial nerve**

A31.1   Intracranial stereotactic neurolysis of optic nerve (ii)
A31.2   Intracranial stereotactic neurolysis of oculomotor nerve (iii)
         Includes: Intracranial stereotactic neurolysis of trochlear nerve (iv)
         *   Intracranial stereotactic neurolysis of abducens nerve (vi)*
A31.3   Intracranial stereotactic neurolysis of trigeminal nerve (v)
A31.4   Intracranial stereotactic neurolysis of facial nerve (vii)
A31.5   Intracranial stereotactic neurolysis of acoustic nerve (viii)
A31.6   Intracranial stereotactic neurolysis of glossopharyngeal nerve (ix)
A31.7   Intracranial stereotactic neurolysis of vagus nerve (x)
A31.8   Intracranial stereotactic neurolysis of specified cranial nerve NEC
         Includes: Intracranial stereotactic neurolysis of accessory nerve (xi)
         *   Intracranial stereotactic neurolysis of hypoglossal nerve (xii)*
A31.9   Unspecified

A32   **Other decompression of cranial nerve**

A32.1   Decompression of optic nerve (ii)
A32.2   Decompression of oculomotor nerve (iii)
         Includes: Decompression of trochlear nerve (iv)
         *   Decompression of abducens nerve (vi)*
A32.3   Decompression of trigeminal nerve (v)
A32.4   Decompression of facial nerve (vii)
A32.5   Decompression of acoustic nerve (viii)
A32.6   Decompression of glossopharyngeal nerve (ix)
A32.7   Decompression of vagus nerve (x)
A32.8   Decompression of specified cranial nerve NEC
         Includes: Decompression of accessory nerve (xi)
         *   Decompression of hypoglossal nerve (xii)*
A32.9   Unspecified

A33   **Neurostimulation of cranial nerve**

A33.1   Introduction of neurostimulator into cranial nerve
A33.2   Maintenance of neurostimulator in cranial nerve
A33.3   Removal of neurostimulator from cranial nerve
A33.4   Insertion of neurostimulator electrodes into the cranial nerve
A33.8   Other specified
A33.9   Unspecified

A34   **Exploration of cranial nerve**

A34.1   Exploration of optic nerve (ii)
A34.2   Exploration of oculomotor nerve (iii)
         Includes: Exploration of trochlear nerve (iv)
         *   Exploration of abducens nerve (vi)*
A34.3   Exploration of trigeminal nerve (v)
A34.4   Exploration of facial nerve (vii)
A34.5   Exploration of acoustic nerve (viii)
A34.6   Exploration of glossopharyngeal nerve (ix)
A34.7   Exploration of vagus nerve (x)
A34.8   Exploration of specified cranial nerve NEC
         Includes: Exploration of accessory nerve (xi)
         *   Exploration of hypoglossal nerve (xii)*
A34.9   Unspecified

A36   **Other operations on cranial nerve**

A36.1   Hypoglossofacial anastomosis
A36.2   Anastomosis of cranial nerve NEC
A36.3   Biopsy of lesion of cranial nerve
                Includes: Biopsy of cranial nerve
A36.4   Radial optic neurotomy (ii)
A36.5   Denervation of trigeminal nerve (v)
A36.8   Other specified
A36.9   Unspecified

A38   **Extirpation of lesion of meninges of brain**
                Note: Principal category, extended at A43

A38.1   Extirpation of lesion of meninges of cortex of brain
A38.2   Extirpation of lesion of meninges of sphenoidal ridge of cranium
A38.3   Extirpation of lesion of meninges of subfrontal region of brain
A38.4   Extirpation of lesion of meninges of parasagittal region of brain
A38.5   Extirpation of lesion of falx cerebri
A38.6   Extirpation of lesion of tentorium cerebelli
A38.8   Other specified
A38.9   Unspecified

A39   **Repair of dura**

A39.1   Repair of meningoencephalocele
                Excludes: Repair of post-traumatic meningoencephalocele (A06.4)
A39.2   Repair of dura of anterior fossa of cranium
A39.3   Repair of dura of middle fossa of cranium
A39.4   Repair of dura of posterior fossa of cranium
A39.5   Repair of dura of vault of cranium
A39.8   Other specified
A39.9   Unspecified

A40   **Drainage of extradural space**

A40.1   Evacuation of extradural haematoma
A40.8   Other specified
A40.9   Unspecified

A41   **Drainage of subdural space**

A41.1   Evacuation of subdural haematoma
A41.2   Drainage of abscess of subdural space
A41.8   Other specified
A41.9   Unspecified

A42   **Other operations on meninges of brain**

A42.1   Creation of anastomosis of dura
A42.2   Biopsy of lesion of meninges of brain
                Includes: Biopsy of meninges of brain
A42.8   Other specified
A42.9   Unspecified

A43   **Other extirpation of lesion of meninges of brain**
                    Note: Principal A38

A43.1   Extirpation of lesion of meninges of skull base
A43.2   Extirpation of lesion of meninges of skull clivus
A43.8   Other specified
A43.9   Unspecified

A44   **Partial extirpation of spinal cord**

A44.1   Chordectomy of spinal cord
A44.2   Extirpation of lesion of spinal cord NEC
A44.3   Excision of lesion of intradural intramedullary spinal cord
A44.4   Excision of lesion of extradural spinal cord
A44.5   Excision of lesion of intradural extramedullary spinal cord
A44.8   Other specified
A44.9   Unspecified

A45   **Other open operations on spinal cord**
                    Includes: Spinal tract

A45.1   Stereotactic chordotomy of spinal cord
A45.2   Open chordotomy of spinal cord NEC
A45.3   Myelotomy of spinal cord
A45.4   Open biopsy of lesion of spinal cord
                    Includes: Open biopsy of spinal cord
A45.5   Removal of foreign body from spinal cord
A45.6   Open aspiration of lesion of spinal cord
A45.8   Other specified
A45.9   Unspecified

A47   **Other destruction of spinal cord**

A47.1   Needle destruction of substantia gelatinosa of cervical spinal cord
A47.2   Radiofrequency controlled thermal destruction of spinothalamic tract
A47.3   Percutaneous chordotomy of spinal cord
A47.8   Other specified
A47.9   Unspecified

A48   **Other operations on spinal cord**

A48.1   Biopsy of lesion of spinal cord NEC
                    Includes: Biopsy of spinal cord NEC
A48.2   Aspiration of lesion of spinal cord
A48.3   Insertion of neurostimulator adjacent to spinal cord
A48.4   Attention to neurostimulator adjacent to spinal cord NEC
A48.5   Reprogramming of neurostimulator adjacent to spinal cord
A48.6   Removal of neurostimulator adjacent to spinal cord
A48.7   Insertion of neurostimulator electrodes into the spinal cord
A48.8   Other specified
A48.9   Unspecified

A49	**Repair of spina bifida**

A49.1	Freeing of spinal tether NEC
	*Includes:	Division of tethered filum terminale*
A49.2	Closure of spinal myelomeningocele
A49.3	Closure of spinal meningocele
A49.4	Complex freeing of spinal tether
	*Includes:	Complex reduction of abnormal tissue to free spinal cord*
A49.8	Other specified
A49.9	Unspecified

A51	**Other operations on meninges of spinal cord**

A51.1	Extirpation of lesion of meninges of spinal cord
A51.2	Freeing of adhesions of meninges of spinal cord
A51.3	Biopsy of lesion of meninges of spinal cord
	*Includes:	Biopsy of meninges of spinal cord*
A51.4	Endoscopic division of epidural adhesions
A51.8	Other specified
A51.9	Unspecified

A52	**Therapeutic epidural injection**
	*Excludes:	Epidural anaesthetic procedures (Y81)*

A52.1	Therapeutic lumbar epidural injection
A52.2	Therapeutic sacral epidural injection
	*Includes:	Caudal epidural*
A52.3	Epidural blood patch
A52.8	Other specified
A52.9	Unspecified

A53	**Drainage of spinal canal**

A53.1	Cerebrospinal syringostomy
A53.2	Creation of thecoperitoneal shunt
A53.3	Creation of syringoperitoneal shunt
A53.4	Creation of lumboperitoneal shunt
A53.5	Drainage of cerebrospinal fluid NEC
A53.6	Creation of lumbar subcutaneous shunt
A53.8	Other specified
A53.9	Unspecified

A54	**Therapeutic spinal puncture**

A54.1	Injection of destructive substance into cerebrospinal fluid
A54.2	Injection of therapeutic substance into cerebrospinal fluid
A54.3	Implantation of intrathecal drug delivery device adjacent to spinal cord
A54.4	Attention to intrathecal drug delivery device adjacent to spinal cord
A54.5	Removal of intrathecal drug delivery device adjacent to spinal cord
A54.8	Other specified
A54.9	Unspecified

A55   **Diagnostic spinal puncture**

A55.1   Radiculography
A55.2   Spinal myelography NEC
A55.3   Spinal manometry
A55.8   Other specified
A55.9   Unspecified
        Includes: Lumbar puncture NEC

A57   **Operations on spinal nerve root**
        Includes: Spinal nerve root ganglion

A57.1   Extirpation of lesion of spinal nerve root
A57.2   Rhizotomy of spinal nerve root
A57.3   Radiofrequency controlled thermal destruction of spinal nerve root
A57.4   Injection of destructive substance into spinal nerve root
A57.5   Destruction of spinal nerve root NEC
A57.6   Reimplantation of spinal nerves into spinal cord
A57.7   Injection of therapeutic substance around spinal nerve root
A57.8   Other specified
A57.9   Unspecified

A59   **Excision of peripheral nerve**

A59.1   Total sacrifice of peripheral nerve
A59.2   Partial sacrifice of peripheral nerve
A59.8   Other specified
A59.9   Unspecified
        Includes: Neurectomy NEC

A60   **Destruction of peripheral nerve**

A60.1   Enucleation of peripheral nerve
A60.2   Avulsion of peripheral nerve
A60.3   Transection of peripheral nerve
A60.4   Radiofrequency controlled thermal destruction of peripheral nerve
A60.5   Injection of destructive substance into peripheral nerve
A60.6   Selective denervation of peripheral nerve
        Includes: Denervation of peripheral nerve NEC
A60.8   Other specified
A60.9   Unspecified

A61   **Extirpation of lesion of peripheral nerve**

A61.1   Excision of lesion of peripheral nerve
A61.2   Cryotherapy to lesion of peripheral nerve
A61.3   Radiotherapy to lesion of peripheral nerve
        Note: Use an additional code to specify radiotherapy delivery (X65)
A61.4   Destruction of lesion of peripheral nerve NEC
A61.8   Other specified
A61.9   Unspecified

A62   **Microsurgical repair of peripheral nerve**

A62.1   Primary microsurgical graft to peripheral nerve
A62.2   Secondary microsurgical graft to peripheral nerve
A62.3   Microsurgical graft to peripheral nerve NEC
A62.4   Primary microsurgical repair of peripheral nerve NEC
A62.5   Secondary microsurgical repair of peripheral nerve NEC
A62.6   Microsurgical graft to multiple peripheral nerves NEC
A62.7   Microsurgical repair of multiple peripheral nerves NEC
A62.8   Other specified
A62.9   Unspecified

A63   **Other graft to peripheral nerve**

A63.1   Primary graft to peripheral nerve NEC
A63.2   Secondary graft to peripheral nerve NEC
A63.8   Other specified
A63.9   Unspecified

A64   **Other repair of peripheral nerve**

A64.1   Primary approximation of peripheral nerve
A64.2   Primary repair of peripheral nerve NEC
A64.3   Secondary repair of peripheral nerve and mobilisation of peripheral nerve
A64.4   Secondary repair of peripheral nerve NEC
A64.8   Other specified
A64.9   Unspecified

A65   **Release of entrapment of peripheral nerve at wrist**

A65.1   Carpal tunnel release
A65.2   Canal of Guyon release
A65.8   Other specified
A65.9   Unspecified

A66   **Release of entrapment of peripheral nerve at ankle**

A66.1   Tarsal tunnel release
A66.8   Other specified
A66.9   Unspecified

A67   **Release of entrapment of peripheral nerve at other site**

A67.1   Cubital tunnel release
A67.2   Release of entrapment of lateral cutaneous nerve of thigh
A67.3   Release of entrapment of plantar digital nerve
A67.8   Other specified
A67.9   Unspecified

A68   **Other release of peripheral nerve**

A68.1   Primary neurolysis of peripheral nerve and transposition of peripheral nerve
A68.2   Secondary neurolysis of peripheral nerve and transposition of peripheral nerve
A68.3   Neurolysis of peripheral nerve and transposition of peripheral nerve NEC
A68.4   Primary neurolysis of peripheral nerve NEC
A68.5   Secondary neurolysis of peripheral nerve NEC
A68.8   Other specified
A68.9   Unspecified
          Includes: Neurolysis of peripheral nerve NEC

A69   **Revision of release of peripheral nerve**

A69.1   Revision of neurolysis of peripheral nerve and transposition of peripheral nerve
A69.2   Revision of carpal tunnel release
A69.3   Revision of tarsal tunnel release
A69.8   Other specified
A69.9   Unspecified
          Includes: Revision of release of peripheral nerve NEC

A70   **Neurostimulation of peripheral nerve**

A70.1   Implantation of neurostimulator into peripheral nerve
A70.2   Maintenance of neurostimulator in peripheral nerve
A70.3   Removal of neurostimulator from peripheral nerve
A70.4   Insertion of neurostimulator electrodes into peripheral nerve
A70.5   Electroacupuncture
A70.6   Acupuncture NEC
A70.7   Application of transcutaneous electrical nerve stimulator
A70.8   Other specified
A70.9   Unspecified

A73   **Other operations on peripheral nerve**

A73.1   Biopsy of lesion of peripheral nerve
          Includes: Biopsy of peripheral nerve
A73.2   Freeing of adhesions of peripheral nerve NEC
A73.3   Decompression of peripheral nerve NEC
A73.4   Exploration of peripheral nerve
A73.5   Injection of therapeutic substance around peripheral nerve
          Includes: Pain relieving plexus block of peripheral nerve
A73.6   Transfer and reimplantation of peripheral nerve NEC
A73.8   Other specified
A73.9   Unspecified

A75   **Excision of sympathetic nerve**

A75.1   Excision of cervical sympathetic nerve
A75.2   Excision of thoracic sympathetic nerve
A75.3   Excision of lumbar sympathetic nerve
A75.4   Excision of perivascular sympathetic nerve
A75.5   Excision of splanchnic sympathetic nerve
A75.8   Other specified
A75.9   Unspecified
          Includes: Sympathectomy NEC

A76 **Chemical destruction of sympathetic nerve**

A76.1 Chemical destruction of cervical sympathetic nerve
A76.2 Chemical destruction of thoracic sympathetic nerve
A76.3 Chemical destruction of lumbar sympathetic nerve
A76.4 Chemical destruction of perivascular sympathetic nerve
A76.5 Chemical destruction of splanchnic sympathetic nerve
A76.8 Other specified
A76.9 Unspecified
Includes: Chemical sympathectomy NEC

A77 **Cryotherapy to sympathetic nerve**

A77.1 Cryotherapy to cervical sympathetic nerve
A77.2 Cryotherapy to thoracic sympathetic nerve
A77.3 Cryotherapy to lumbar sympathetic nerve
A77.4 Cryotherapy to perivascular sympathetic nerve
A77.5 Cryotherapy to splanchnic sympathetic nerve
A77.8 Other specified
A77.9 Unspecified

A78 **Radiofrequency controlled thermal destruction of sympathetic nerve**

A78.1 Radiofrequency controlled thermal destruction of cervical sympathetic nerve
A78.2 Radiofrequency controlled thermal destruction of thoracic sympathetic nerve
A78.3 Radiofrequency controlled thermal destruction of lumbar sympathetic nerve
A78.4 Radiofrequency controlled thermal destruction of perivascular sympathetic nerve
A78.5 Radiofrequency controlled thermal destruction of splanchnic sympathetic nerve
A78.8 Other specified
A78.9 Unspecified

A79 **Other destruction of sympathetic nerve**

A79.1 Destruction of cervical sympathetic nerve NEC
A79.2 Destruction of thoracic sympathetic nerve NEC
A79.3 Destruction of lumbar sympathetic nerve NEC
A79.4 Destruction of perivascular sympathetic nerve NEC
A79.5 Destruction of splanchnic sympathetic nerve NEC
A79.8 Other specified
A79.9 Unspecified

A81 **Other operations on sympathetic nerve**

A81.1 Stellate ganglion blockade
A81.2 Injection of therapeutic substance around sympathetic nerve
A81.8 Other specified
A81.9 Unspecified

A83 **Electroconvulsive therapy**

A83.8 Other specified
A83.9 Unspecified

A84   **Neurophysiological operations**

A84.1   Electroencephalography NEC
             Includes: Ambulatory electroencephalography
             Excludes: Placement of electrodes for electroencephalography (A11)
             *   Electroencephalograph telemetry (U22.1)*
A84.2   Electromyography
A84.3   Nerve conduction studies
A84.4   Evoked potential recording
A84.5   Electroretinography NEC
A84.6   Pattern electroretinography
A84.7   Sleep studies NEC
             Includes: Full polysomnography
A84.8   Other specified
A84.9   Unspecified

CHAPTER B
ENDOCRINE SYSTEM AND BREAST
(CODES B01–B40)

Note: *Use a subsidiary code for minimal access approach (Y74–Y76)*
Use a subsidiary code to identify method of image control (Y53)

B01 **Excision of pituitary gland**

B01.1 Transethmoidal hypophysectomy
B01.2 Trans-sphenoidal hypophysectomy
B01.3 Trans-septal hypophysectomy
B01.4 Transcranial hypophysectomy
B01.8 Other specified
B01.9 Unspecified
Includes: *Hypophysectomy NEC*

B02 **Destruction of pituitary gland**

B02.1 Cryotherapy to pituitary gland
B02.2 Implantation of radioactive substance into pituitary gland
Note: *Use an additional code to specify radiotherapy delivery (X65)*
B02.3 Injection of destructive substance into pituitary gland NEC
B02.8 Other specified
B02.9 Unspecified

B04 **Other operations on pituitary gland**
Includes: *Pituitary stalk (B04.5)*

B04.1 Excision of lesion of pituitary gland
B04.2 Biopsy of lesion of pituitary gland
Includes: *Biopsy of pituitary gland*
B04.3 Decompression of pituitary gland
B04.4 Exploration of pituitary gland
B04.5 Operations on pituitary stalk
B04.8 Other specified
B04.9 Unspecified

B06 **Operations on pineal gland**

B06.1 Excision of pineal gland
B06.8 Other specified
B06.9 Unspecified

B08 **Excision of thyroid gland**

B08.1 Total thyroidectomy
B08.2 Subtotal thyroidectomy
B08.3 Hemithyroidectomy
B08.4 Lobectomy of thyroid gland NEC
B08.5 Isthmectomy of thyroid gland
B08.6 Partial thyroidectomy NEC
B08.8 Other specified
B08.9 Unspecified
Includes: *Thyroidectomy NEC*

B09   **Operations on aberrant thyroid tissue**

B09.1   Excision of substernal thyroid tissue
B09.2   Excision of sublingual thyroid tissue
B09.8   Other specified
B09.9   Unspecified

B10   **Operations on thyroglossal tissue**

B10.1   Excision of thyroglossal cyst
B10.2   Excision of thyroglossal tract
B10.3   Biopsy of lesion of thyroglossal tract
            Includes: Biopsy of thyroglossal tract
B10.4   Incision of thyroglossal cyst
B10.8   Other specified
B10.9   Unspecified

B12   **Other operations on thyroid gland**

B12.1   Excision of lesion of thyroid gland
B12.2   Biopsy of lesion of thyroid gland
            Includes: Biopsy of thyroid gland
            Note: Use a subsidiary code for fine needle aspiration (Y20.4)
B12.3   Incision of lesion of thyroid gland
B12.4   Exploration of thyroid gland
B12.8   Other specified
B12.9   Unspecified

B14   **Excision of parathyroid gland**

B14.1   Global parathyroidectomy and transposition of parathyroid tissue
B14.2   Global parathyroidectomy NEC
B14.3   Partial parathyroidectomy and transposition of parathyroid tissue
B14.4   Partial parathyroidectomy NEC
B14.5   Excision of lesion of parathyroid gland
B14.8   Other specified
B14.9   Unspecified
            Includes: Parathyroidectomy NEC

B16   **Other operations on parathyroid gland**

B16.1   Modification of transposed parathyroid gland
B16.2   Biopsy of lesion of parathyroid gland
            Includes: Biopsy of parathyroid gland
B16.3   Exploration of parathyroid gland
B16.4   Parathyroid washout
B16.8   Other specified
B16.9   Unspecified

B17   **Transplantation of thymus gland**

B17.1   Allotransplantation of thymus gland
B17.8   Other specified
B17.9   Unspecified

B18   **Excision of thymus gland**

B18.1   Trans-sternal thymectomy
B18.2   Transcervical thymectomy
B18.8   Other specified
B18.9   Unspecified
         Includes: Thymectomy NEC

B20   **Other operations on thymus gland**

B20.1   Biopsy of lesion of thymus gland
         Includes: Biopsy of thymus gland
B20.2   Exploration of thymus gland
B20.8   Other specified
B20.9   Unspecified

B22   **Excision of adrenal gland**

B22.1   Bilateral adrenalectomy and transposition of adrenal tissue
B22.2   Bilateral adrenalectomy NEC
B22.3   Unilateral adrenalectomy
         Includes: Adrenalectomy NEC
B22.4   Partial adrenalectomy
B22.8   Other specified
B22.9   Unspecified

B23   **Operations on aberrant adrenal tissue**

B23.1   Excision of lesion of aberrant adrenal tissue
B23.2   Exploration of aberrant adrenal tissue
B23.8   Other specified
B23.9   Unspecified

B25   **Other operations on adrenal gland**

B25.1   Excision of lesion of adrenal gland
B25.2   Biopsy of lesion of adrenal gland NEC
         Includes: Biopsy of adrenal gland NEC
B25.3   Embolisation of adrenal gland
B25.4   Exploration of adrenal gland
B25.8   Other specified
B25.9   Unspecified

B27   **Total excision of breast**
         Note: Use a supplementary code for removal of lymph node (T85–T87)

B27.1   Total mastectomy and excision of both pectoral muscles and part of chest wall
B27.2   Total mastectomy and excision of both pectoral muscles NEC
B27.3   Total mastectomy and excision of pectoralis minor muscle
B27.4   Total mastectomy NEC
         Includes: Simple mastectomy
B27.5   Subcutaneous mastectomy
B27.6   Skin sparing mastectomy
B27.8   Other specified
B27.9   Unspecified
         Includes: Mastectomy NEC

B28   **Other excision of breast**

            Note: *Use a supplementary code for removal of lymph node (T85–T87)*

B28.1   Quadrantectomy of breast

B28.2   Partial excision of breast NEC

            Includes: *Wedge excision of breast NEC*

                           Wide excision of breast NEC

B28.3   Excision of lesion of breast NEC

            Includes: *Lumpectomy of breast NEC*

B28.4   Re-excision of breast margins

B28.5   Wire guided partial excision of breast

            Includes: *Wire guided wedge excision of breast*

                           Wire guided wide excision of breast

B28.6   Excision of accessory breast tissue

B28.7   Wire guided excision of lesion of breast

            Includes: *Wire guided lumpectomy of breast*

B28.8   Other specified

B28.9   Unspecified

B29   **Reconstruction of breast**

            Excludes: *Reconstruction of breast using flap of skin of buttock (B38)*

                         Reconstruction of breast using abdominal flap (B39)

            Note: *Use a supplementary code for insertion of prosthesis for breast (B30.1)*

B29.1   Reconstruction of breast using myocutaneous flap of latissimus dorsi muscle

B29.2   Reconstruction of breast using local flap of skin NEC

B29.3   Reconstruction of breast using flap of skin of abdomen NEC

B29.4   Reconstruction of breast using distant flap of skin NEC

B29.5   Revision of reconstruction of breast

B29.8   Other specified

B29.9   Unspecified

B30   **Prosthesis for breast**

            Excludes: *Augmentation mammoplasty (B31.2)*

B30.1   Insertion of prosthesis for breast

B30.2   Revision of prosthesis for breast

B30.3   Removal of prosthesis for breast

B30.4   Renewal of prosthesis for breast

B30.8   Other specified

B30.9   Unspecified

B31   **Other plastic operations on breast**

B31.1   Reduction mammoplasty

B31.2   Augmentation mammoplasty

B31.3   Mastopexy

B31.4   Revision of mammoplasty

B31.8   Other specified

B31.9   Unspecified

B32   **Biopsy of breast**

B32.1   Percutaneous biopsy of lesion of breast
          Includes: Percutaneous biopsy of breast
B32.2   Biopsy of lesion of breast NEC
B32.3   Wire guided biopsy of lesion of breast
B32.8   Other specified
B32.9   Unspecified

B33   **Incision of breast**

B33.1   Drainage of lesion of breast
B33.2   Capsulotomy of breast
B33.3   Exploration of breast
B33.8   Other specified
B33.9   Unspecified

B34   **Operations on duct of breast**

B34.1   Subareolar excision of mammary duct
B34.2   Excision of mammary duct NEC
B34.3   Excision of lesion of mammary duct
B34.4   Microdochotomy
B34.5   Exploration of mammary duct NEC
B34.8   Other specified
B34.9   Unspecified

B35   **Operations on nipple**
          Includes: Skin of nipple
             Note: Codes from Chapter S may be used to enhance these codes

B35.1   Transposition of nipple
B35.2   Excision of nipple
B35.3   Extirpation of lesion of nipple
B35.4   Plastic operations on nipple
B35.5   Biopsy of lesion of nipple
          Includes: Biopsy of nipple
B35.6   Eversion of nipple
B35.8   Other specified
B35.9   Unspecified

B36   **Reconstruction of nipple and areola**
          Includes: Skin of nipple
             Note: Codes from Chapter S may be used to enhance these codes

B36.1   Reconstruction of nipple
B36.2   Nipple sharing using other tissue
B36.3   Nipple sharing NEC
B36.4   Tattooing of nipple
B36.8   Other specified
B36.9   Unspecified

B37	**Other operations on breast**
B37.1	Aspiration of lesion of breast
	Includes: Aspiration of breast
	Note: Use a subsidiary code for fine needle aspiration (Y20.4)
B37.2	Injection into breast
B37.3	Extraction of milk from breast
B37.4	Capsulectomy of breast
B37.5	Lipofilling of breast
B37.8	Other specified
B37.9	Unspecified
B38	**Reconstruction of breast using flap of skin of buttock**
	Note: Use a supplementary code for insertion of prosthesis for breast (B30.1)
B38.1	Reconstruction of breast using free superior gluteal artery perforator flap
B38.2	Reconstruction of breast using free inferior gluteal artery perforator flap
B38.8	Other specified
B38.9	Unspecified
B39	**Reconstruction of breast using abdominal flap**
	Excludes: Reconstruction of breast using flap of skin of abdomen NEC (B29.3)
	Note: Use a supplementary code for insertion of prosthesis for breast (B30.1)
B39.1	Reconstruction of breast using free transverse rectus abdominis myocutaneous flap
B39.2	Reconstruction of breast using pedicled transverse rectus abdominis myocutaneous flap
B39.3	Reconstruction of breast using free deep inferior epigastric perforator flap
B39.4	Reconstruction of breast using pedicled omental flap
B39.5	Reconstruction of breast using free omental flap
B39.8	Other specified
B39.9	Unspecified
B40	**Destruction of lesion of breast**
B40.1	Interstitial laser destruction of lesion of breast
B40.8	Other specified
B40.9	Unspecified

CHAPTER C
EYE
(CODES C01–C90)

Note: *Use a subsidiary code for minimal access approach (Y76.3–Y76.9)*

Use a subsidiary code to identify method of image control (Y53)

C01   **Excision of eye**
      Note: *Use an additional code as necessary for concurrent insertion of prosthetic replacement of eye (C03)*

C01.1   Exenteration of orbit
C01.2   Enucleation of eye
      Includes: Enucleation of eyeball
C01.3   Evisceration of eye
      Includes: Evisceration of contents of eyeball
C01.8   Other specified
C01.9   Unspecified

C02   **Extirpation of lesion of orbit**

C02.1   Excision of lesion of orbit
C02.2   Destruction of lesion of orbit
C02.8   Other specified
C02.9   Unspecified

C03   **Insertion of prosthesis of eye**
      Includes: Orbital implant
      Note: Use as a secondary code when associated with concurrent excision of eye (C01)

C03.1   Insertion of prosthetic replacement for orbit
      Includes: Insertion of orbital wall prosthesis
C03.2   Insertion of prosthetic replacement for eyeball
      Includes: Insertion of central orbital prosthesis
C03.8   Other specified
C03.9   Unspecified

C04   **Attention to prosthesis of eye**
      Includes: Orbital implant

C04.1   Revision of prosthetic replacement for orbit
      Includes: Revision of prosthetic replacement for orbital wall
C04.2   Revision of prosthetic replacement for eyeball
      Includes: Revision of central orbital prosthesis
                 Repair of extruding central orbital implant
C04.3   Removal of prosthetic replacement for orbit
      Includes: Removal of prosthetic replacement for orbital wall
C04.4   Removal of prosthetic replacement for eyeball
      Includes: Removal of central orbital prosthesis
C04.8   Other specified
C04.9   Unspecified

C05   **Plastic repair of orbit**
> *Note: Use a subsidiary code to identify harvest of skin and fat (Y67.2)*

C05.1   Reconstruction of cavity of orbit
C05.2   Plastic repair of cavity of orbit
C05.3   Enlargement of cavity of orbit
C05.8   Other specified
C05.9   Unspecified

C06   **Incision of orbit**

C06.1   Biopsy of lesion of orbit
> *Includes: Biopsy of orbit*

C06.2   Drainage of orbit
C06.3   Decompression of orbit
C06.4   Removal of foreign body from orbit
C06.5   Exploration of orbit
C06.8   Other specified
C06.9   Unspecified
> *Includes: Orbitotomy NEC*

C08   **Other operations on orbit**

C08.1   Transposition of ligament of orbit
C08.2   Open reduction of fracture of orbit
C08.3   Removal of fixation from fracture of orbit
C08.4   Retrobulbar injection into orbit
> *Excludes: Peribulbar injection of therapeutic substance (C86.7)*

C08.5   Internal fixation of fracture of orbit
C08.8   Other specified
C08.9   Unspecified

C09   **Replacement of canthal tendon**
> *Excludes: When associated with correction of ectropion (C15.1) or correction of entropion (C15.2)*

C09.1   Replacement of lateral canthal tendon using tarsal strip
C09.2   Replacement of lateral canthal tendon using periosteal strip
C09.3   Replacement of medial canthal tendon using periosteal strip
C09.8   Other specified
C09.9   Unspecified

C10   **Operations on eyebrow**
> *Includes: Skin of eyebrow*
> *Note: Codes from Chapter S may be used to enhance these codes*

C10.1   Excision of lesion of eyebrow
C10.2   Hair bearing flap to eyebrow
C10.3   Hair bearing graft to eyebrow
C10.4   Suture of eyebrow
C10.5   Incision of lesion of eyebrow
C10.6   Biopsy of lesion of eyebrow
C10.8   Other specified
C10.9   Unspecified

C11 Operations on canthus

Excludes: Replacement of canthal tendon (C09)
Medial canthoplasty for correction of ectropion (C15.1)
Note: Codes from Chapter S may be used to enhance these codes

C11.1   Excision of lesion of canthus
C11.2   Destruction of lesion of canthus
C11.3   Correction of epicanthus
C11.4   Correction of telecanthus
C11.5   Graft of skin to canthus
C11.6   Canthotomy
C11.7   Biopsy of lesion of canthus
C11.8   Other specified
C11.9   Unspecified

C12 Extirpation of lesion of eyelid

Includes: Skin of eyelid
Note: Codes from Chapter S may be used to enhance these codes

C12.1   Excision of lesion of eyelid NEC
C12.2   Cauterisation of lesion of eyelid
C12.3   Cryotherapy to lesion of eyelid
C12.4   Curettage of lesion of eyelid
C12.5   Destruction of lesion of eyelid NEC
C12.6   Wedge excision of lesion of eyelid
C12.8   Other specified
C12.9   Unspecified

C13 Excision of redundant skin of eyelid

Includes: Excision of orbital fat

C13.1   Blepharoplasty of both eyelids
C13.2   Blepharoplasty of upper eyelid
C13.3   Blepharoplasty of lower eyelid
C13.4   Blepharoplasty NEC
C13.8   Other specified
C13.9   Unspecified

C14 Reconstruction of eyelid

Note: Use a subsidiary code to identify harvest of tissue (Y54–Y69)

C14.1   Flap of skin to eyelid
C14.2   Graft of skin to eyelid
C14.3   Graft of cartilage to eyelid
C14.4   Graft of skin and fat to eyelid
          Includes: Dermis fat graft to eyelid
C14.5   Graft of fascia to eyelid
C14.8   Other specified
C14.9   Unspecified

C15   **Correction of deformity of eyelid**

C15.1   Correction of ectropion NEC
               Includes: Medial canthoplasty for correction of ectropion
C15.2   Correction of entropion NEC
C15.3   Correction of trichiasis
C15.4   Correction of cicatricial ectropion
C15.5   Correction of cicatricial entropion
C15.8   Other specified
C15.9   Unspecified

C16   **Other plastic repair of eyelid**
               Excludes: Protective tarsorrhaphy (C20)

C16.1   Central tarsorrhaphy
C16.2   Lateral tarsorrhaphy
C16.3   Medial tarsorrhaphy
C16.4   Tarsorrhaphy NEC
C16.5   Revision of tarsorrhaphy
C16.8   Other specified
C16.9   Unspecified

C17   **Other repair of eyelid**
               Includes: Skin of eyelid
                    Note: Codes from Chapter S may be used to enhance these codes

C17.1   Suture of eyelid
               Excludes: Protective suture of eyelid (C20)
C17.2   Recession of upper eyelid HFQ
C17.3   Recession of lower eyelid HFQ
C17.8   Other specified
C17.9   Unspecified

C18   **Correction of ptosis of eyelid**

C18.1   Correction of ptosis of eyelid using levator muscle technique
C18.2   Correction of ptosis of eyelid using frontalis muscle technique
C18.3   Correction of ptosis of eyelid using sling of fascia
C18.4   Correction of ptosis of eyelid using superior rectus muscle technique
C18.5   Tarsomullerectomy
C18.6   Correction of ptosis of eyelid using aponeurosis technique
C18.8   Other specified
C18.9   Unspecified

C19   **Incision of eyelid**
               Includes: Skin of eyelid
                    Note: Codes from Chapter S may be used to enhance these codes

C19.1   Drainage of lesion of eyelid
C19.8   Other specified
C19.9   Unspecified

C20   **Protective suture of eyelid**
Includes: *Protective tarsorrhaphy*

C20.1   Complete protective suture of eyelid
C20.2   Central protective suture of eyelid
C20.3   Lateral protective suture of eyelid
C20.4   Medial protective suture of eyelid
C20.5   Removal of protective suture from eyelid
C20.8   Other specified
C20.9   Unspecified

C22   **Other operations on eyelid**
Includes: *Skin of eyelid*
     Note: **Principal category, extended at C23**
              Codes from Chapter S may be used to enhance these codes

C22.1   Avulsion of nerve of eyelid
C22.2   Biopsy of lesion of eyelid
        Includes: *Biopsy of eyelid*
C22.3   Removal of foreign body from eyelid
C22.4   Injection into eyelid
C22.5   Exploration of eyelid
C22.6   Epilation of eyelash
C22.7   Denervation of nerve of eyelid
C22.8   Other specified
C22.9   Unspecified

C23   **Operations on eyelid**
Includes: *Skin of eyelid*
     Note: **Principal C22**
              Codes from Chapter S may be used to enhance these codes

C23.1   Insertion of weight into upper eyelid
        Includes: *Insertion of gold weight into upper eyelid*
                      Insertion of platinum chain into upper eyelid
C23.2   Renewal of weight into upper eyelid
        Includes: *Renewal of gold weight into upper eyelid*
                      Renewal of platinum chain into upper eyelid
C23.3   Removal of weight from upper eyelid
        Includes: *Removal of gold weight from upper eyelid*
                      Removal of platinum chain from upper eyelid
C23.8   Other specified
C23.9   Unspecified

C24   **Operations on lacrimal gland**

C24.1   Excision of lacrimal gland
C24.2   Radiotherapy to lacrimal gland
     Note: **Use an additional code to specify radiotherapy delivery (X65)**
C24.3   Destruction of lacrimal gland NEC
C24.4   Biopsy of lesion of lacrimal gland
        Includes: *Biopsy of lacrimal gland*
C24.5   Incision of lacrimal gland
C24.8   Other specified
C24.9   Unspecified

C25   **Connection between lacrimal apparatus and nose**

C25.1   Canaliculodacryocystorhinostomy
C25.2   Conjunctivodacryocystorhinostomy
C25.3   Dacryocystorhinostomy and insertion of tube HFQ
C25.4   Dacryocystorhinostomy NEC
C25.5   Revision of anastomosis between lacrimal apparatus and nose
C25.8   Other specified
C25.9   Unspecified

C26   **Other operations on lacrimal sac**

C26.1   Excision of lacrimal sac
C26.2   Destruction of lesion of lacrimal sac
C26.3   Biopsy of lesion of lacrimal sac
        Includes: Biopsy of lacrimal sac
C26.4   Incision of lacrimal sac
C26.8   Other specified
C26.9   Unspecified

C27   **Operations on nasolacrimal duct**

C27.1   Drainage of nasolacrimal duct
        Includes: Insertion of tube into nasolacrimal duct
                    Insertion of canalicular stent
C27.2   Dilation of nasolacrimal duct
C27.3   Irrigation of nasolacrimal duct
        Includes: Syringing of nasolacrimal duct
C27.4   Removal of tube from nasolacrimal duct
C27.5   Probing of nasolacrimal duct NEC
C27.8   Other specified
C27.9   Unspecified

C29   **Other operations on lacrimal apparatus**

C29.1   Repair of canaliculus
C29.2   Enlargement of lacrimal punctum
C29.3   Occlusion of lacrimal punctum
        Includes: Insertion of punctal plug
C29.4   Marsupialisation of canaliculus
C29.5   Canaliculotomy
C29.8   Other specified
C29.9   Unspecified

C31   **Combined operations on muscles of eye**
        Note: Use an additional code for insertion of adjustable suture into muscle of eye (C35.3)

C31.1   Recession of medial rectus muscle and resection of lateral rectus muscle of eye
C31.2   Bilateral recession of medial recti muscles of eyes
C31.3   Bilateral resection of medial recti muscles of eyes
C31.4   Bilateral recession of lateral recti muscles of eyes
C31.5   Bilateral resection of lateral recti muscles of eyes
C31.6   Recession of lateral rectus muscle and resection of medial rectus muscle of eye
C31.8   Other specified
C31.9   Unspecified

C32   **Recession of muscle of eye**
Excludes: Combined operations on muscles of eye (C31)
> ***Note: Use an additional code for insertion of adjustable suture into muscle of eye (C35.3)***

C32.1   Recession of medial rectus muscle of eye NEC
C32.2   Recession of lateral rectus muscle of eye NEC
C32.3   Recession of superior rectus muscle of eye
C32.4   Recession of inferior rectus muscle of eye
C32.5   Recession of superior oblique muscle of eye
C32.6   Recession of inferior oblique muscle of eye
C32.7   Recession of combinations of muscles of eye
C32.8   Other specified
C32.9   Unspecified

C33   **Resection of muscle of eye**
Includes: Advancement of muscle of eye
            Plication of muscle of eye
            Tucking of muscle of eye
Excludes: Combined operations on muscles of eye (C31)
> ***Note: Use an additional code for insertion of adjustable suture into muscle of eye (C35.3)***

C33.1   Resection of medial rectus muscle of eye NEC
C33.2   Resection of lateral rectus muscle of eye NEC
C33.3   Resection of superior rectus muscle of eye
C33.4   Resection of inferior rectus muscle of eye
C33.5   Resection of superior oblique muscle of eye
C33.6   Resection of inferior oblique muscle of eye
C33.7   Resection of combinations of muscles of eye
C33.8   Other specified
C33.9   Unspecified

C34   **Partial division of tendon of muscle of eye**
> ***Note: Use an additional code for insertion of adjustable suture into muscle of eye (C35.3)***

C34.1   Tenotomy of medial rectus muscle of eye
C34.2   Tenotomy of lateral rectus muscle of eye
C34.3   Tenotomy of superior rectus muscle of eye
C34.4   Tenotomy of inferior rectus muscle of eye
C34.5   Tenotomy of superior oblique muscle of eye
C34.6   Tenotomy of inferior oblique muscle of eye
C34.7   Tenotomy of combinations of muscles of eye
C34.8   Other specified
C34.9   Unspecified
        Includes: Tenotomy of muscle of eye NEC

C35   **Other adjustment to muscle of eye**

C35.1   Transposition of muscle of eye NEC
C35.2   Lengthening of muscle of eye by muscle slide
C35.3   Insertion of adjustable suture into muscle of eye
> ***Note: Use as an additional code when associated with concurrent procedures on muscle of the eye (C31–C37)***

C35.8   Other specified
C35.9   Unspecified

C37   **Other operations on muscle of eye**
> *Note:* *Use an additional code for insertion of adjustable suture into muscle of eye (C35.3)*

C37.1   Excision of lesion of muscle of eye
C37.2   Freeing of adhesions of muscle of eye
C37.3   Biopsy of lesion of muscle of eye
> *Includes:* *Biopsy of muscle of eye*

C37.4   Repair of muscle of eye NEC
C37.8   Other specified
C37.9   Unspecified

C39   **Extirpation of lesion of conjunctiva**

C39.1   Excision of lesion of conjunctiva
C39.2   Cauterisation of lesion of conjunctiva
C39.3   Cryotherapy to lesion of conjunctiva
C39.4   Curettage of lesion of conjunctiva
C39.5   Radiotherapy to lesion of conjunctiva
> *Note:* *Use an additional code to specify radiotherapy delivery (X65)*

C39.8   Other specified
C39.9   Unspecified

C40   **Repair of conjunctiva**

C40.1   Mucosal graft to conjunctiva
C40.2   Amniotic graft to conjunctiva
C40.3   Sliding graft to conjunctiva
C40.4   Prosthetic replacement of conjunctiva
C40.5   Suture of conjunctiva
C40.8   Other specified
C40.9   Unspecified

C41   **Incision of conjunctiva**

C41.1   Peritomy
C41.8   Other specified
C41.9   Unspecified

C43   **Other operations on conjunctiva**

C43.1   Division of adhesions of conjunctiva
C43.2   Biopsy of lesion of conjunctiva
> *Includes:* *Biopsy of conjunctiva*

C43.3   Removal of foreign body from conjunctiva
C43.4   Subconjunctival injection
> *Excludes:* *Injection of bleb (C65.2)*

C43.5   Exploration of conjunctiva
C43.6   Creation of hood of conjunctiva
C43.7   Transplantation of conjunctiva
C43.8   Other specified
C43.9   Unspecified

C44   **Other plastic operations on cornea**
          Note: Principal C46

C44.1   Hydrogel prosthetic keratoplasty
C44.2   Laser in situ keratomileusis
C44.3   Endothelial graft to cornea
          Includes: Endothelial keratoplasty
C44.4   Photorefractive keratectomy
C44.5   Laser subepithelial keratomileusis
C44.8   Other specified
C44.9   Unspecified

C45   **Extirpation of lesion of cornea**

C45.1   Superficial keratectomy
          Includes: Laser keratectomy
          ***Note: For laser keratectomy use a subsidiary code to identify laser modification of
          organ (Y08.5)***
C45.2   Excision of lesion of cornea NEC
C45.3   Cauterisation of lesion of cornea
C45.4   Cryotherapy to lesion of cornea
C45.5   Radiotherapy to lesion of cornea
          Note: Use an additional code to specify radiotherapy delivery (X65)
C45.6   Destruction of lesion of cornea NEC
C45.7   Debridement of lesion of cornea
C45.8   Other specified
C45.9   Unspecified

C46   **Plastic operations on cornea**
          Note: Principal category, extended at C44

C46.1   Refractive keratoplasty
C46.2   Lamellar graft to cornea NEC
          Includes: Lamellar keratoplasty NEC
C46.3   Penetrating graft to cornea
          Includes: Penetrating keratoplasty
C46.4   Insertion of prosthesis into cornea
          Excludes: Insertion of therapeutic contact lens (C51.5)
C46.5   Deep lamellar graft to cornea
          Includes: Deep lamellar keratoplasty
C46.6   Amniotic membrane graft to cornea
C46.7   Transplant of corneal limbal cells
          Note: Use a subsidiary code to identify type of graft (Y27)
C46.8   Other specified
C46.9   Unspecified

C47   **Closure of cornea**

C47.1   Suture of cornea
C47.2   Adjustment to suture of cornea
C47.3   Removal of suture from cornea
C47.4   Gluing of cornea
C47.8   Other specified
C47.9   Unspecified

C48   **Removal of foreign body from cornea**

C48.1   Surgical removal of foreign body from cornea
C48.2   Magnetic extraction of foreign body from cornea
C48.8   Other specified
C48.9   Unspecified

C49   **Incision of cornea**

C49.1   Section of cornea
C49.2   Trephine of cornea
C49.3   Radial keratotomy
C49.8   Other specified
C49.9   Unspecified

C51   **Other operations on cornea**

C51.1   Biopsy of lesion of cornea
            Includes: Biopsy of cornea
C51.2   Chelation of cornea
C51.3   Exploration of cornea
C51.4   Tattooing of cornea
C51.5   Placement of therapeutic contact lens on to cornea
            Includes: Insertion of therapeutic contact lens
C51.8   Other specified
C51.9   Unspecified

C52   **Excision of sclera**
            Excludes: Excision of lesion of sclera NEC (C53.2)

C52.1   Deep sclerectomy with spacer
C52.2   Deep sclerectomy without spacer
            Includes: Deep sclerectomy NEC
C52.8   Other specified
C52.9   Unspecified

C53   **Extirpation of lesion of sclera**

C53.1   Punch resection of sclera
C53.2   Excision of lesion of sclera NEC
C53.3   Cauterisation of lesion of sclera
C53.4   Destruction of lesion of sclera NEC
C53.8   Other specified
C53.9   Unspecified

C54	**Buckling operations for attachment of retina**

C54.1   Overlay scleroplasty
C54.2   Imbrication of sclera
C54.3   Buckling of sclera and implant HFQ
C54.4   Buckling of sclera and local or encircling explant HFQ
             Includes: *Buckling of sclera using tyres, bands or plombs*
C54.5   Buckling of sclera NEC
C54.6   Removal of implant or explant from sclera
C54.7   Maintenance of implant or explant in sclera
             Includes: *Renewal of implant or explant in sclera*
                         Revision of implant or explant in sclera
C54.8   Other specified
C54.9   Unspecified

C55	**Incision of sclera**

C55.1   Drainage of lesion of sclera
C55.2   Corneoscleral trephine
C55.3   Drainage of subretinal fluid through sclera
             Excludes: Drainage of subretinal fluid through retina (C84.5)
C55.4   Expansion of sclera
C55.8   Other specified
C55.9   Unspecified
             Includes: *Sclerotomy NEC*

C57	**Other operations on sclera**

C57.1   Biopsy of lesion of sclera
             Includes: *Biopsy of sclera*
C57.2   Repair of sclera
C57.3   Graft to sclera
C57.4   Suture of sclera
C57.8   Other specified
C57.9   Unspecified

C59	**Excision of iris**

C59.1   Iridocyclectomy
C59.2   Surgical iridectomy
             Includes: *Iridectomy NEC*
C59.8   Other specified
C59.9   Unspecified

C60	**Filtering operations on iris**

C60.1   Trabeculectomy
C60.2   Inclusion of iris
C60.3   Fixation of iris
C60.4   Iridoplasty NEC
             Includes: *Pupilloplasty*
C60.5   Insertion of tube into anterior chamber of eye to assist drainage of aqueous humour
C60.6   Viscocanulostomy
C60.8   Other specified
C60.9   Unspecified

C61   **Other operations on trabecular meshwork of eye**

C61.1   Laser trabeculoplasty
C61.2   Trabeculotomy
C61.3   Goniotomy
C61.4   Goniopuncture
C61.5   Viscogonioplasty

> *Note:*   *Use as a supplementary code when associated with concurrent extraction of lens (C71–C74)*

C61.8   Other specified
C61.9   Unspecified

C62   **Incision of iris**

C62.1   Iridosclerotomy
C62.2   Surgical iridotomy

> *Includes:*   *Iridotomy NEC*

C62.3   Laser iridotomy
C62.4   Correction iridodialysis NEC
C62.8   Other specified
C62.9   Unspecified

C64   **Other operations on iris**

C64.1   Excision of prolapsed iris
C64.2   Excision of lesion of iris
C64.3   Destruction of lesion of iris
C64.4   Biopsy of lesion of iris

> *Includes:*   *Biopsy of iris*

C64.5   Removal of foreign body from iris
C64.6   Stretching of iris
C64.7   Insertion of iris hooks

> *Note:*   *Use as a supplementary code when associated with concurrent extraction of lens (C71–C74)*

C64.8   Other specified
C64.9   Unspecified

C65   **Operations following glaucoma surgery**

C65.1   Needling of bleb
C65.2   Injection of bleb
C65.3   Revision of bleb NEC
C65.4   Removal of releasable suture following glaucoma surgery
C65.5   Laser suture lysis following glaucoma surgery
C65.8   Other specified
C65.9   Unspecified

C66   **Extirpation of ciliary body**

C66.1   Excision of ciliary body

> *Includes:*   *Excision of lesion of ciliary body*

C66.2   Cauterisation of ciliary body
C66.3   Cryotherapy to ciliary body
C66.4   Laser photocoagulation of ciliary body
C66.5   Destruction of ciliary body NEC
C66.8   Other specified
C66.9   Unspecified

C

C67 Other operations on ciliary body

C67.1 Separation of ciliary body
Includes: Cyclodialysis
C67.8 Other specified
C67.9 Unspecified

C69 Other operations on anterior chamber of eye

C69.1 Reformation of anterior chamber of eye
C69.2 Paracentesis of anterior chamber of eye
C69.3 Injection into anterior chamber of eye
C69.4 Irrigation of anterior chamber of eye
Includes: Washout of anterior chamber of eye
C69.8 Other specified
C69.9 Unspecified

C71 Extracapsular extraction of lens
Note: Use as an additional code when associated with concurrent insertion of prosthetic replacement for lens (C75.1)
Use a supplementary code for concurrent insertion of iris hooks (C64.7)
Use a supplementary code for concurrent insertion of capsule tension ring (C77.6)

C71.1 Simple linear extraction of lens
Includes: Needling of lens for cataract
C71.2 Phacoemulsification of lens
C71.3 Aspiration of lens
C71.8 Other specified
C71.9 Unspecified

C72 Intracapsular extraction of lens
Note: Use as an additional code when associated with concurrent insertion of prosthetic replacement for lens (C75.1)
Use a supplementary code for concurrent insertion of iris hooks (C64.7)
Use a supplementary code for concurrent insertion of capsule tension ring (C77.6)

C72.1 Forceps extraction of lens
C72.2 Suction extraction of lens
C72.3 Cryoextraction of lens
C72.8 Other specified
C72.9 Unspecified

C73 Incision of capsule of lens
Note: Use as an additional code when associated with concurrent insertion of prosthetic replacement for lens (C75.1)
Use a supplementary code for concurrent insertion of iris hooks (C64.7)
Use a supplementary code for concurrent insertion of capsule tension ring (C77.6)
Use a subsidiary code to identify laser incision of organ (Y08.6)

C73.1 Membranectomy of lens
C73.2 Capsulotomy of anterior lens capsule
C73.3 Capsulotomy of posterior lens capsule
C73.4 Capsulotomy of lens NEC
C73.8 Other specified
C73.9 Unspecified

C74   **Other extraction of lens**
        Note: *Use as an additional code when associated with concurrent insertion of prosthetic replacement for lens (C75.1)*
                Use a supplementary code for concurrent insertion of iris hooks (C64.7)
                Use a supplementary code for concurrent insertion of capsule tension ring (C77.6)

C74.1   Curettage of lens
C74.2   Discission of cataract
C74.3   Mechanical lensectomy
         Includes: *Pars plana lensectomy*
C74.8   Other specified
C74.9   Unspecified

C75   **Prosthesis of lens**
        Excludes: *Placement of therapeutic contact lens on to cornea (C51.5)*
           Note: *Use a supplementary code to identify method of concurrent extraction of lens (C71–C74)*

C75.1   Insertion of prosthetic replacement for lens NEC
C75.2   Revision of prosthetic replacement for lens
C75.3   Removal of prosthetic replacement for lens
C75.4   Insertion of prosthetic replacement for lens using suture fixation
         Includes: *Suture fixation of lens implant*
C75.8   Other specified
C75.9   Unspecified

C77   **Other operations on lens**

C77.1   Capsulectomy
C77.2   Couching of lens
C77.3   Biopsy of lesion of lens
         Includes: *Biopsy of lens*
C77.4   Surgical removal of foreign body from lens
C77.5   Magnetic extraction of foreign body from lens
C77.6   Insertion of capsule tension ring
           Note: *Use as a supplementary code when associated with concurrent extraction of lens (C71–C74)*
C77.8   Other specified
C77.9   Unspecified

C79 Operations on vitreous body

C79.1 Vitrectomy using anterior approach
Includes: *Destruction of vitreous body using anterior approach*
   Note: Use a supplementary code for concurrent tamponade of retina (C79.5, C79.6)

C79.2 Vitrectomy using pars plana approach
Includes: *Vitrectomy NEC*
   Destruction of vitreous body using pars plana approach
   Destruction of vitreous body NEC
   Note: Use a supplementary code for concurrent tamponade of retina (C79.5, C79.6)

C79.3 Injection of vitreous substitute into vitreous body NEC
Excludes: *Internal tamponade of retina using gas (C79.5)*
   Internal tamponade of retina using liquid (C79.6)

C79.4 Injection into vitreous body NEC

C79.5 Internal tamponade of retina using gas
Includes: *Internal tamponade of retina using air*
   Note: Use as a secondary code when associated with vitrectomy (C79.1, C79.2)

C79.6 Internal tamponade of retina using liquid
Includes: *Internal tamponade of retina using oil or heavy liquids*
   Note: Use as a secondary code when associated with vitrectomy (C79.1, C79.2)

C79.7 Removal of internal tamponade agent from vitreous body
C79.8 Other specified
C79.9 Unspecified

C80 Operations on retinal membrane
Includes: *Macula*
Excludes: *Epiretinal dissection (C84.1)*
   Excision of lesion of retina NEC (C84.2)

C80.1 Peel of epiretinal fibroglial membrane
Includes: *Peel of epiretinal membrane*
C80.2 Peel of internal limiting membrane
C80.3 Delamination of epiretinal fibrovascular membrane
C80.4 Segmentation of epiretinal fibrovascular membrane
C80.5 Removal of subretinal vascular membrane
C80.6 Removal of subretinal membrane NEC
Includes: *Removal of subretinal band*
C80.8 Other specified
C80.9 Unspecified

C81 Photocoagulation of retina for detachment
C81.1 Xenon photocoagulation of retina for detachment
C81.2 Laser photocoagulation of retina for detachment
Includes: *Laser retinopexy for detachment*
C81.8 Other specified
C81.9 Unspecified

C82   **Destruction of lesion of retina**
Includes: Destruction of retina
Excludes: Destruction of subretinal lesion (C88)

C82.1   Cauterisation of lesion of retina
Includes: Photocoagulation of lesion of retina NEC
             Electrocoagulation of lesion of retina NEC

C82.2   Cryotherapy to lesion of retina

C82.3   External beam radiotherapy to lesion of retina
Includes: Radiotherapy to lesion of retina NEC
     Note: Use an additional code to specify radiotherapy delivery (X65)

C82.4   Plaque radiotherapy to lesion of retina
     Note: Use an additional code to specify radiotherapy delivery (X65)

C82.5   Panretinal laser photocoagulation to lesion of retina
Excludes: Laser photocoagulation of retina for detachment (C81.2)
     Note: Panretinal applies when more than a quadrant of the retina is treated

C82.6   Laser photocoagulation to lesion of retina NEC
Excludes: Laser photocoagulation of retina for detachment (C81.2)

C82.8   Other specified
C82.9   Unspecified

C83   **Translocation of retina**
Includes: Pigment epithelium
             Macula

C83.1   Pigment epithelium translocation of retina
C83.2   Macular translocation three hundred and sixty degrees
C83.3   Limited macular translocation
Includes: Macular translocation NEC

C83.8   Other specified
C83.9   Unspecified

C84   **Other operations on retina**
Includes: Choroid

C84.1   Epiretinal dissection
Excludes: Operations on retinal membrane (C80)

C84.2   Excision of lesion of retina NEC
C84.3   Biopsy of lesion of retina
Includes: Biopsy of retina

C84.4   Retinal vascular sheathotomy
C84.5   Drainage of subretinal fluid through retina
Excludes: Drainage of subretinal fluid through sclera (C55.3)

C84.6   Retinotomy NEC
Includes: Relieving retinectomy

C84.8   Other specified
C84.9   Unspecified

C85   **Fixation of retina**
            Excludes: Laser retinopexy for retinal detachment (C81.2)

C85.1   Retinopexy using cryotherapy
C85.2   Retinopexy using diathermy
C85.3   Retinopexy using mechanical tacks
C85.4   Retinopexy using tissue adhesive
C85.5   Retinopexy NEC
C85.8   Other specified
C85.9   Unspecified

C86   **Other operations on eye**

C86.1   Biopsy of lesion of eye NEC
            Includes: Biopsy of eye NEC
C86.2   Repair of globe
            Includes: Repair of penetrating injury to eye
C86.3   Suture of eye NEC
C86.4   Removal of foreign body from eye NEC
C86.5   Fluorescein angiography of eye
            Includes: Fluorescein angiography of retina
C86.6   Examination of eye under anaesthetic
C86.7   Injection of therapeutic substance around the eye
            Includes: Peribulbar injection of therapeutic substance
            *   Subtenons injection of therapeutic substance*
            Excludes: Retrobulbar injection into orbit (C08.4)
            *   Subconjunctival Injection (C43.4)*
            *   Injection into posterior segment of eye (C89.3)*
C86.8   Other specified
C86.9   Unspecified

C87   **Evaluation of retina**
            Excludes: Examination of eye under anaesthetic (C86.6)
            *   Fluorescein angiography of eye (C86.5)*
            *   Electroretinography (A84.5)*

C87.1   Digital imaging of retina
C87.2   Indocyanine angiography evaluation of retina
C87.3   Tomography evaluation of retina
C87.4   Ultrasonic evaluation of retina
C87.5   Scanning laser ophthalmoscopy evaluation of retina
C87.8   Other specified
C87.9   Unspecified

C88   **Destruction of subretinal lesion**

C88.1   Transpupillary thermotherapy to subretinal lesion
            Includes: Transpupillary thermotherapy to retinal lesion
C88.2   Photodynamic therapy to subretinal lesion
            Includes: Photodynamic therapy to retinal lesion
C88.8   Other specified
C88.9   Unspecified

C89   **Operations on posterior segment of eye**
>   *Note: Operations on named sites within the posterior segment are usually classified elsewhere*

C89.1   Insertion of sustained release device into posterior segment of eye
C89.2   Injection of steroid into posterior segment of eye
C89.3   Injection of therapeutic substance into posterior segment of eye NEC
>   *Excludes: Injection of therapeutic substance around the eye (C86.7)*

C89.8   Other specified
C89.9   Unspecified

C90   **Local anaesthetics for ophthalmology procedures**
>   *Excludes: General anaesthetic (Y80)*

C90.1   Topical anaesthetic
C90.2   Subconjunctival anaesthetic
C90.3   Subtenons anaesthetic
C90.4   Peribulbar anaesthetic
C90.5   Retrobulbar anaesthetic
C90.8   Other specified
C90.9   Unspecified

CHAPTER D
EAR
(CODES D01–D28)

Note: *Use a subsidiary code for minimal access approach (Y74–Y76)*
Use a subsidiary code to identify method of image control (Y53)

D01   **Excision of external ear**

D01.1   Total excision of external ear
D01.2   Partial excision of external ear
D01.3   Excision of preauricular abnormality
D01.8   Other specified
D01.9   Unspecified

D02   **Extirpation of lesion of external ear**
            Includes: *Skin of external ear*
                Note: *Codes from Chapter S may be used to enhance these codes*

D02.1   Excision of lesion of external ear
D02.2   Destruction of lesion of external ear
D02.8   Other specified
D02.9   Unspecified

D03   **Plastic operations on external ear**
            Note at D02 applies
            Includes: *Skin of external ear*
            Excludes: *Replantation of ear (X03.1)*

D03.1   Reconstruction of external ear using graft
D03.2   Reconstruction of external ear NEC
D03.3   Pinnaplasty
            Includes: *Correction of prominent ear*
D03.4   Meatoplasty of external ear
D03.8   Other specified
D03.9   Unspecified

D04   **Drainage of external ear**
            Note at D02 applies
            Includes: *Skin of external ear*

D04.1   Drainage of haematoma of external ear
D04.2   Drainage of abscess of external ear
D04.8   Other specified
D04.9   Unspecified

D05   **Attachment of auricular prosthesis**
            Excludes: *Attachment of bone anchored hearing prosthesis (D13)*

D05.1   First stage insertion of fixtures for auricular prosthesis
D05.2   Second stage insertion of fixtures for auricular prosthesis
D05.3   Reduction of soft tissue for auricular prosthesis
D05.4   Attention to fixtures for auricular prosthesis
D05.5   Placement of hearing implant in external ear
D05.6   Attention to hearing implant in external ear
D05.7   Removal of hearing implant from external ear
D05.8   Other specified
D05.9   Unspecified

D06   **Other operations on external ear**
               Note at D02 applies
              Includes: Skin of external ear

D06.1   Biopsy of lesion of external ear
              Includes: Biopsy of external ear
D06.2   Repair of lobe of external ear
D06.3   Repair of external ear NEC
D06.8   Other specified
D06.9   Unspecified

D07   **Clearance of external auditory canal**

D07.1   Irrigation of external auditory canal for removal of wax
              Includes: Syringing of ear for removal of wax
                          Washout of ear for removal of wax
D07.2   Removal of wax from external auditory canal NEC
D07.3   Removal of foreign body from external auditory canal
D07.8   Other specified
D07.9   Unspecified

D08   **Other operations on external auditory canal**

D08.1   Extirpation of lesion of external auditory canal
D08.2   Reconstruction of external auditory canal
D08.3   Drainage of external auditory canal
D08.4   Incision of external auditory canal
D08.5   Irrigation of external auditory canal NEC
D08.6   Blind sac closure of external auditory canal
D08.8   Other specified
D08.9   Unspecified

D10   **Exenteration of mastoid air cells**

D10.1   Radical mastoidectomy NEC
D10.2   Modified radical mastoidectomy
D10.3   Cortical mastoidectomy
D10.4   Simple mastoidectomy
              Includes: Mastoidectomy NEC
D10.5   Excision of lesion of mastoid
D10.6   Revision of mastoidectomy
D10.8   Other specified
D10.9   Unspecified

D12   **Other operations on mastoid**
              Includes: Attic

D12.1   Obliteration of mastoid
D12.2   Atticotomy
D12.3   Biopsy of mastoid
D12.4   Exploration of mastoid
D12.5   Removal of pack from mastoid
D12.7   Atticoantrostomy
D12.8   Other specified
D12.9   Unspecified

D13 **Attachment of bone anchored hearing prosthesis**
Excludes: Attachment of auricular prosthesis (D05)

D13.1 First stage insertion of fixtures for bone anchored hearing prosthesis
D13.2 Second stage insertion of fixtures for bone anchored hearing prosthesis
D13.3 Reduction of soft tissue for bone anchored hearing prosthesis
D13.4 Attention to fixtures for bone anchored hearing prosthesis
D13.5 One stage insertion of fixtures for bone anchored hearing prosthesis
D13.6 Fitting of external hearing prosthesis to bone anchored fixtures
D13.8 Other specified
D13.9 Unspecified

D14 **Repair of eardrum**

D14.1 Tympanoplasty using graft
Includes: Myringoplasty using graft
D14.2 Tympanoplasty NEC
Includes: Myringoplasty NEC
Note: Use as a supplementary code when associated with prosthetic replacement of ossicular chain (D16.1)
D14.3 Revision of tympanoplasty
Includes: Revision of myringoplasty
D14.4 Combined approach tympanoplasty
D14.8 Other specified
D14.9 Unspecified

D15 **Drainage of middle ear**

D15.1 Myringotomy with insertion of ventilation tube through tympanic membrane
Includes: Insertion of ventilation tube through tympanic membrane
Insertion of grommet through tympanic membrane
D15.2 Suction clearance of middle ear
D15.3 Incision of ear drum NEC
Includes: Myringotomy
Tympanotomy NEC
Exploration of middle ear
Excludes: Myringotomy with insertion of ventilation tube through tympanic membrane (D15.1)
D15.8 Other specified
D15.9 Unspecified

D16 **Reconstruction of ossicular chain**
Note: Use a supplementary code for other concurrent operations on ossicle of ear (D17)

D16.1 Prosthetic replacement of ossicular chain
Note: Use a supplementary code for concurrent tympanoplasty (D14.2)
D16.2 Graft replacement of ossicular chain
D16.8 Other specified
D16.9 Unspecified

D17   **Other operations on ossicle of ear**
> *Note:*   *Use as a supplementary code when associated with reconstruction of ossicular chain (D16)*

D17.1   Stapedectomy
D17.2   Revision of stapedectomy
D17.3   Division of adhesions of ossicle of ear
D17.8   Other specified
D17.9   Unspecified

D19   **Extirpation of lesion of middle ear**

D19.1   Excision of lesion of middle ear
D19.2   Destruction of lesion of middle ear
D19.8   Other specified
D19.9   Unspecified

D20   **Other operations on middle ear**

D20.1   Biopsy of lesion of middle ear
> *Includes:*   *Biopsy of middle ear*

D20.2   Maintenance of ventilation tube through tympanic membrane
> *Includes:*   *Maintenance of grommet through tympanic membrane*

D20.3   Removal of ventilation tube from tympanic membrane
> *Includes:*   *Removal of grommet from tympanic membrane*

D20.4   Placement of hearing implant in middle ear
D20.5   Attention to hearing implant in middle ear
D20.6   Removal of hearing implant in middle ear
D20.7   Transtympanic injection to middle ear
D20.8   Other specified
D20.9   Unspecified

D22   **Operations on eustachian canal**

D22.1   Graft to eustachian canal
D22.2   Intubation of eustachian canal
D22.3   Insufflation of eustachian canal
D22.8   Other specified
D22.9   Unspecified

D23   **Operations on inner ear**

D23.1   Transtympanic injection to inner ear
D23.8   Other specified
D23.9   Unspecified

D24   **Operations on cochlea**

D24.1   Implantation of intracochlear prosthesis
D24.2   Implantation of extracochlear prosthesis
D24.3   Attention to cochlear prosthesis
D24.4   Neurectomy of cochlea
D24.5   Transtympanic electrocochleography
D24.6   Removal of cochlear prosthesis
D24.8   Other specified
D24.9   Unspecified

D26	**Operations on vestibular apparatus**
D26.1	Operations on endolymphatic sac
D26.2	Membranous labyrinthectomy
D26.3	Osseous labyrinthectomy
D26.4	Neurectomy of vestibular apparatus
D26.8	Other specified
D26.9	Unspecified

D28	**Other operations on ear**
D28.1	Biopsy of lesion of ear NEC
	Includes: Biopsy of ear NEC
D28.2	Examination of ear under anaesthetic
D28.8	Other specified
D28.9	Unspecified

CHAPTER E
RESPIRATORY TRACT
(CODES E01–E98)

Excludes:	CHEST WALL	(Chapter T)
	PLEURA	(Chapter T)
	PLEURAL CAVITY	(Chapter T)

Note: Use a subsidiary code for minimal access approach (Y74–Y76)

Use a subsidiary code to identify method of image control (Y53)

E01 **Excision of nose**

E01.1 Total excision of nose
E01.8 Other specified
E01.9 Unspecified

E02 **Plastic operations on nose**
Excludes: Replantation of nose (X03.2)
Note: Principal category, extended at E07
Codes from Chapter S may be used to enhance these codes

E02.1 Total reconstruction of nose
E02.2 Reconstruction of nose NEC
E02.3 Septorhinoplasty using implant
Excludes: Septorhinoplasty NEC (E07.3)
E02.4 Septorhinoplasty using graft
Excludes: Septorhinoplasty NEC (E07.3)
E02.5 Reduction rhinoplasty
E02.6 Rhinoplasty NEC
E02.7 Alar reconstruction with cartilage graft
E02.8 Other specified
E02.9 Unspecified

E03 **Operations on septum of nose**

E03.1 Submucous excision of septum of nose
E03.2 Excision of lesion of septum of nose
E03.3 Biopsy of lesion of septum of nose
Includes: Biopsy of septum of nose
E03.4 Closure of perforation of septum of nose NEC
E03.5 Incision of septum of nose
E03.6 Septoplasty of nose NEC
E03.7 Septal reconstruction with cartilage graft
E03.8 Other specified
E03.9 Unspecified

E04 **Operations on turbinate of nose**

E04.1 Submucous diathermy to turbinate of nose
E04.2 Excision of turbinate of nose NEC
Includes: Reduction of turbinate of nose NEC
E04.3 Excision of lesion of turbinate of nose NEC
E04.4 Division of adhesions of turbinate of nose
E04.5 Biopsy of lesion of turbinate of nose
Includes: Biopsy of turbinate of nose
E04.6 Cauterisation of turbinate of nose
E04.7 Surgical outfracture of turbinate of nose
E04.8 Other specified
E04.9 Unspecified

E05   **Surgical arrest of bleeding from internal nose**
Includes: Surgical arrest of spontaneous bleeding from internal nose

E05.1   Cauterisation of internal nose
E05.2   Ligation of artery of internal nose
E05.3   Embolisation of artery of internal nose
E05.4   Laser therapy of internal nose
E05.8   Other specified
E05.9   Unspecified

E06   **Packing of cavity of nose**

E06.1   Packing of posterior cavity of nose NEC
E06.2   Packing of anterior cavity of nose NEC
E06.3   Removal of packing from cavity of nose
E06.4   Balloon packing of cavity of nose
E06.8   Other specified
E06.9   Unspecified

E07   **Other plastic operations on nose**
Note: Principal E02
Codes from Chapter S may be used to enhance these codes

E07.1   Correction of stenosis of nasal pyriform aperture
E07.2   Septodermoplasty
E07.3   Septorhinoplasty NEC
E07.8   Other specified
E07.9   Unspecified

E08   **Other operations on internal nose**

E08.1   Polypectomy of internal nose
E08.2   Extirpation of lesion of internal nose NEC
E08.3   Correction of congenital atresia of choana
E08.4   Division of adhesions of internal nose
E08.5   Removal of foreign body from cavity of nose
E08.6   Surgical closure of anterior nares
E08.7   Surgical reopening of anterior nares
E08.8   Other specified
E08.9   Unspecified

E09   **Operations on external nose**
Includes: Skin of external nose
Note: Codes from Chapter S may be used to enhance these codes

E09.1   Excision of lesion of external nose
E09.2   Destruction of lesion of external nose NEC
E09.3   Suture of external nose
E09.4   Shave of skin of nose
E09.5   Biopsy of lesion of external nose
Includes: Biopsy of external nose
E09.6   Laser destruction of lesion of external nose
E09.8   Other specified
E09.9   Unspecified

E10   **Other operations on nose**

E10.1   Biopsy of lesion of nose NEC
               Includes: Biopsy of nose NEC
E10.8   Other specified
E10.9   Unspecified

E11   **Operations on fixtures for nasal prosthesis**

E11.1   One stage attachment of fixtures for nasal prosthesis NEC
E11.2   First stage attachment of fixtures for nasal prosthesis
E11.3   Second stage attachment of fixtures for nasal prosthesis
E11.4   Revision of fixtures for attachment of nasal prosthesis
E11.5   Removal of fixtures for attachment of nasal prosthesis
E11.6   Attachment of nasal prosthesis
E11.8   Other specified
E11.9   Unspecified

E12   **Operations on maxillary antrum using sublabial approach**

E12.1   Ligation of maxillary artery using sublabial approach
E12.2   Drainage of maxillary antrum using sublabial approach
E12.3   Irrigation of maxillary antrum using sublabial approach
               Includes: Washout of maxillary antrum using sublabial approach
E12.4   Transantral neurectomy of vidian nerve using sublabial approach
               Excludes: Neurectomy of vidian nerve NEC (E13.7)
E12.8   Other specified
E12.9   Unspecified

E13   **Other operations on maxillary antrum**

E13.1   Drainage of maxillary antrum NEC
E13.2   Excision of lesion of maxillary antrum
E13.3   Intranasal antrostomy
E13.4   Biopsy of lesion of maxillary antrum
               Includes: Biopsy of maxillary antrum
E13.5   Closure of fistula between maxillary antrum and mouth
E13.6   Puncture of maxillary antrum
               Includes: Irrigation of maxillary antrum NEC
E13.7   Neurectomy of vidian nerve NEC
               Excludes: Transantral neurectomy of vidian nerve using sublabial approach (E12.4)
E13.8   Other specified
E13.9   Unspecified

E14   **Operations on frontal sinus**
               Note: Principal category, extended at E16

E14.1   External frontoethmoidectomy
E14.2   Intranasal ethmoidectomy
E14.3   External ethmoidectomy
E14.4   Transantral ethmoidectomy
E14.5   Bone flap to frontal sinus
E14.6   Trephine of frontal sinus
E14.7   Median drainage of frontal sinus
               Excludes: Drainage of frontal sinus NEC (E16.2)
E14.8   Other specified
E14.9   Unspecified

E15   **Operations on sphenoid sinus**

E15.1   Drainage of sphenoid sinus
E15.2   Puncture of sphenoid sinus
E15.3   Repair of sphenoidal sinus
E15.4   Excision of lesion of sphenoid sinus
E15.8   Other specified
E15.9   Unspecified

E16   **Other operations on frontal sinus**
             Includes: Ethmoid sinus
                       Note: Principal E14

E16.1   Frontal sinus osteoplasty
E16.2   Drainage of frontal sinus NEC
             Excludes: Median drainage of frontal sinus (E14.7)
E16.8   Other specified
E16.9   Unspecified

E17   **Operations on unspecified nasal sinus**

E17.1   Excision of nasal sinus NEC
E17.2   Excision of lesion of nasal sinus NEC
E17.3   Biopsy of lesion of nasal sinus NEC
             Includes: Biopsy of nasal sinus NEC
E17.4   Lateral rhinotomy into nasal sinus NEC
E17.8   Other specified
E17.9   Unspecified

E19   **Excision of pharynx**
             Includes: Nasopharynx

E19.1   Total pharyngectomy
             Note: Use a supplementary code for concurrent laryngectomy (E29)
E19.2   Partial pharyngectomy
             Includes: Pharyngectomy NEC
             Note: Use a supplementary code for concurrent laryngectomy (E29)
E19.8   Other specified
E19.9   Unspecified

E20   **Operations on adenoid**

E20.1   Total adenoidectomy
             Includes: Excision of adenoid
                       Adenoidectomy
             Note: Use as a secondary code when associated with excision of tonsil (F34, F36.6)

E20.2   Biopsy of adenoid
             Includes: Biopsy of lesion of adenoid
E20.3   Surgical arrest of postoperative bleeding of adenoid
E20.4   Suction diathermy adenoidectomy
             Note: Use as a secondary code when associated with excision of tonsil (F34, F36.6)
E20.8   Other specified
E20.9   Unspecified

E21 **Repair of pharynx**
Includes: Nasopharynx

E21.1 Pharyngoplasty using posterior pharyngeal implant
E21.2 Pharyngoplasty using posterior pharyngeal flap
E21.3 Pharyngoplasty using lateral pharyngeal flap
E21.4 Plastic repair of pharynx NEC
E21.8 Other specified
E21.9 Unspecified

E23 **Other open operations on pharynx**
Includes: Nasopharynx

E23.1 Open excision of lesion of pharynx
E23.2 Operations on pharyngeal pouch
E23.8 Other specified
E23.9 Unspecified

E24 **Therapeutic endoscopic operations on pharynx**
Includes: Nasopharynx
Excludes: Therapeutic endoscopic operations on nasal cavity (E64)
> **Note:** **It is not necessary to code additionally any mention of diagnostic endoscopic examination of nasopharynx (E25.3) or pharynx NEC (E25.9)**

E24.1 Endoscopic extirpation of lesion of nasopharynx
E24.2 Endoscopic extirpation of lesion of pharynx NEC
E24.3 Endoscopic operations on pharyngeal pouch
E24.8 Other specified
E24.9 Unspecified

E25 **Diagnostic endoscopic examination of pharynx**
Includes: Nasopharynx
Excludes: Endoscopic examination of nasal cavity (E65)

E25.1 Diagnostic endoscopic examination of nasopharynx and biopsy of lesion of nasopharynx
Includes: Diagnostic endoscopic examination of nasopharynx and biopsy of nasopharynx
Endoscopic biopsy of lesion of nasopharynx
Endoscopic biopsy of nasopharynx
Biopsy of lesion of nasopharynx NEC
Biopsy of nasopharynx NEC
E25.2 Diagnostic endoscopic examination of pharynx and biopsy of lesion of pharynx NEC
Includes: Diagnostic endoscopic examination of pharynx and biopsy of pharynx NEC
Endoscopic biopsy of lesion of pharynx NEC
Endoscopic biopsy of pharynx NEC
Biopsy of lesion of pharynx NEC
Biopsy of pharynx NEC
E25.3 Diagnostic endoscopic examination of nasopharynx NEC
Includes: Nasopharyngoscopy NEC
E25.8 Other specified
E25.9 Unspecified
Includes: Pharyngoscopy NEC

E27   **Other operations on pharynx**
            Includes: Nasopharynx

E27.1   Open biopsy of lesion of pharynx
            Includes: Open biopsy of pharynx
E27.2   Drainage of retropharyngeal abscess
            Includes: Drainage of parapharyngeal abscess
E27.3   Incision of pharynx NEC
E27.4   Removal of foreign body from pharynx
E27.5   Dilation of pharynx
E27.6   Examination of pharynx under anaesthetic
E27.8   Other specified
E27.9   Unspecified

E28   **Operations on cricopharyngeus muscle**

E28.1   Cricopharyngeal myotomy
E28.8   Other specified
E28.9   Unspecified

E29   **Excision of larynx**
            Note: Use as a supplementary code when associated with pharyngectomy (E19)

E29.1   Total laryngectomy
E29.2   Partial horizontal laryngectomy
E29.3   Partial vertical laryngectomy
E29.4   Partial laryngectomy NEC
E29.5   Laryngofissure and chordectomy of vocal chord
E29.6   Laryngectomy NEC
E29.8   Other specified
E29.9   Unspecified

E30   **Open extirpation of lesion of larynx**

E30.1   Excision of lesion of larynx using thyrotomy as approach
E30.2   Excision of lesion of larynx using lateral pharyngotomy as approach
E30.3   Open destruction of lesion of larynx
E30.8   Other specified
E30.9   Unspecified

E31   **Reconstruction of larynx**

E31.1   Laryngotracheal reconstruction using cartilage graft
E31.2   Laryngotracheoplasty NEC
E31.3   Division of stenosis of larynx and insertion of prosthesis into larynx
E31.4   Implantation of artificial voice box into larynx
E31.5   Attention to artificial voice box in larynx
E31.8   Other specified
E31.9   Unspecified

E33 **Other open operations on larynx**

E33.1 External arytenoidectomy

E33.2 Chordopexy of vocal chord

E33.3 Operations on cartilage of larynx NEC
Includes: Chondroplasty of larynx

E33.4 Open biopsy of lesion of larynx
Includes: Open biopsy of larynx

E33.5 Vocal cord medialisation using implant
Includes: Thyroplasty using implant

E33.6 Vocal cord medialisation using biological material
Includes: Thyroplasty using biological material

E33.8 Other specified

E33.9 Unspecified

E34 **Microtherapeutic endoscopic operations on larynx**
Note: It is not necessary to code additionally any mention of diagnostic endoscopic examination of larynx (E36.9) or diagnostic microendoscopic examination of larynx (E37.9)

E34.1 Microtherapeutic endoscopic extirpation of lesion of larynx using laser

E34.2 Microtherapeutic endoscopic resection of lesion of larynx NEC

E34.3 Microtherapeutic endoscopic destruction of lesion of larynx NEC

E34.8 Other specified

E34.9 Unspecified

E35 **Other therapeutic endoscopic operations on larynx**
Note: It is not necessary to code additionally any mention of diagnostic endoscopic examination of larynx (E36.9) or diagnostic microendoscopic examination of larynx (E37.9)

E35.1 Endoscopic arytenoidectomy

E35.2 Endoscopic resection of lesion of larynx

E35.3 Endoscopic destruction of lesion of larynx

E35.4 Endoscopic removal of prosthesis from larynx

E35.5 Endoscopic removal of foreign body from larynx

E35.6 Endoscopic partial laryngectomy

E35.7 Endoscopic vocal cord medialisation

E35.8 Other specified

E35.9 Unspecified

E36 **Diagnostic endoscopic examination of larynx**
Excludes: Diagnostic microendoscopic examination of larynx (E37)

E36.1 Diagnostic endoscopic examination of larynx and biopsy of lesion of larynx
Includes: Diagnostic endoscopic examination of larynx and biopsy of larynx
Endoscopic biopsy of lesion of larynx
Endoscopic biopsy of larynx
Biopsy of lesion of larynx NEC
Biopsy of larynx NEC

E36.8 Other specified

E36.9 Unspecified
Includes: Laryngoscopy NEC

E37   **Diagnostic microendoscopic examination of larynx**
Excludes: Diagnostic endoscopic examination of larynx (E36)

E37.1   Diagnostic microendoscopic examination of larynx and biopsy of lesion of larynx
Includes: Microendoscopic examination of larynx and biopsy of larynx
Microendoscopic biopsy of lesion of larynx
Microendoscopic biopsy of larynx

E37.8   Other specified
E37.9   Unspecified
Includes: Microlaryngoscopy NEC

E38   **Other operations on larynx**

E38.1   Injection into larynx
E38.8   Other specified
E38.9   Unspecified

E39   **Partial excision of trachea**
Note: Use an additional code for excision of carina as necessary (E44.1)

E39.1   Open excision of lesion of trachea
Includes: Excision of lesion of trachea NEC

E39.8   Other specified
E39.9   Unspecified

E40   **Plastic operations on trachea**
Note: Use an additional code for reconstruction of carina as necessary (E44.2)

E40.1   Reconstruction of trachea and anastomosis HFQ
E40.2   Reconstruction of trachea using graft
E40.3   Reconstruction of trachea NEC
E40.8   Other specified
E40.9   Unspecified

E41   **Open placement of prosthesis in trachea**
Excludes: Placement of tracheostomy tube (E42)

E41.1   Open insertion of tubal prosthesis in trachea
E41.2   Open renewal of tubal prosthesis in trachea
E41.3   Open removal of tubal prosthesis from trachea
E41.4   Tracheo-oesophageal puncture with insertion of speech prosthesis
E41.8   Other specified
E41.9   Unspecified

E42   **Exteriorisation of trachea**

E42.1   Permanent tracheostomy
E42.2   Cricothyroidostomy
E42.3   Temporary tracheostomy
             Includes: *Tracheostomy NEC*
                           Tracheostomy
                           Placement of tracheostomy tube
E42.4   Revision of tracheostomy
E42.5   Closure of tracheostomy
E42.6   Replacement of tracheostomy tube
E42.7   Removal of tracheostomy tube
             Includes: *Decannulation of tracheostomy*
E42.8   Other specified
E42.9   Unspecified

E43   **Other open operations on trachea**

E43.1   Open destruction of lesion of trachea
E43.2   Tracheorrhaphy
E43.3   Tracheopexy
E43.4   Open biopsy of lesion of trachea
             Includes: *Open biopsy of trachea*
E43.5   Closure of tracheocutaneous fistula
E43.8   Other specified
E43.9   Unspecified

E44   **Open operations on carina**

E44.1   Excision of carina
             Excludes: *When associated with reconstruction of carina (E44.2)*
                Note: ***Use as a secondary code in association with excision of trachea (E39) bronchus***
                          (E46) or lung (E54) as necessary
E44.2   Reconstruction of carina
             Includes: *Excision of carina and reconstruction HFQ*
                Note: ***Use as a secondary code in association with plastic operations on trachea (E40)***
E44.3   Open biopsy of lesion of carina
             Includes: *Open biopsy of carina*
E44.8   Other specified
E44.9   Unspecified

E45   **Code deleted**

E46   **Partial extirpation of bronchus**
                Note: ***Use an additional code for excision of carina as necessary (E44.1)***

E46.1   Sleeve resection of bronchus and anastomosis HFQ
E46.2   Excision of cyst of bronchus
E46.3   Excision of lesion of bronchus NEC
E46.4   Open destruction of lesion of bronchus
E46.8   Other specified
E46.9   Unspecified

E47　　　**Other open operations on bronchus**

E47.1　　Open biopsy of lesion of bronchus NEC
　　　　　Includes:　Open biopsy of bronchus NEC
E47.2　　Closure of fistula of bronchus
E47.3　　Repair of bronchus NEC
E47.8　　Other specified
E47.9　　Unspecified

E48　　　**Therapeutic fibreoptic endoscopic operations on lower respiratory tract**
　　　　　Includes:　Therapeutic endoscopic operations on lower respiratory tract NEC
　　　　　　　　　　Trachea
　　　　　　　　　　Carina
　　　　　　　　　　Bronchus
　　　　　　　　　　Lung
　　　　　Note:　It is not necessary to code additionally any mention of diagnostic fibreoptic endoscopic examination of lower respiratory tract (E49.9)
　　　　　　　　　Use a subsidiary site code as necessary

E48.1　　Fibreoptic endoscopic snare resection of lesion of lower respiratory tract
E48.2　　Fibreoptic endoscopic laser destruction of lesion of lower respiratory tract
E48.3　　Fibreoptic endoscopic destruction of lesion of lower respiratory tract NEC
E48.4　　Fibreoptic endoscopic aspiration of lower respiratory tract
E48.5　　Fibreoptic endoscopic removal of foreign body from lower respiratory tract
E48.6　　Fibreoptic endoscopic irrigation of lower respiratory tract
　　　　　Includes:　Fibreoptic endoscopic lavage of lower respiratory tract
E48.7　　Fibreoptic endoscopic photodynamic therapy of lesion of lower respiratory tract
E48.8　　Other specified
E48.9　　Unspecified

E49 **Diagnostic fibreoptic endoscopic examination of lower respiratory tract**

Includes: *Diagnostic endoscopic examination of lower respiratory tract NEC*
Trachea
Carina
Bronchus
Lung

Note: **Use a supplementary code for concurrent biopsy of mediastinal lymph node (T87.4)**
Use a subsidiary site code as necessary

E49.1 Diagnostic fibreoptic endoscopic examination of lower respiratory tract and biopsy of lesion of lower respiratory tract
Includes: *Diagnostic fibreoptic endoscopic examination of lower respiratory tract and biopsy of lower respiratory tract*
Fibreoptic endoscopic biopsy of lesion of lower respiratory tract
Fibreoptic endoscopic biopsy of lower respiratory tract
Biopsy of lesion of lower respiratory tract
Biopsy of lower respiratory tract NEC

E49.2 Diagnostic fibreoptic endoscopic examination of lower respiratory tract and lavage of lesion of lower respiratory tract
Includes: *Diagnostic fibreoptic endoscopic examination of lower respiratory tract and lavage of lower respiratory tract*

E49.3 Diagnostic fibreoptic endoscopic examination of lower respiratory tract and brush cytology of lesion of lower respiratory tract
Includes: *Diagnostic fibreoptic endoscopic examination of lower respiratory tract and brush cytology of lower respiratory tract*

E49.4 Diagnostic fibreoptic endoscopic examination of lower respiratory tract with lavage and brush cytology of lesion of lower respiratory tract
Includes: *Diagnostic fibreoptic endoscopic examination of lower respiratory tract with lavage and brush cytology of lower respiratory tract*

E49.5 Diagnostic fibreoptic endoscopic examination of lower respiratory tract with biopsy, lavage and brush cytology of lesion of lower respiratory tract
Includes: *Diagnostic fibreoptic endoscopic examination of lower respiratory tract with biopsy, lavage and brush cytology of lower respiratory tract*

E49.8 Other specified
E49.9 Unspecified
Includes: *Fibreoptic bronchoscopy NEC*
Tracheoscopy NEC
Bronchoscopy NEC
Tracheobronchoscopy NEC

E50   **Therapeutic endoscopic operations on lower respiratory tract using rigid bronchoscope**

       Includes: *Trachea*
                          Carina
                          Bronchus
                          Lung

       Note: ***It is not necessary to code additionally any mention of diagnostic endoscopic examination of lower respiratory tract using rigid bronchoscope (E51.9)***
                Use a subsidiary site code as necessary

E50.1   Endoscopic snare resection of lesion of lower respiratory tract using rigid bronchoscope
E50.2   Endoscopic laser destruction of lesion of lower respiratory tract using rigid bronchoscope
E50.3   Endoscopic destruction of lesion of lower respiratory tract using rigid bronchoscope NEC
E50.4   Endoscopic aspiration of lower respiratory tract using rigid bronchoscope
E50.5   Endoscopic removal of foreign body from lower respiratory tract using rigid bronchoscope
E50.6   Endoscopic irrigation of lower respiratory tract using rigid bronchoscope

       Includes: *Endoscopic lavage of lower respiratory tract using rigid bronchoscope*

E50.8   Other specified
E50.9   Unspecified

E51   **Diagnostic endoscopic examination of lower respiratory tract using rigid bronchoscope**

       Includes: *Trachea*
                          Carina
                          Bronchus
                          Lung

       Note: ***Use a subsidiary site code as necessary***

E51.1   Diagnostic endoscopic examination of lower respiratory tract and biopsy of lesion of lower respiratory tract using rigid bronchoscope

       Includes: *Diagnostic endoscopic examination of lower respiratory tract and biopsy of lower respiratory tract using rigid bronchoscope*
                   Endoscopic biopsy of lesion of lower respiratory tract using rigid bronchoscope
                   Endoscopic biopsy of lower respiratory tract using rigid bronchoscope

       Excludes: *Biopsy of lesion of lung NEC (E59)*
                   Biopsy of lung NEC (E59)
                   Biopsy of lesion of lower respiratory tract (E49.1)
                   Biopsy of lower respiratory tract NEC (E49.1)

E51.8   Other specified
E51.9   Unspecified

E52   **Other operations on bronchus**

       Includes: *Trachea*

E52.1   Irrigation of bronchus NEC

       Includes: *Lavage of bronchus NEC*

E52.2   Aspiration of bronchus NEC

       Includes: *Clearance of airway*

E52.8   Other specified
E52.9   Unspecified

E53	**Transplantation of lung**

Excludes: Transplantation of heart and lung (K01)

E53.1	Double lung transplant
E53.2	Single lung transplant
E53.3	Single lobe lung transplant
E53.8	Other specified
E53.9	Unspecified

E54	**Excision of lung**

Note: Use an additional code for excision of carina as necessary (E44.1)

E54.1	Total pneumonectomy
	Includes: Pneumonectomy NEC
E54.2	Bilobectomy of lung
E54.3	Lobectomy of lung
E54.4	Excision of segment of lung
E54.5	Partial lobectomy of lung NEC
E54.6	Reduction of lung volume
E54.8	Other specified
E54.9	Unspecified

E55	**Open extirpation of lesion of lung**

E55.1	Open decortication of lesion of lung
E55.2	Open excision of lesion of lung
	Includes: Excision of lesion of lung NEC
	Excision of bulla of lung
E55.3	Open cauterisation of lesion of lung
E55.4	Open destruction of lesion of lung NEC
E55.8	Other specified
E55.9	Unspecified

E57	**Other open operations on lung**

E57.1	Repair of lung
E57.2	Ligation of bulla of lung
E57.3	Deflation of bulla of lung
E57.4	Incision of lung NEC
E57.8	Other specified
E57.9	Unspecified

E59	**Other operations on lung**

E59.1	Needle biopsy of lesion of lung
	Includes: Needle biopsy of lung
E59.2	Aspiration biopsy of lesion of lung
	Includes: Aspiration biopsy of lung
E59.3	Biopsy of lesion of lung NEC
	Includes: Biopsy of lung NEC
E59.4	Drainage of lung
E59.5	Percutaneous radiofrequency ablation of lesion of lung
E59.8	Other specified
E59.9	Unspecified

E61   **Open operations on mediastinum**

E61.1   Open excision of lesion of mediastinum
E61.2   Open biopsy of lesion of mediastinum
          Includes: Open biopsy of mediastinum
E61.3   Open drainage of mediastinum
E61.4   Mediastinotomy NEC
E61.5   Exploration of mediastinum NEC
E61.8   Other specified
E61.9   Unspecified

E62   **Therapeutic endoscopic operations on mediastinum**
          Note: It is not necessary to code additionally any mention of diagnostic endoscopic examination of mediastinum (E63.9)

E62.1   Endoscopic extirpation of lesion of mediastinum
E62.8   Other specified
E62.9   Unspecified

E63   **Diagnostic endoscopic examination of mediastinum**
          Note: Use a supplementary code for concurrent biopsy of mediastinal lymph nodes (T87.4)

E63.1   Diagnostic endoscopic examination of mediastinum and biopsy of lesion of mediastinum
          Includes: Diagnostic endoscopic examination of mediastinum and biopsy of mediastinum
                        Endoscopic biopsy of lesion of mediastinum
                        Endoscopic biopsy of mediastinum
                        Biopsy of lesion of mediastinum NEC
                        Biopsy of mediastinum NEC
E63.2   Endobronchial ultrasound examination of mediastinum
E63.3   Endo-oesophageal ultrasound examination of mediastinum
E63.8   Other specified
E63.9   Unspecified
          Includes: Cervical mediastinoscopy NEC
                        Mediastinoscopy NEC

E64   **Therapeutic endoscopic operations on nasal cavity**
          Excludes: Therapeutic endoscopic operations on pharynx (E24)
          Note: It is not necessary to code additionally any mention of diagnostic endoscopic examination of nasal cavity (E65.9)

E64.1   Endoscopic extirpation of lesion of nasal cavity
E64.8   Other specified
E64.9   Unspecified

E65   **Diagnostic endoscopic examination of nasal cavity**
          Excludes: Diagnostic endoscopic examination of pharynx (E25)

E65.1   Diagnostic endoscopic examination of nasal cavity and biopsy of lesion of nasal cavity
          Includes: Diagnostic endoscopic examination of nasal cavity and biopsy of nasal cavity
                        Endoscopic biopsy of lesion of nasal cavity
                        Endoscopic biopsy of nasal cavity
                        Biopsy of lesion of nasal cavity NEC
                        Biopsy of nasal cavity NEC
E65.8   Other specified
E65.9   Unspecified
          Includes: Nasendoscopy NEC

E85   **Ventilation support**

E85.1   Invasive ventilation
             Includes: Endotracheal intermittent positive pressure ventilation
E85.2   Non-invasive ventilation NEC
             Includes: Continuous positive airway pressure
             *   Intermittent positive pressure ventilation NEC*
             *   Negative pressure ventilation*
             *   Bilevel positive airway pressure*
             *   High flow continuous positive airway pressure*
E85.3   Improving efficiency of ventilation
E85.4   Bag valve mask ventilation
E85.5   Nebuliser ventilation
             Excludes: Nebuliser therapy (E89.3)
E85.8   Other specified
E85.9   Unspecified

E87   **Oxygen therapy support**
             Excludes: Oxygen therapy (X52)

E87.1   Home oxygen support
E87.2   Long term oxygen assessment
E87.3   Ambulatory oxygen assessment
E87.4   Diagnostic assessment of circulatory oxygenation using reduced oxygen air
             Includes: Flight assessment
E87.8   Other specified
E87.9   Unspecified

E89   **Other respiratory support**

E89.1   Clearance of secretions of respiratory tract
E89.2   Expectoration of induced sputum from respiratory tract
E89.3   Nebuliser therapy
             Includes: Nebuliser NEC
             Excludes: Nebuliser ventilation (E85.5)
E89.4   Control of respiration
E89.8   Other specified
E89.9   Unspecified

E91   **Oximetry testing**

E91.1   Oximetry assessment
E91.2   Continuous pulse oximetry
E91.3   Overnight oximetry
             Includes: Measurement of oxygen desaturation index
E91.8   Other specified
E91.9   Unspecified

E92   **Respiratory tests**

E92.1   Carbon monoxide transfer factor test
E92.2   Distribution of ventilation test
E92.3   Measurement of alveolar carbon monoxide
E92.4   Blood gas analysis
          Includes: Arterial blood gas analysis
          Capillary blood gas analysis
E92.5   Complex lung function exercise test
          Includes: Progressive cycle test with measure of gas exchange
          Progressive treadmill test with measure of gas exchange
          Stage 2–4 Jones test
E92.6   Simple lung function exercise test
          Includes: Exercise induced asthma test
          Shuttle walk test
          6 minute walk test
          Step test
E92.8   Other specified
E92.9   Unspecified

E93   **Respiratory measurements**

E93.1   Measurement of peak expiratory flow rate
          Excludes: Bronchodilator response to inhaled therapy using peak flow rate (E94.1)
E93.2   Spirometry
          Excludes: Bronchodilator response to inhaled therapy using spirometry (E94.1)
E93.3   Body plethysmographic measurement of airways resistance
          Excludes: Bronchodilator response to inhaled therapy using body plethysmography
          airway resistance (E94.2)
E93.4   Measurement of airways resistance using forced oscillation technique
          Excludes: Bronchodilator response to inhaled therapy using forced oscillation
          technique (E94.2)
E93.5   Measurement of static lung volume
E93.6   Measurement of respiratory muscle strength
E93.7   Measurement of maximum expiratory and inspiratory flow volume loop
E93.8   Other specified
E93.9   Unspecified

E94   **Bronchial reaction studies**

E94.1   Bronchodilator response to inhaled therapy using simple measures of airflow
          Includes: Bronchodilator response to inhaled therapy using peak flow rate
          Bronchodilator response to inhaled therapy using spirometry
          Bronchodilator response to inhaled therapy using flow volume
E94.2   Bronchodilator response to inhaled therapy using complex measures of airflow
          Includes: Bronchodilator response to inhaled therapy using body plethysmography
          airway resistance
          Bronchodilator response to inhaled therapy using forced oscillation technique
E94.3   Bronchial reactivity
          Includes: Bronchial reactivity to histamine or metacholine
E94.4   Bronchial challenge
          Includes: Allergen challenge
          Occupational respiratory sensitising agents
E94.8   Other specified
E94.9   Unspecified

E95   **Tuberculosis support**

E95.1   Heaf test
E95.2   Administration of Bacillus Calmette-Guerin vaccine
E95.3   Directly observed therapy
E95.4   Contact tracing
E95.5   Mantoux test
E95.8   Other specified
E95.9   Unspecified

E97   **Respiratory education**
            Includes: Demonstration and guidance of respiratory education

E97.1   Education for inhaled therapy
            Includes: Nebuliser technique
                          Inhaler technique
                          Determination of optimal inhaler device
E97.2   Education for peak flow technique
E97.3   Education for self-management of respiratory health
            Includes: Education for initiation of continuous positive airways pressure
E97.8   Other specified
E97.9   Unspecified

E98   **Smoking cessation therapy**

E98.1   Nicotine replacement therapy using nicotine patches
E98.2   Nicotine replacement therapy using nicotine gum
E98.3   Nicotine replacement therapy using nicotine inhalator
E98.4   Nicotine replacement therapy using nicotine lozenges
E98.8   Other specified
E98.9   Unspecified

CHAPTER F
MOUTH
(CODES F01–F63)

F01 Partial excision of lip
Includes: *Skin of lip*
Note: *Codes from Chapter S may be used to enhance these codes*

F01.1 Excision of vermilion border of lip and advancement of mucosa of lip
F01.8 Other specified
F01.9 Unspecified

F02 Extirpation of lesion of lip
Note at F01 applies
Includes: *Skin of lip*
Mucosa of lip

F02.1 Excision of lesion of lip
F02.2 Destruction of lesion of lip
F02.8 Other specified
F02.9 Unspecified

F03 Correction of deformity of lip
Note at F01 applies
Includes: *Skin of lip*
Excludes: *Transcranial repair of craniofacial cleft and reconstruction of cranial and facial bones HFQ (V12.3)*
Subcranial repair of craniofacial cleft and reconstruction of cranial and facial bones HFQ (V12.4)

F03.1 Primary closure of cleft lip
F03.2 Revision of primary closure of cleft lip
F03.3 Adjustment to vermilion border of lip NEC
F03.8 Other specified
F03.9 Unspecified

F04 Other reconstruction of lip
Note at F01 applies
Includes: *Skin of lip*

F04.1 Reconstruction of lip using tongue flap
F04.2 Reconstruction of lip using skin flap
F04.8 Other specified
F04.9 Unspecified

F05 Other repair of lip
Note at F01 applies
Includes: *Skin of lip*

F05.1 Excision of excess mucosa from lip
Includes: *Frenectomy of lip*
F05.2 Advancement of mucosa of lip NEC
F05.3 Suture of lip
F05.4 Removal of suture from lip
F05.8 Other specified
F05.9 Unspecified

F06   **Other operations on lip**
                      Note at F01 applies
                   Includes: *Skin of lip*
                                       Mucosa of lip

F06.1   Division of adhesions of lip
F06.2   Biopsy of lesion of lip
                   Includes: *Biopsy of lip*
F06.3   Shave of lip
F06.8   Other specified
F06.9   Unspecified

F08   **Implantation of tooth**

F08.1   Allotransplantation of tooth
F08.2   Autotransplantation of tooth
F08.3   Replantation of tooth
F08.4   Repositioning of tooth
F08.8   Other specified
F08.9   Unspecified

F09   **Surgical removal of tooth**

F09.1   Surgical removal of impacted wisdom tooth
F09.2   Surgical removal of impacted tooth NEC
F09.3   Surgical removal of wisdom tooth NEC
F09.4   Surgical removal of tooth NEC
F09.5   Surgical removal of retained root of tooth
F09.8   Other specified
F09.9   Unspecified

F10   **Simple extraction of tooth**
                   Excludes: Extraction of wisdom tooth (F09)

F10.1   Full dental clearance
                   Includes: Dental clearance NEC
F10.2   Upper dental clearance
F10.3   Lower dental clearance
F10.4   Extraction of multiple teeth NEC
F10.8   Other specified
F10.9   Unspecified
                   Includes: Extraction of single tooth

F11   **Preprosthetic oral surgery**
                   Excludes: Reduction of fracture of alveolus (V15.1)

F11.1   Oral alveoplasty
F11.2   Augmentation of alveolar ridge using autobone graft
F11.3   Augmentation of alveolar ridge NEC
F11.4   Vestibuloplasty of mouth
F11.5   Endosseous implantation into jaw
F11.6   Subperiosteal implantation into jaw
F11.8   Other specified
F11.9   Unspecified

F12   Surgery on apex of tooth

F12.1   Apicectomy of tooth
F12.2   Root canal therapy to tooth
F12.8   Other specified
F12.9   Unspecified

F13   Restoration of tooth
Excludes: Specific procedures as part of restoration of crown or bridge (F17)

F13.1   Full restoration of crown of tooth
F13.2   Partial restoration of crown of tooth
F13.3   Restoration of crown of tooth NEC
F13.4   Restoration of part of tooth using inlay NEC
F13.5   Restoration of part of tooth using filling NEC
F13.6   Bleaching of teeth
F13.8   Other specified
F13.9   Unspecified

F14   Orthodontic operations
Note: Principal category, extended at F15

F14.1   Insertion of fixed orthodontic appliance
F14.2   Insertion of movable orthodontic appliance
F14.3   Insertion of orthodontic appliance NEC
F14.4   Removal of orthodontic appliance NEC
F14.5   Surgical exposure of tooth
F14.6   Insertion of orthodontic anchorage
              Includes: Insertion of orthodontic screw
                                Insertion of orthodontic mini screw
                                Insertion of orthodontic micro screw
F14.7   Removal of orthodontic anchorage
              Includes: Removal of orthodontic screw
                                  Removal of orthodontic mini screw
                                  Removal of orthodontic micro screw
F14.8   Other specified
F14.9   Unspecified

F15   Other orthodontic operations
Note: Principal F14

F15.1   Creation of orthodontic impression
F15.2   Fitting of orthodontic bracket
F15.3   Fitting of orthodontic headgear
F15.4   Fitting of orthodontic separators
F15.5   Adjustment of orthodontic device
F15.6   Repair of orthodontic appliance
F15.7   Debonding of orthodontic bracket
F15.8   Other specified
F15.9   Unspecified

F16   **Other operations on tooth**

F16.1   Drainage of abscess of alveolus of tooth
F16.2   Surgical arrest of postoperative bleeding from tooth socket
F16.3   Packing of tooth socket
F16.4   Scaling of tooth
F16.5   Application of fissure sealant
F16.6   Application of topical fluoride
F16.7   Polishing teeth
F16.8   Other specified
F16.9   Unspecified

F17   **Operations on teeth using dental crown or bridge**
             Excludes: Restoration of tooth (F13)

F17.1   Preparation of tooth for dental crown
F17.2   Creation of impression of tooth for dental crown
F17.3   Fitting of dental crown on tooth
F17.4   Adjustment of dental crown on tooth
F17.5   Removal of dental crown from tooth
F17.6   Preparation of teeth for bridge
F17.7   Fitting of bridge on teeth
F17.8   Other specified
F17.9   Unspecified

F18   **Excision of dental lesion of jaw**

F18.1   Enucleation of dental cyst of jaw
             Includes: Dental cystectomy
F18.2   Marsupialisation of dental lesion of jaw
F18.8   Other specified
F18.9   Unspecified

F20   **Operations on gingiva**

F20.1   Excision of gingiva
             Includes: Gingivectomy NEC
F20.2   Excision of lesion of gingiva
F20.3   Biopsy of lesion of gingiva
             Includes: Biopsy of gingiva
F20.4   Gingivoplasty
F20.5   Suture of gingiva
F20.8   Other specified
F20.9   Unspecified

F22   **Excision of tongue**

F22.1   Total glossectomy
F22.2   Partial glossectomy
F22.8   Other specified
F22.9   Unspecified
             Includes: Glossectomy NEC

F23   **Extirpation of lesion of tongue**

F23.1   Excision of lesion of tongue
F23.2   Destruction of lesion of tongue
F23.8   Other specified
F23.9   Unspecified

F24   **Incision of tongue**

F24.1   Biopsy of lesion of tongue
           Includes: Biopsy of tongue
F24.2   Removal of foreign body from tongue
F24.3   Glossotomy
F24.8   Other specified
F24.9   Unspecified

F26   **Other operations on tongue**

F26.1   Commissurectomy of tongue
F26.2   Excision of frenulum of tongue
           Includes: Frenectomy of tongue
F26.3   Incision of frenulum of tongue
           Includes: Frenotomy of tongue
F26.4   Freeing of adhesions of tongue
F26.5   Suture of tongue
F26.8   Other specified
F26.9   Unspecified

F28   **Extirpation of lesion of palate**

F28.1   Excision of lesion of palate
F28.2   Destruction of lesion of palate
F28.8   Other specified
F28.9   Unspecified

F29   **Correction of deformity of palate**
           *Excludes: Transcranial repair of craniofacial cleft and reconstruction of cranial and facial
                        bones HFQ (V12.3)
                        Subcranial repair of craniofacial cleft and reconstruction of cranial and facial
                        bones HFQ (V12.4)*

F29.1   Primary repair of cleft palate
F29.2   Revision of repair of cleft palate
F29.8   Other specified
F29.9   Unspecified

F30   **Other repair of palate**

F30.1   Plastic repair of palate using flap of palate
F30.2   Plastic repair of palate using flap of skin
F30.3   Plastic repair of palate using flap of tongue
F30.4   Plastic repair of palate using graft of skin
F30.5   Plastic repair of palate using flap of mucosa
F30.6   Plastic repair of palate using graft of mucosa
F30.7   Suture of palate
F30.8   Other specified
F30.9   Unspecified

F32　　**Other operations on palate**
　　　　　　Includes:　Uvula (F32.4)

F32.1　　Biopsy of lesion of palate
　　　　　Includes:　Biopsy of palate
F32.2　　Removal of foreign body from palate
F32.3　　Incision of palate
F32.4　　Operations on uvula NEC
F32.5　　Uvulopalatopharyngoplasty
F32.6　　Uvulopalatoplasty
F32.8　　Other specified
F32.9　　Unspecified

F34　　**Excision of tonsil**
　　　　　　Note:　Use a supplementary code for concurrent excision of adenoid (E20.1, E20.4)

F34.1　　Bilateral dissection tonsillectomy
F34.2　　Bilateral guillotine tonsillectomy
F34.3　　Bilateral laser tonsillectomy
F34.4　　Bilateral excision of tonsil NEC
　　　　　Includes:　Bilateral tonsillectomy NEC
F34.5　　Excision of remnant of tonsil
F34.6　　Excision of lingual tonsil
F34.7　　Bilateral coblation tonsillectomy
F34.8　　Other specified
F34.9　　Unspecified
　　　　　Includes:　Tonsillectomy NEC

F36　　**Other operations on tonsil**
　　　　　　Includes:　Peritonsillar region

F36.1　　Destruction of tonsil
　　　　　Includes:　Destruction of lesion of tonsil
F36.2　　Biopsy of lesion of tonsil
　　　　　Includes:　Biopsy of tonsil
F36.3　　Drainage of abscess of peritonsillar region
F36.4　　Removal of foreign body from tonsil
F36.5　　Surgical arrest of postoperative bleeding from tonsillar bed
F36.6　　Excision of lesion of tonsil
　　　　　Note:　Use a supplementary code for concurrent excision of adenoid (E20.1, E20.4)
F36.8　　Other specified
F36.9　　Unspecified

F38　　**Extirpation of lesion of other part of mouth**
　　　　　　Includes:　Unspecified part of mouth

F38.1　　Excision of lesion of floor of mouth
F38.2　　Excision of lesion of mouth NEC
F38.3　　Destruction of lesion of floor of mouth
F38.4　　Destruction of lesion of mouth NEC
F38.8　　Other specified
F38.9　　Unspecified

F39   **Reconstruction of other part of mouth**
Includes: Unspecified part of mouth

F39.1   Reconstruction of mouth using flap NEC
F39.2   Reconstruction of mouth using graft NEC
F39.8   Other specified
F39.9   Unspecified

F40   **Other repair of other part of mouth**
Includes: Unspecified part of mouth

F40.1   Revision of repair of mouth NEC
F40.2   Graft of skin to mouth NEC
F40.3   Graft of mucosa to mouth NEC
F40.4   Suture of mouth NEC
F40.5   Removal of suture from mouth NEC
F40.8   Other specified
F40.9   Unspecified

F42   **Other operations on mouth**

F42.1   Biopsy of lesion of mouth NEC
Includes: Biopsy of mouth NEC
F42.2   Incision of mouth NEC
F42.3   Removal of excess mucosa from mouth NEC
F42.4   Photography of mouth
F42.5   Recording of jaw relationships
F42.8   Other specified
F42.9   Unspecified

F43   **Other examinations of mouth**

F43.1   Smear of buccal mucosa
F43.8   Other specified
F43.9   Unspecified

F44   **Excision of salivary gland**

F44.1   Total excision of parotid gland
F44.2   Partial excision of parotid gland
F44.3   Excision of parotid gland NEC
F44.4   Excision of submandibular gland
F44.5   Excision of sublingual gland
F44.8   Other specified
F44.9   Unspecified

F45   **Extirpation of lesion of salivary gland**

F45.1   Excision of lesion of parotid gland
F45.2   Excision of lesion of submandibular gland
F45.3   Excision of lesion of sublingual gland
F45.4   Excision of lesion of salivary gland NEC
F45.5   Destruction of lesion of salivary gland
F45.8   Other specified
F45.9   Unspecified

F46 **Incision of salivary gland**

F46.1   Incision of parotid gland
F46.2   Incision of submandibular gland
F46.3   Incision of sublingual gland
F46.8   Other specified
F46.9   Unspecified

F48 **Other operations on salivary gland**

F48.1   Biopsy of lesion of salivary gland
         Includes: Biopsy of salivary gland
F48.2   Closure of fistula of salivary gland
F48.3   Repair of salivary gland NEC
F48.4   Sialography
F48.5   Injection of therapeutic substance into salivary gland
F48.8   Other specified
F48.9   Unspecified

F50 **Transposition of salivary duct**

F50.1   Transposition of parotid duct
F50.2   Transposition of submandibular duct
F50.8   Other specified
F50.9   Unspecified

F51 **Open extraction of calculus from salivary duct**

F51.1   Open extraction of calculus from parotid duct
F51.2   Open extraction of calculus from submandibular duct
F51.8   Other specified
F51.9   Unspecified

F52 **Ligation of salivary duct**

F52.1   Ligation of parotid duct
F52.2   Ligation of submandibular duct
F52.8   Other specified
F52.9   Unspecified

F53 **Other open operations on salivary duct**

F53.1   Open operations on parotid duct NEC
F53.2   Open operations on submandibular duct NEC
F53.8   Other specified
F53.9   Unspecified

F55 **Dilation of salivary duct**

F55.1   Dilation of parotid duct
F55.2   Dilation of submandibular duct
F55.8   Other specified
F55.9   Unspecified

F56 **Manipulative removal of calculus from salivary duct**

F56.1   Manipulative removal of calculus from parotid duct
F56.2   Manipulative removal of calculus from submandibular duct
F56.8   Other specified
F56.9   Unspecified

F58 **Other operations on salivary duct**

F58.1   Operations on parotid duct NEC
F58.2   Operations on submandibular duct NEC
F58.8   Other specified
F58.9   Unspecified

F63 **Insertion of dental prosthesis**

F63.1   Creating of impression for denture or obturator
F63.2   Fitting of denture or obturator
F63.3   Adjustment of denture or obturator
F63.4   Repair of denture or obturator
F63.5   Splinting of teeth
F63.8   Other specified
F63.9   Unspecified

CHAPTER G
UPPER DIGESTIVE TRACT
(CODES G01–G82)

Note: *Use a subsidiary code for minimal access approach (Y74–Y76)*
Use a subsidiary code to identify method of image control (Y53)

G01   **Excision of oesophagus and stomach**

G01.1   Oesophagogastrectomy and anastomosis of oesophagus to stomach
G01.2   Oesophagogastrectomy and anastomosis of oesophagus to transposed jejunum
G01.3   Oesophagogastrectomy and anastomosis of oesophagus to jejunum NEC
G01.8   Other specified
G01.9   Unspecified

G02   **Total excision of oesophagus**

G02.1   Total oesophagectomy and anastomosis of pharynx to stomach
G02.2   Total oesophagectomy and interposition of microvascularly attached jejunum
G02.3   Total oesophagectomy and interposition of jejunum NEC
G02.4   Total oesophagectomy and interposition of microvascularly attached colon
G02.5   Total oesophagectomy and interposition of colon NEC
G02.8   Other specified
G02.9   Unspecified

G03   **Partial excision of oesophagus**

G03.1   Partial oesophagectomy and end to end anastomosis of oesophagus
            Includes: *Partial oesophagectomy and reanastomosis of oesophagus to stomach*
G03.2   Partial oesophagectomy and interposition of microvascularly attached jejunum
G03.3   Partial oesophagectomy and anastomosis of oesophagus to transposed jejunum
G03.4   Partial oesophagectomy and anastomosis of oesophagus to jejunum NEC
G03.5   Partial oesophagectomy and interposition of microvascularly attached colon
G03.6   Partial oesophagectomy and interposition of colon NEC
G03.8   Other specified
G03.9   Unspecified
            Includes: *Oesophagectomy NEC*

G04   **Open extirpation of lesion of oesophagus**

G04.1   Excision of lesion of oesophagus
G04.2   Open laser destruction of lesion of oesophagus
G04.3   Open destruction of lesion of oesophagus NEC
G04.8   Other specified
G04.9   Unspecified

G05   **Bypass of oesophagus**
            Includes: *Anastomosis or interposition of oesophagus without mention of bypass*
            Excludes: *When associated with excision of oesophagus (G01–G03)*

G05.1   Bypass of oesophagus by anastomosis of oesophagus to oesophagus
G05.2   Bypass of oesophagus by anastomosis of oesophagus to stomach
G05.3   Bypass of oesophagus by interposition of microvascularly attached jejunum
G05.4   Bypass of oesophagus by interposition of jejunum NEC
G05.5   Bypass of oesophagus by interposition of microvascularly attached colon
G05.6   Bypass of oesophagus by interposition of colon NEC
G05.8   Other specified
G05.9   Unspecified

G06   **Attention to connection of oesophagus**

G06.1   Revision of interposition anastomosis of oesophagus
G06.2   Revision of anastomosis of oesophagus NEC
         Includes: Revision of bypass of oesophagus NEC
G06.3   Removal of bypass of oesophagus
         Includes: Conversion of interposition anastomosis to direct anastomosis of oesophagus
G06.4   Closure of bypass of oesophagus NEC
G06.8   Other specified
G06.9   Unspecified
G06.0   Conversion from previous direct anastomosis of oesophagus
         Note: For use as a subsidiary code when associated with construction of interposition anastomosis of oesophagus (G05)

G07   **Repair of oesophagus**

G07.1   Closure of tracheo-oesophageal fistula
         Includes: Excision of tracheo-oesophageal fistula
G07.2   Closure of fistula of oesophagus NEC
         Includes: Excision of fistula of oesophagus NEC
G07.3   Correction of congenital atresia of oesophagus
G07.4   Repair of rupture of oesophagus
G07.8   Other specified
G07.9   Unspecified

G08   **Artificial opening into oesophagus**

G08.1   Exteriorisation of pouch of oesophagus
G08.2   External fistulisation of oesophagus NEC
G08.3   Tube oesophagostomy
         Includes: Insertion of feeding tube through artificial opening of oesophagus
G08.8   Other specified
G08.9   Unspecified
         Includes: Oesophagostomy NEC

G09   **Incision of oesophagus**

G09.1   Cardiomyotomy
G09.2   Oesophagomyotomy NEC
G09.3   Division of web of oesophagus
G09.4   Drainage of oesophagus
         Includes: Drainage of perioesophageal tissue
G09.8   Other specified
G09.9   Unspecified

G10   **Open operations on varices of oesophagus**
         Excludes: Portal decompression operations (L77)

G10.1   Disconnection of azygos vein
G10.2   Transection of oesophagus using staple gun
G10.3   Transection of oesophagus NEC
G10.4   Local ligation of varices of oesophagus
G10.5   Open injection sclerotherapy to varices of oesophagus
G10.8   Other specified
G10.9   Unspecified

G11 Open placement of prosthesis in oesophagus

G11.1   Insertion of tubal prosthesis into oesophagus through stomach
G11.2   Open insertion of tubal prosthesis into oesophagus NEC
G11.3   Open revision of tubal prosthesis in oesophagus
G11.4   Open removal of tubal prosthesis from oesophagus
G11.8   Other specified
G11.9   Unspecified

G13 Other open operations on oesophagus

G13.1   Open biopsy of lesion of oesophagus
         Includes: Open biopsy of oesophagus
G13.2   Open removal of foreign body from oesophagus
G13.8   Other specified
G13.9   Unspecified

G14 Fibreoptic endoscopic extirpation of lesion of oesophagus

Includes: Endoscopic extirpation of lesion of oesophagus NEC
Excludes: When associated with general fibreoptic endoscopic examination of upper gastrointestinal tract (G42,G43)
Note: It is not necessary to code diagnostic fibreoptic endoscopic examination limited to oesophagus (G16.9)

G14.1   Fibreoptic endoscopic snare resection of lesion of oesophagus
G14.2   Fibreoptic endoscopic laser destruction of lesion of oesophagus
G14.3   Fibreoptic endoscopic cauterisation of lesion of oesophagus
G14.4   Fibreoptic endoscopic injection sclerotherapy to varices of oesophagus
G14.5   Fibreoptic endoscopic destruction of lesion of oesophagus NEC
G14.6   Fibreoptic endoscopic submucosal resection of lesion of oesophagus
G14.7   Fibreoptic endoscopic photodynamic therapy of lesion of oesophagus
G14.8   Other specified
G14.9   Unspecified

G15 Other therapeutic fibreoptic endoscopic operations on oesophagus

Includes: Therapeutic endoscopic operations on oesophagus NEC
Excludes: When associated with general fibreoptic endoscopic examination of upper gastrointestinal tract (G44, G46)
Note: It is not necessary to code diagnostic fibreoptic endoscopic examination limited to oesophagus (G16.9)

G15.1   Fibreoptic endoscopic removal of foreign body from oesophagus
         Includes: Removal of foreign body from oesophagus NEC
G15.2   Fibreoptic endoscopic balloon dilation of oesophagus
G15.3   Fibreoptic endoscopic dilation of oesophagus NEC
G15.4   Fibreoptic endoscopic insertion of tubal prosthesis into oesophagus
G15.5   Fibreoptic endoscopic dilation of web of oesophagus
G15.6   Fibreoptic endoscopic insertion of expanding metal stent into oesophagus NEC
G15.7   Fibreoptic endoscopic insertion of expanding covered metal stent into oesophagus
G15.8   Other specified
G15.9   Unspecified

G16   **Diagnostic fibreoptic endoscopic examination of oesophagus**
Includes: *Diagnostic endoscopic examination of oesophagus NEC*
Biopsy of lesion of oesophagus NEC
Biopsy of oesophagus NEC
Excludes: *When not limited to oesophagus (G45)*

G16.1   Diagnostic fibreoptic endoscopic examination of oesophagus and biopsy of lesion of oesophagus
Includes: *Diagnostic fibreoptic endoscopic examination of oesophagus and biopsy of oesophagus*
Fibreoptic endoscopic biopsy of lesion of oesophagus
Fibreoptic endoscopic biopsy of oesophagus
Biopsy of lesion of oesophagus NEC
Biopsy of oesophagus NEC

G16.2   Diagnostic fibreoptic endoscopic ultrasound examination of oesophagus
G16.3   Diagnostic fibreoptic insertion of Bravo pH capsule into oesophagus
Excludes: *When associated with general fibreoptic examination of upper gastrointestinal tract (G45.3)*

G16.8   Other specified
G16.9   Unspecified
Includes: *Fibreoptic oesophagoscopy NEC*
Oesophagoscopy NEC

G17   **Endoscopic extirpation of lesion of oesophagus using rigid oesophagoscope**
Includes: *Endoscopic extirpation of lesion of stomach using rigid gastroscope*
Excludes: *Endoscopic extirpation of lesion of stomach NEC (G42, G43)*
   Note: ***It is not necessary to code diagnostic endoscopic examination of oesophagus using rigid oesophagoscope (G19.9)***

G17.1   Endoscopic snare resection of lesion of oesophagus using rigid oesophagoscope
G17.2   Endoscopic laser destruction of lesion of oesophagus using rigid oesophagoscope
G17.3   Endoscopic cauterisation of lesion of oesophagus using rigid oesophagoscope
G17.4   Endoscopic injection sclerotherapy to varices of oesophagus using rigid oesophagoscope
G17.8   Other specified
G17.9   Unspecified

G18   **Other therapeutic endoscopic operations on oesophagus using rigid oesophagoscope**
Includes: *Therapeutic endoscopic operations on stomach using rigid gastroscope NEC*
Excludes: *Therapeutic endoscopic operations on stomach NEC (G44, G46)*
   Note: ***It is not necessary to code diagnostic endoscopic examination of oesophagus using rigid oesophagoscope (G19.9)***

G18.1   Endoscopic removal of foreign body from oesophagus using rigid oesophagoscope
G18.2   Endoscopic balloon dilation of oesophagus using rigid oesophagoscope
G18.3   Endoscopic dilation of oesophagus using rigid oesophagoscope NEC
G18.4   Endoscopic insertion of tubal prosthesis into oesophagus using rigid oesophagoscope
G18.5   Dilation of web of oesophagus using rigid oesophagoscope
G18.8   Other specified
G18.9   Unspecified

G19   **Diagnostic endoscopic examination of oesophagus using rigid oesophagoscope**
        Includes: *Diagnostic endoscopic examination of stomach using rigid gastroscope*
        Excludes: *Diagnostic endoscopic examination of stomach NEC (G45)*

G19.1   Diagnostic endoscopic examination of oesophagus and biopsy of lesion of oesophagus using rigid oesophagoscope
        Includes: *Diagnostic endoscopic examination of oesophagus and biopsy of oesophagus using rigid oesophagoscope*
                  Endoscopic biopsy of lesion of oesophagus using rigid oesophagoscope
                  Biopsy of lesion of oesophagus using rigid oesophagoscope NEC
                  Biopsy of oesophagus using rigid oesophagoscope NEC
        Excludes: *Biopsy of lesion of stomach NEC (G45.1)*
                  Biopsy of stomach NEC (G45.1)

G19.2   Diagnostic endoscopic insertion of Bravo pH capsule using rigid oesophagoscope
        Excludes: *When associated with general fibreoptic examination of upper gastrointestinal tract (G45.3)*

G19.8   Other specified

G19.9   Unspecified

G21   **Other operations on oesophagus**

G21.1   Intubation of oesophagus for pH manometry

G21.2   Intubation of oesophagus for pressure manometry

G21.3   Intubation of oesophagus and instillation of acid or alkali HFQ

G21.4   Intubation of oesophagus NEC

G21.5   Insertion of stent into oesophagus NEC

G21.8   Other specified

G21.9   Unspecified

G23   **Repair of diaphragmatic hernia**

G23.1   Repair of oesophageal hiatus using thoracic approach

G23.2   Repair of diaphragmatic hernia using thoracic approach NEC

G23.3   Repair of oesophageal hiatus using abdominal approach

G23.4   Repair of diaphragmatic hernia using abdominal approach NEC

G23.8   Other specified

G23.9   Unspecified

G24   **Antireflux operations**

G24.1   Antireflux fundoplication using thoracic approach

G24.2   Antireflux operation using thoracic approach NEC

G24.3   Antireflux fundoplication using abdominal approach

G24.4   Antireflux gastropexy

G24.5   Gastroplasty and antireflux procedure HFQ

G24.6   Insertion of Angelchick prosthesis

G24.8   Other specified

G24.9   Unspecified

G25   **Revision of antireflux operations**

G25.1   Revision of fundoplication of stomach

G25.2   Adjustment to Angelchick prosthesis

G25.3   Removal of Angelchick prosthesis

G25.8   Other specified

G25.9   Unspecified

G26   **Transplantation of stomach**

G26.1   Allotransplantation of stomach
G26.8   Other specified
G26.9   Unspecified

G27   **Total excision of stomach**

G27.1   Total gastrectomy and excision of surrounding tissue
                   Note: ***Use an additional code as necessary for excision of lymph node (T87)***
G27.2   Total gastrectomy and anastomosis of oesophagus to duodenum
G27.3   Total gastrectomy and interposition of jejunum
G27.4   Total gastrectomy and anastomosis of oesophagus to transposed jejunum
G27.5   Total gastrectomy and anastomosis of oesophagus to jejunum NEC
G27.8   Other specified
G27.9   Unspecified

G28   **Partial excision of stomach**

G28.1   Partial gastrectomy and anastomosis of stomach to duodenum
G28.2   Partial gastrectomy and anastomosis of stomach to transposed jejunum
G28.3   Partial gastrectomy and anastomosis of stomach to jejunum NEC
G28.4   Sleeve gastrectomy and duodenal switch
                   Excludes: Duodenal switch (G71.6)
G28.5   Sleeve gastrectomy NEC
G28.8   Other specified
G28.9   Unspecified
                   Includes: Gastrectomy NEC

G29   **Open extirpation of lesion of stomach**

G29.1   Open excision of polyp of stomach
G29.2   Open excision of lesion of stomach NEC
G29.3   Open laser destruction of lesion of stomach
G29.4   Diathermy to lesion of stomach
G29.5   Cryotherapy to lesion of stomach
G29.8   Other specified
G29.9   Unspecified

G30   **Plastic operations on stomach**

G30.1   Gastroplasty NEC
G30.2   Partitioning of stomach NEC
G30.3   Partitioning of stomach using band
G30.4   Partitioning of stomach using staples
G30.5   Maintenance of gastric band
                   Excludes: Removal of gastric band (G38.7)
G30.8   Other specified
G30.9   Unspecified

G31   **Connection of stomach to duodenum**
            Includes: Gastroduodenostomy
            Excludes: Connection of stomach to duodenum when associated with concurrent
            *   excision of stomach (G27.2, G28.1)*

G31.1   Bypass of stomach by anastomosis of oesophagus to duodenum
G31.2   Bypass of stomach by anastomosis of stomach to duodenum
G31.3   Revision of anastomosis of stomach to duodenum
G31.4   Conversion to anastomosis of stomach to duodenum
            Note: Use a subsidiary conversion from code as necessary
G31.5   Closure of connection of stomach to duodenum
G31.6   Attention to connection of stomach to duodenum
            Excludes: Revision of anastomosis of stomach to duodenum (G31.3)
            *   Closure of connection of stomach to duodenum (G31.5)*
G31.8   Other specified
G31.9   Unspecified
G31.0   Conversion from previous anastomosis of stomach to duodenum

G32   **Connection of stomach to transposed jejunum**
            Excludes: Connection of stomach to transposed jejunum when associated with
            *   concurrent excision of stomach (G27.4, G28.2)*

G32.1   Bypass of stomach by anastomosis of stomach to transposed jejunum
G32.2   Revision of anastomosis of stomach to transposed jejunum
G32.3   Conversion to anastomosis of stomach to transposed jejunum
            Note: Use a subsidiary conversion from code as necessary
G32.4   Closure of connection of stomach to transposed jejunum
G32.5   Attention to connection of stomach to transposed jejunum
            Excludes: Revision of anastomosis of stomach to transposed jejunum (G32.2)
            *   Closure of anastomosis of stomach to transposed jejunum (G32.4)*
G32.8   Other specified
G32.9   Unspecified
G32.0   Conversion from previous anastomosis of stomach to transposed jejunum

G33   **Other connection of stomach to jejunum**
            Includes: Gastroenterostomy NEC
            Excludes: Connection of stomach to jejunum when associated with concurrent excision
            *   of stomach NEC (G27.5, G28.3)*

G33.1   Bypass of stomach by anastomosis of stomach to jejunum NEC
            Note: Use as a secondary code when associated with concurrent vagotomy (A27)
G33.2   Revision of anastomosis of stomach to jejunum NEC
G33.3   Conversion to anastomosis of stomach to jejunum NEC
            Note: Use a subsidiary conversion from code as necessary
G33.4   Open reduction of intussusception of gastroenterostomy
G33.5   Closure of connection of stomach to jejunum NEC
G33.6   Attention to connection of stomach to jejunum
            Excludes: Revision of anastomosis of stomach to jejunum NEC (G33.2)
            *   Closure of anastomosis of stomach to jejunum NEC (G33.5)*
G33.8   Other specified
G33.9   Unspecified
G33.0   Conversion from previous anastomosis of stomach to jejunum NEC

G34   **Artificial opening into stomach**

G34.1   Creation of permanent gastrostomy
G34.2   Creation of temporary gastrostomy
              Includes: Creation of gastrostomy NEC
G34.3   Reconstruction of gastrostomy
G34.4   Closure of gastrostomy
G34.5   Attention to gastrostomy tube
G34.8   Other specified
G34.9   Unspecified

G35   **Operations on ulcer of stomach**

G35.1   Closure of perforated ulcer of stomach
G35.2   Closure of ulcer of stomach NEC
              Includes: Suture of ulcer of stomach NEC
G35.8   Other specified
G35.9   Unspecified

G36   **Other repair of stomach**

G36.1   Gastropexy NEC
G36.2   Closure of perforation of stomach NEC
G36.3   Closure of abnormal opening of stomach NEC
G36.8   Other specified
G36.9   Unspecified

G38   **Other open operations on stomach**

G38.1   Open biopsy of lesion of stomach
              Includes: Open biopsy of stomach
G38.2   Open insertion of prosthesis into stomach
G38.3   Open insertion of feeding tube into stomach
G38.4   Open removal of foreign body from stomach
G38.5   Incision of stomach NEC
              Includes: Gastrotomy NEC
G38.6   Reduction of volvulus of stomach
G38.7   Removal of gastric band
G38.8   Other specified
G38.9   Unspecified

G40   **Incision of pylorus**

G40.1   Pyloromyotomy
              Note: *Use as a secondary code when associated with concurrent vagotomy (A27)*
G40.2   Repair of congenital atresia of pylorus
G40.3   Pyloroplasty NEC
              Note: *Use as a secondary code when associated with concurrent vagotomy (A27)*
G40.4   Revision of pyloroplasty
G40.5   Closure of pyloroplasty
G40.6   Open dilation of pylorus
G40.8   Other specified
G40.9   Unspecified

G41   **Other operations on pylorus**

G41.1   Open biopsy of lesion of pylorus
               Includes: Open biopsy of pylorus
G41.2   Repair of perforation of pylorus
G41.8   Other specified
G41.9   Unspecified

G42   **Other fibreoptic endoscopic extirpation of lesion of upper gastrointestinal tract**
               Includes: Endoscopic extirpation of lesion of upper gastrointestinal tract NEC
                              Oesophagus
                              Stomach
                              Pylorus
                              Proximal duodenum
               Excludes: When associated with endoscopic examination limited to oesophagus
                              (G14, G17)
                              When associated with endoscopic examination limited to duodenum (G54.1)
               Note: Principal G43
                              It is not necessary to code diagnostic endoscopic examination of upper
                              gastrointestinal tract (G45.9)
                              Use a subsidiary site code as necessary

G42.1   Fibreoptic endoscopic submucosal resection of lesion of upper gastrointestinal tract
G42.2   Fibreoptic endoscopic photodynamic therapy of lesion of upper gastrointestinal tract
G42.8   Other specified
G42.9   Unspecified

G43   **Fibreoptic endoscopic extirpation of lesion of upper gastrointestinal tract**
               Includes: Endoscopic extirpation of lesion of upper gastrointestinal tract NEC
                              Oesophagus
                              Stomach
                              Pylorus
                              Proximal duodenum
               Excludes: When associated with endoscopic examination limited to oesophagus
                              (G14, G17)
                              When associated with endoscopic examination limited to duodenum (G54.1)
               Note: Principal category, extended at G42
                              It is not necessary to code diagnostic endoscopic examination of upper
                              gastrointestinal tract (G45.9)
                              Use a subsidiary site code as necessary

G43.1   Fibreoptic endoscopic snare resection of lesion of upper gastrointestinal tract
G43.2   Fibreoptic endoscopic laser destruction of lesion of upper gastrointestinal tract
G43.3   Fibreoptic endoscopic cauterisation of lesion of upper gastrointestinal tract
G43.4   Fibreoptic endoscopic sclerotherapy to lesion of upper gastrointestinal tract
G43.5   Fibreoptic endoscopic destruction of lesion of upper gastrointestinal tract NEC
G43.6   Fibreoptic endoscopic injection therapy to lesion of upper gastrointestinal tract NEC
G43.7   Fibreoptic endoscopic rubber band ligation of upper gastrointestinal tract varices
G43.8   Other specified
G43.9   Unspecified

G44   **Other therapeutic fibreoptic endoscopic operations on upper gastrointestinal tract**

         Includes: *Therapeutic endoscopic operations on upper gastrointestinal tract NEC*
                       Oesophagus
                       Stomach
                       Pylorus
                       Proximal duodenum

         Excludes: *When associated with endoscopic examination limited to oesophagus (G15, G18)*
                       When associated with endoscopic examination limited to duodenum (G54)

            Note: **Principal category, extended at G46**
                       It is not necessary to code additionally any mention of diagnostic endoscopic examination of upper gastrointestinal tract (G45.9)
                       Use a subsidiary site code as necessary

G44.1   Fibreoptic endoscopic insertion of prosthesis into upper gastrointestinal tract
         Includes: *Endoscopic insertion of expanding metal stent into upper gastrointestinal tract*

G44.2   Fibreoptic endoscopic removal of foreign body from upper gastrointestinal tract

G44.3   Fibreoptic endoscopic dilation of upper gastrointestinal tract NEC

G44.4   Fibreoptic endoscopic reduction of intussusception of gastroenterostomy

G44.5   Fibreoptic endoscopic percutaneous insertion of gastrostomy

G44.6   Fibreoptic endoscopic pressure controlled balloon dilation of lower oesophageal sphincter

G44.7   Fibreoptic endoscopic removal of gastrostomy tube

G44.8   Other specified

G44.9   Unspecified

G45   **Diagnostic fibreoptic endoscopic examination of upper gastrointestinal tract**

         Includes: *Diagnostic endoscopic examination of upper gastrointestinal tract NEC*
                       Oesophagus
                       Stomach
                       Pylorus
                       Proximal duodenum

         Excludes: *When associated with examination limited to oesophagus (G16)*
                       When associated with examination limited to duodenum (G55)

            Note: **Use a subsidiary site code as necessary**

G45.1   Fibreoptic endoscopic examination of upper gastrointestinal tract and biopsy of lesion of upper gastrointestinal tract
         Includes: *Fibreoptic endoscopic examination of upper gastrointestinal tract and biopsy of upper gastrointestinal tract*
                       Biopsy of lesion of upper gastrointestinal tract NEC
                       Biopsy of upper gastrointestinal tract NEC

G45.2   Fibreoptic endoscopic ultrasound examination of upper gastrointestinal tract
         Includes: *Endoscopic ultrasound examination of upper gastrointestinal tract NEC*

G45.3   Fibreoptic endoscopic insertion of Bravo pH capsule into upper gastrointestinal tract
         Excludes: *When associated with examination limited to oesophagus (G16.3, G19.2)*

G45.4   Fibreoptic endoscopic examination of upper gastrointestinal tract and staining of gastric mucosa
         Includes: *Staining of gastric mucosa NEC*

G45.8   Other specified

G45.9   Unspecified
         Includes: *Fibreoptic gastroscopy NEC*
                       Gastroscopy NEC

G46   **Therapeutic fibreoptic endoscopic operations on upper gastrointestinal tract**
   Includes: *Therapeutic endoscopic operations on upper gastrointestinal tract NEC*
            Oesophagus
            Stomach
            Pylorus
            Proximal duodenum
   Excludes: *When associated with endoscopic examination limited to oesophagus*
            (G15, G18)
            When associated with endoscopic examination limited to duodenum (G54)
      Note: Principal G44
            It is not necessary to code additionally any mention of diagnostic endoscopic
            examination of upper gastrointestinal tract (G45.9)
            Use a subsidiary site code as necessary

G46.1   Fibreoptic endoscopic endoluminal plication of gastro-oesophageal junction
G46.8   Other specified
G46.9   Unspecified

G47   **Intubation of stomach**

G47.1   Intubation of stomach for pH manometry
G47.2   Intubation of stomach for pressure manometry
G47.3   Irrigation of stomach
      Includes: *Lavage of stomach*
               Washout of stomach
G47.4   Intubation of stomach for study of gastric secretion
G47.8   Other specified
G47.9   Unspecified

G48   **Other operations on stomach**

G48.1   Insertion of gastric bubble
G48.2   Attention to gastric bubble
G48.3   Induction of emesis
G48.4   Administration of activated charcoal
G48.5   Insertion of gastric balloon
G48.6   Attention to gastric balloon
G48.8   Other specified
G48.9   Unspecified

G49   **Excision of duodenum**
   Excludes: Pancreaticoduodenectomy (J56)

G49.1   Gastroduodenectomy
G49.2   Total excision of duodenum
G49.3   Partial excision of duodenum
G49.8   Other specified
G49.9   Unspecified
      Includes: Duodenectomy NEC

G50   **Open extirpation of lesion of duodenum**

G50.1   Excision of lesion of duodenum
G50.2   Open destruction of lesion of duodenum
G50.8   Other specified
G50.9   Unspecified

G51   **Bypass of duodenum**

G51.1   Bypass of duodenum by anastomosis of stomach to jejunum
G51.2   Bypass of duodenum by anastomosis of duodenum to duodenum
G51.3   Bypass of duodenum by anastomosis of duodenum to jejunum
G51.4   Bypass of duodenum by anastomosis of duodenum to colon
G51.8   Other specified
G51.9   Unspecified

G52   **Operations on ulcer of duodenum**

G52.1   Closure of perforated ulcer of duodenum
G52.2   Suture of ulcer of duodenum NEC
G52.3   Oversew of blood vessel of duodenal ulcer
G52.8   Other specified
G52.9   Unspecified

G53   **Other open operations on duodenum**

G53.1   Open biopsy of lesion of duodenum
                 Includes: *Open biopsy of duodenum*
G53.2   Closure of perforation of duodenum NEC
G53.3   Open removal of foreign body from duodenum
G53.4   Open insertion of tubal prosthesis into duodenum
G53.5   Incision of duodenum NEC
                 Includes: *Duodenotomy NEC*
G53.6   Correction of malrotation of duodenum
G53.8   Other specified
G53.9   Unspecified

G54   **Therapeutic endoscopic operations on duodenum**
                 Excludes: *When associated with general endoscopic examination of upper*
                                 gastrointestinal tract (G42, G43, G44, G46)
                                 When associated with endoscopic examination of biliary and pancreatic ducts
                                 (J40–J42)
               Note: **It is not necessary to code additionally any mention of diagnostic endoscopic**
                                 examination limited to duodenum (G55.9)

G54.1   Endoscopic extirpation of lesion of duodenum
                 Includes: *Snare resection of duodenum*
G54.2   Endoscopic dilation of duodenum
G54.3   Endoscopic insertion of tubal prosthesis into duodenum
G54.8   Other specified
G54.9   Unspecified

G55   **Diagnostic endoscopic examination of duodenum**
                 Excludes: *When not limited to duodenum (G45)*

G55.1   Diagnostic endoscopic examination of duodenum and biopsy of lesion of duodenum
                 Includes: *Diagnostic endoscopic examination of duodenum and biopsy of duodenum*
                                 Endoscopic biopsy of lesion of duodenum
                                 Endoscopic biopsy of duodenum
                                 Biopsy of lesion of duodenum NEC
                                 Biopsy of duodenum NEC
G55.8   Other specified
G55.9   Unspecified
                 Includes: *Duodenoscopy NEC*

G57   **Other operations on duodenum**

G57.1   Intubation of duodenum for studies of pancreatic function HFQ
G57.2   Intubation of duodenum NEC
G57.8   Other specified
G57.9   Unspecified

G58   **Excision of jejunum**

G58.1   Total jejunectomy and anastomosis of stomach to ileum
G58.2   Total jejunectomy and anastomosis of duodenum to ileum
G58.3   Total jejunectomy and anastomosis of duodenum to colon
G58.4   Partial jejunectomy and anastomosis of jejunum to ileum
         Includes: Jejunectomy and anastomosis of jejunum to jejunum
G58.5   Partial jejunectomy and anastomosis of duodenum to colon
G58.8   Other specified
G58.9   Unspecified
         Includes: Jejunectomy NEC

G59   **Extirpation of lesion of jejunum**

G59.1   Excision of lesion of jejunum
G59.2   Open destruction of lesion of jejunum
G59.8   Other specified
G59.9   Unspecified

G60   **Artificial opening into jejunum**

G60.1   Creation of jejunostomy
G60.2   Refashioning of jejunostomy
G60.3   Closure of jejunostomy
G60.8   Other specified
G60.9   Unspecified

G61   **Bypass of jejunum**

G61.1   Bypass of jejunum by anastomosis of jejunum to jejunum
G61.2   Bypass of jejunum by anastomosis of jejunum to ileum
G61.3   Bypass of jejunum by anastomosis of jejunum to colon
G61.8   Other specified
G61.9   Unspecified

G62   **Open endoscopic operations on jejunum**

G62.1   Open jejunoscopy
         Includes: Operative jejunoscopy
G62.8   Other specified
G62.9   Unspecified

G63   **Other open operations on jejunum**

G63.1   Open biopsy of lesion of jejunum
              Includes: Open biopsy of jejunum
              Biopsy of lesion of jejunum NEC
              Biopsy of jejunum NEC
G63.2   Incision of jejunum
G63.3   Closure of perforation of jejunum
G63.4   Open intubation of jejunum
G63.8   Other specified
G63.9   Unspecified

G64   **Therapeutic endoscopic operations on jejunum**
              *Note: **It is not necessary to code additionally any mention of diagnostic endoscopic***
              examination of jejunum (G65.9)

G64.1   Endoscopic extirpation of lesion of jejunum
G64.2   Endoscopic dilation of jejunum
G64.3   Endoscopic insertion of tubal prosthesis into jejunum
G64.8   Other specified
G64.9   Unspecified

G65   **Diagnostic endoscopic examination of jejunum**

G65.1   Diagnostic endoscopic examination of jejunum and biopsy of lesion of jejunum
              Includes: Diagnostic endoscopic examination of jejunum and biopsy of jejunum
              Endoscopic biopsy of lesion of jejunum
              Endoscopic biopsy of jejunum
G65.8   Other specified
G65.9   Unspecified
              Includes: Jejunoscopy NEC

G67   **Other operations on jejunum**

G67.1   Intubation of jejunum for decompression of intestine
G67.2   Intubation of jejunum for measurement of intestinal function
G67.3   Passage of Crosby capsule into jejunum for biopsy of mucosa of jejunum
G67.4   Intubation of jejunum NEC
G67.8   Other specified
G67.9   Unspecified

G68   **Transplantation of ileum**
              Includes: Small intestine NEC

G68.1   Allotransplantation of ileum
G68.8   Other specified
G68.9   Unspecified

G69   **Excision of ileum**
              Includes: Small intestine NEC

G69.1   Ileectomy and anastomosis of stomach to ileum
G69.2   Ileectomy and anastomosis of duodenum to ileum
G69.3   Ileectomy and anastomosis of ileum to ileum
G69.4   Ileectomy and anastomosis of ileum to colon
G69.8   Other specified
G69.9   Unspecified
              Includes: Ileectomy NEC

G70   **Open extirpation of lesion of ileum**
              Includes: Small intestine NEC

G70.1   Excision of Meckel's diverticulum
G70.2   Excision of lesion of ileum NEC
G70.3   Open destruction of lesion of ileum
G70.8   Other specified
G70.9   Unspecified

G71   **Bypass of ileum**
              Includes: Small intestine NEC

G71.1   Bypass of ileum by anastomosis of jejunum to ileum
G71.2   Bypass of ileum by anastomosis of ileum to ileum
G71.3   Bypass of ileum by anastomosis of ileum to caecum
G71.4   Bypass of ileum by anastomosis of ileum to transverse colon
G71.5   Bypass of ileum by anastomosis of ileum to colon NEC
              Includes: Bypass of ileum by anastomosis of ileum to rectum
G71.6   Duodenal switch
              Excludes: Duodenal switch associated with concurrent sleeve gastrectomy (G28.4)
G71.7   Reversal of duodenal switch
G71.8   Other specified
G71.9   Unspecified

G72   **Other connection of ileum**
              Includes: Small intestine NEC
              Excludes: When associated with concurrent excision of ileum (G69)

G72.1   Anastomosis of ileum to caecum
G72.2   Anastomosis of ileum to transverse colon
G72.3   Anastomosis of ileum to colon NEC
G72.4   Anastomosis of ileum to rectum
G72.5   Anastomosis of ileum to anus and creation of pouch HFQ
G72.8   Other specified
G72.9   Unspecified

G73   **Attention to connection of ileum**
Includes: *Small intestine NEC*

G73.1   Revision of anastomosis of ileum
Includes: *Revision of ileocolic anastomosis*
                     Revision of anastomosis of small intestine NEC
G73.2   Closure of anastomosis of ileum
G73.3   Resection of ileostomy
G73.4   Resection of ileocolic anastomosis
G73.8   Other specified
G73.9   Unspecified

G74   **Creation of artificial opening into ileum**
Includes: *Small intestine NEC*

G74.1   Creation of continent ileostomy
G74.2   Creation of temporary ileostomy
G74.3   Creation of defunctioning ileostomy
Includes: *Creation of split ileostomy*
G74.8   Other specified
G74.9   Unspecified

G75   **Attention to artificial opening into ileum**
Includes: *Small intestine NEC*

G75.1   Refashioning of ileostomy
G75.2   Repair of prolapse of ileostomy
G75.3   Closure of ileostomy
G75.4   Dilation of ileostomy
G75.5   Reduction of prolapse of ileostomy
G75.6   Resiting of ileostomy
G75.8   Other specified
G75.9   Unspecified

G76   **Intra-abdominal manipulation of ileum**
Includes: *Small intestine NEC*

G76.1   Open reduction of intussusception of ileum
G76.2   Open relief of strangulation of ileum
G76.3   Open relief of obstruction of ileum NEC
G76.4   Plication of ileum
G76.8   Other specified
G76.9   Unspecified

G78   **Other open operations on ileum**
Includes: Small intestine NEC

G78.1   Open biopsy of lesion of ileum
Includes: Open biopsy of ileum
Biopsy of lesion of ileum NEC
Biopsy of ileum NEC

G78.2   Strictureplasty of ileum
G78.3   Removal of foreign body from ileum
G78.4   Closure of perforation of ileum
G78.5   Exclusion of segment of ileum
G78.6   Open intubation of ileum
G78.8   Other specified
G78.9   Unspecified

G79   **Therapeutic endoscopic operations on ileum**
Includes: Small intestine NEC
    Note: **It is not necessary to code additionally any mention of diagnostic endoscopic examination of ileum (G80.9)**

G79.1   Endoscopic extirpation of lesion of ileum
G79.2   Endoscopic dilation of ileum
G79.3   Endoscopic insertion of tubal prosthesis into ileum
G79.8   Other specified
G79.9   Unspecified

G80   **Diagnostic endoscopic examination of ileum**
Includes: Small intestine NEC

G80.1   Diagnostic endoscopic examination of ileum and biopsy of lesion of ileum
Includes: Diagnostic endoscopic examination of ileum and biopsy of ileum
Endoscopic biopsy of lesion of ileum
Endoscopic biopsy of ileum

G80.2   Wireless capsule endoscopy
Includes: Capsule endoscopy NEC

G80.3   Diagnostic endoscopic balloon examination of ileum
G80.8   Other specified
G80.9   Unspecified
Includes: Ileoscopy NEC
Enteroscopy NEC

G82   **Other operations on ileum**
Includes: Small intestine NEC

G82.1   Radiological reduction of intussusception of ileum using barium enema
G82.2   Intubation of ileum for decompression of intestine
G82.3   Intubation of ileum for studies on function HFQ
G82.4   Intubation of ileum NEC
G82.8   Other specified
G82.9   Unspecified

CHAPTER H
LOWER DIGESTIVE TRACT
(CODES H01–H70)

Note: *Use a subsidiary code for minimal access approach (Y74–Y76)*

Use a subsidiary code to identify method of image control (Y53)

H01   **Emergency excision of appendix**

H01.1   Emergency excision of abnormal appendix and drainage HFQ
H01.2   Emergency excision of abnormal appendix NEC
H01.3   Emergency excision of normal appendix
H01.8   Other specified
H01.9   Unspecified
           Includes: Emergency appendicectomy NEC

H02   **Other excision of appendix**

H02.1   Interval appendicectomy
H02.2   Planned delayed appendicectomy NEC
H02.3   Prophylactic appendicectomy NEC
H02.4   Incidental appendicectomy
           Includes: Appendicectomy performed during course of other abdominal operation
                   Note: Use as a secondary code when performed during creation of caecostomy (H14.9)
H02.8   Other specified
H02.9   Unspecified
           Includes: Appendicectomy NEC

H03   **Other operations on appendix**

H03.1   Drainage of abscess of appendix
H03.2   Drainage of appendix NEC
H03.3   Exteriorisation of appendix
           Includes: Appendicostomy
H03.8   Other specified
H03.9   Unspecified

H04   **Total excision of colon and rectum**
           Excludes: Subtotal excision of colon (H29)

H04.1   Panproctocolectomy and ileostomy
           Includes: Proctocolectomy NEC
H04.2   Panproctocolectomy and anastomosis of ileum to anus and creation of pouch HFQ
H04.3   Panproctocolectomy and anastomosis of ileum to anus NEC
H04.8   Other specified
H04.9   Unspecified

H05   **Total excision of colon**
           Excludes: Subtotal excision of colon (H29)

H05.1   Total colectomy and anastomosis of ileum to rectum
H05.2   Total colectomy and ileostomy and creation of rectal fistula HFQ
H05.3   Total colectomy and ileostomy NEC
H05.8   Other specified
H05.9   Unspecified

H06　　　**Extended excision of right hemicolon**

Includes:　Excision of right colon and other segment of ileum or colon and surrounding tissue

Caecum

H06.1　Extended right hemicolectomy and end to end anastomosis
H06.2　Extended right hemicolectomy and anastomosis of ileum to colon
H06.3　Extended right hemicolectomy and anastomosis NEC
H06.4　Extended right hemicolectomy and ileostomy HFQ
H06.5　Extended right hemicolectomy and end to side anastomosis
H06.8　Other specified
H06.9　Unspecified

H07　　　**Other excision of right hemicolon**

Includes:　Limited excision of caecum and terminal ileum caecum

H07.1　Right hemicolectomy and end to end anastomosis of ileum to colon
　　　　Includes:　Ileocaecal resection
H07.2　Right hemicolectomy and side to side anastomosis of ileum to transverse colon
H07.3　Right hemicolectomy and anastomosis NEC
H07.4　Right hemicolectomy and ileostomy HFQ
H07.5　Right hemicolectomy and end to side anastomosis
H07.8　Other specified
H07.9　Unspecified

H08　　　**Excision of transverse colon**

H08.1　Transverse colectomy and end to end anastomosis
H08.2　Transverse colectomy and anastomosis of ileum to colon
H08.3　Transverse colectomy and anastomosis NEC
H08.4　Transverse colectomy and ileostomy HFQ
H08.5　Transverse colectomy and exteriorisation of bowel NEC
　　　　Note:　Use a secondary code for type of exteriorisation of bowel (H14, H15)
H08.6　Transverse colectomy and end to side anastomosis
H08.8　Other specified
H08.9　Unspecified

H09　　　**Excision of left hemicolon**

H09.1　Left hemicolectomy and end to end anastomosis of colon to rectum
H09.2　Left hemicolectomy and end to end anastomosis of colon to colon
H09.3　Left hemicolectomy and anastomosis NEC
H09.4　Left hemicolectomy and ileostomy HFQ
H09.5　Left hemicolectomy and exteriorisation of bowel NEC
　　　　Note:　Use a secondary code for type of exteriorisation of bowel (H14, H15)
H09.6　Left hemicolectomy and end to side anastomosis
H09.8　Other specified
H09.9　Unspecified

H10   **Excision of sigmoid colon**

H10.1   Sigmoid colectomy and end to end anastomosis of ileum to rectum
H10.2   Sigmoid colectomy and anastomosis of colon to rectum
H10.3   Sigmoid colectomy and anastomosis NEC
H10.4   Sigmoid colectomy and ileostomy HFQ
H10.5   Sigmoid colectomy and exteriorisation of bowel NEC
         Note: Use a secondary code for type of exteriorisation of bowel (H14, H15)
H10.6   Sigmoid colectomy and end to side anastomosis
H10.8   Other specified
H10.9   Unspecified

H11   **Other excision of colon**
         Includes: Excision of colon where segment removed is not stated

H11.1   Colectomy and end to end anastomosis of colon to colon NEC
H11.2   Colectomy and side to side anastomosis of ileum to colon NEC
H11.3   Colectomy and anastomosis NEC
H11.4   Colectomy and ileostomy NEC
H11.5   Colectomy and exteriorisation of bowel NEC
         Note: Use a secondary code for type of exteriorisation of bowel (H14, H15)
H11.6   Colectomy and end to side anastomosis NEC
H11.8   Other specified
H11.9   Unspecified
         Includes: Colectomy NEC
                  Hemicolectomy NEC

H12   **Extirpation of lesion of colon**
         Includes: Caecum

H12.1   Excision of diverticulum of colon
H12.2   Excision of lesion of colon NEC
H12.3   Destruction of lesion of colon NEC
H12.8   Other specified
H12.9   Unspecified

H13   **Bypass of colon**
         Includes: Caecum
         Excludes: Bypass of colon when associated with excision of colon (H04–H11)

H13.1   Bypass of colon by anastomosis of ileum to colon
H13.2   Bypass of colon by anastomosis of caecum to sigmoid colon
H13.3   Bypass of colon by anastomosis of transverse colon to sigmoid colon
H13.4   Bypass of colon by anastomosis of transverse colon to rectum
H13.5   Bypass of colon by anastomosis of colon to rectum NEC
H13.8   Other specified
H13.9   Unspecified

H14   **Exteriorisation of caecum**

H14.1   Tube caecostomy
H14.2   Refashioning of caecostomy
H14.3   Closure of caecostomy
H14.4   Appendicocaecostomy
H14.8   Other specified
H14.9   Unspecified
         Includes: Caecostomy NEC

H15   **Other exteriorisation of colon**
               Note: Principal category, extended at H32

H15.1   Loop colostomy
H15.2   End colostomy
H15.3   Refashioning of colostomy
H15.4   Closure of colostomy
H15.5   Dilation of colostomy
H15.6   Reduction of prolapse of colostomy
H15.7   Percutaneous endoscopic sigmoid colostomy
H15.8   Other specified
H15.9   Unspecified
               Includes: Colostomy NEC

H16   **Incision of colon**
               Includes: Caecum

H16.1   Drainage of colon
               Includes: Drainage of pericolonic tissue
H16.2   Caecotomy
H16.3   Colotomy
H16.8   Other specified
H16.9   Unspecified

H17   **Intra-abdominal manipulation of colon**
               Includes: Caecum

H17.1   Open reduction of intussusception of colon
H17.2   Open reduction of volvulus of caecum
H17.3   Open reduction of volvulus of sigmoid colon
H17.4   Open reduction of volvulus of colon NEC
H17.5   Open relief of strangulation of colon
H17.6   Open relief of obstruction of colon NEC
H17.8   Other specified
H17.9   Unspecified

H18   **Open endoscopic operations on colon**
               Includes: Caecum

H18.1   Open colonoscopy
               Includes: Operative colonoscopy
H18.8   Other specified
H18.9   Unspecified

H19   **Other open operations on colon**
               Includes: Caecum
               Excludes: Repair of vesicocolic fistula (M37.2)

H19.1   Open biopsy of lesion of colon
               Includes: Open biopsy of colon
                             Biopsy of lesion of colon
                             Biopsy of colon
H19.2   Fixation of colon
H19.3   Enterorrhaphy of colon   Repair/Suture
H19.4   Open removal of foreign body from colon
H19.8   Other specified
H19.9   Unspecified

H20	**Endoscopic extirpation of lesion of colon**

H20   **Endoscopic extirpation of lesion of colon**

Includes: *Caecum*
               Mucosa of colon
               Mucosa of caecum

Excludes: *Fibreoptic endoscopic extirpation of lesion limited to sigmoid colon (H23)*

       Note: **It is not necessary to code additionally any mention of diagnostic endoscopic examination limited to colon (H22.9)**
                   Use a subsidiary site code as necessary

H20.1   Fibreoptic endoscopic snare resection of lesion of colon
H20.2   Fibreoptic endoscopic cauterisation of lesion of colon
H20.3   Fibreoptic endoscopic laser destruction of lesion of colon
H20.4   Fibreoptic endoscopic destruction of lesion of colon NEC
H20.5   Fibreoptic endoscopic submucosal resection of lesion of colon
H20.6   Fibreoptic endoscopic resection of lesion of colon NEC
H20.8   Other specified
H20.9   Unspecified

H21   **Other therapeutic endoscopic operations on colon**

Includes: *Caecum*
               Mucosa of colon
               Mucosa of caecum

Excludes: *Other therapeutic fibreoptic endoscopic operations limited to sigmoid colon (H24)*

       Note: **It is not necessary to code additionally any mention of diagnostic endoscopic examination limited to colon (H22.9)**
                   Use a subsidiary site code as necessary

H21.1   Fibreoptic endoscopic dilation of colon
H21.2   Fibreoptic endoscopic coagulation of blood vessel of colon
H21.3   Fibreoptic endoscopic removal of foreign body from colon
H21.4   Fibreoptic endoscopic insertion of expanding metal stent into colon
H21.8   Other specified
H21.9   Unspecified

H22   **Diagnostic endoscopic examination of colon**

Includes: *Caecum*
               Mucosa of colon
               Mucosa of caecum

Excludes: *Diagnostic fibreoptic endoscopic examination limited to sigmoid colon (H25)*

       Note: **Use a subsidiary site code as necessary**

H22.1   Diagnostic fibreoptic endoscopic examination of colon and biopsy of lesion of colon

Includes: *Diagnostic fibreoptic endoscopic examination of colon and biopsy of colon*
               Fibreoptic endoscopic biopsy of lesion of colon
               Fibreoptic endoscopic biopsy of colon

H22.8   Other specified
H22.9   Unspecified

Includes: *Colonoscopy NEC*

H23	**Endoscopic extirpation of lesion of lower bowel using fibreoptic sigmoidoscope**

Includes:	Endoscopic extirpation of lesion of lower bowel NEC
		Sigmoid colon
		Colon
		Rectum

Note:	**It is not necessary to code diagnostic endoscopic examination of lower bowel using fibreoptic sigmoidoscope (H25.9)**
		Use a subsidiary site code as necessary

H23.1	Endoscopic snare resection of lesion of lower bowel using fibreoptic sigmoidoscope
H23.2	Endoscopic cauterisation of lesion of lower bowel using fibreoptic sigmoidoscope
H23.3	Endoscopic laser destruction of lesion of lower bowel using fibreoptic sigmoidoscope
H23.4	Endoscopic destruction of lesion of lower bowel using fibreoptic sigmoidoscope NEC
H23.5	Endoscopic submucosal resection of lesion of lower bowel using fibreoptic sigmoidoscope
H23.6	Endoscopic resection of lesion of lower bowel using fibreoptic sigmoidoscope NEC
H23.8	Other specified
H23.9	Unspecified

H24	**Other therapeutic endoscopic operations on lower bowel using fibreoptic sigmoidoscope**

Includes:	Endoscopic operations on lower bowel NEC
		Sigmoid colon
		Colon
		Rectum

Note:	**It is not necessary to code diagnostic endoscopic examination of lower bowel using fibreoptic sigmoidoscope (H25.9)**
		Use a subsidiary site code as necessary

H24.1	Endoscopic dilation of lower bowel using fibreoptic sigmoidoscope
H24.2	Endoscopic coagulation of blood vessel of lower bowel using fibreoptic sigmoidoscope
H24.3	Endoscopic insertion of tubal prosthesis into lower bowel using fibreoptic sigmoidoscope
H24.4	Endoscopic insertion of expanding metal stent into lower bowel using fibreoptic sigmoidoscope
H24.8	Other specified
H24.9	Unspecified

H25	**Diagnostic endoscopic examination of lower bowel using fibreoptic sigmoidoscope**

Includes:	Diagnostic endoscopic examination of lower bowel NEC
		Sigmoid colon
		Colon
		Rectum

Excludes:	General diagnostic examination of colon (H22.9)

Note:	**Use a subsidiary site code as necessary**

H25.1	Diagnostic endoscopic examination of lower bowel and biopsy of lesion of lower bowel using fibreoptic sigmoidoscope
	Includes:	Diagnostic endoscopic examination of lower bowel and biopsy of lower bowel using fibreoptic sigmoidoscope.
			Endoscopic biopsy of lower bowel using fibreoptic sigmoidoscope
H25.2	Diagnostic endoscopic examination of lower bowel and sampling for bacterial overgrowth using fibreoptic sigmoidoscope
	Includes:	Sampling for bacterial overgrowth of lower bowel NEC
H25.8	Other specified
H25.9	Unspecified
	Includes:	Fibreoptic sigmoidoscopy NEC
			Fibrosigmoidoscopy NEC
			Sigmoidoscopy NEC

H26   **Endoscopic extirpation of lesion of sigmoid colon using rigid sigmoidoscope**

        Includes: *Rectum*

        Note: *It is not necessary to code diagnostic endoscopic operations on sigmoid colon using rigid sigmoidoscope (H28.9)*

                    Use a subsidiary site code as necessary

H26.1   Endoscopic snare resection of lesion of sigmoid colon using rigid sigmoidoscope
H26.2   Endoscopic cauterisation of lesion of sigmoid colon using rigid sigmoidoscope
H26.3   Endoscopic laser destruction of lesion of sigmoid colon using rigid sigmoidoscope
H26.4   Endoscopic cryotherapy to lesion of sigmoid colon using rigid sigmoidoscope
H26.5   Endoscopic destruction of lesion of sigmoid colon using rigid sigmoidoscope NEC
H26.6   Endoscopic submucosal resection of lesion of sigmoid colon using rigid sigmoidoscope
H26.7   Endoscopic resection of lesion of sigmoid colon using rigid sigmoidoscope NEC
H26.8   Other specified
H26.9   Unspecified

H27   **Other therapeutic endoscopic operations on sigmoid colon using rigid sigmoidoscope**

        Includes: *Rectum*

        Note: *It is not necessary to code diagnostic endoscopic examination of sigmoid colon using rigid sigmoidoscope (H28.9)*

                    Use a subsidiary site code as necessary

H27.1   Endoscopic dilation of sigmoid colon using rigid sigmoidoscope
H27.2   Endoscopic removal of foreign body from sigmoid colon using rigid sigmoidoscope
H27.3   Endoscopic insertion of tubal prosthesis into sigmoid colon using rigid sigmoidoscope
H27.4   Endoscopic insertion of expanding metal stent into sigmoid colon using rigid sigmoidoscope
H27.8   Other specified
H27.9   Unspecified

H28   **Diagnostic endoscopic examination of sigmoid colon using rigid sigmoidoscope**

        Includes: *Rectum*

        Note: *Use a subsidiary site code as necessary*

H28.1   Diagnostic endoscopic examination of sigmoid colon and biopsy of lesion of sigmoid colon using rigid sigmoidoscope

        Includes: *Diagnostic endoscopic examination of sigmoid colon and biopsy of sigmoid colon using rigid sigmoidoscope*

                    Endoscopic biopsy of lesion of lower bowel using rigid sigmoidoscope

                    Endoscopic biopsy of lower bowel using rigid sigmoidoscope

                    Biopsy of lesion of sigmoid colon using rigid sigmoidoscope

                    Biopsy of sigmoid colon using rigid sigmoidoscope

H28.8   Other specified
H28.9   Unspecified

H29   **Subtotal excision of colon**

H29.1   Subtotal excision of colon and rectum and creation of colonic pouch and anastomosis of colon to anus
H29.2   Subtotal excision of colon and rectum and creation of colonic pouch NEC
H29.3   Subtotal excision of colon and creation of colonic pouch and anastomosis of colon to rectum
H29.4   Subtotal excision of colon and creation of colonic pouch NEC
H29.8   Other specified
H29.9   Unspecified

H30   **Other operations on colon**

H30.1   Radiological reduction of intussusception of colon using barium enema
H30.2   Intubation of colon for pressure manometry
          Includes: Manometry of colon NEC
H30.3   Passage of flatus tube to reduce volvulus of sigmoid colon
H30.4   Intubation of colon NEC
H30.5   Irrigation of colon
          Includes: Lavage of colon
                       Washout of colon
H30.8   Other specified
H30.9   Unspecified

H31   **Image guided colorectal therapeutic operations**

H31.1   Image guided percutaneous occlusion of colorectal fistula
H31.2   Image guided transluminal occlusion of colorectal fistula
H31.3   Image guided balloon dilation of colorectal stricture
H31.4   Image guided insertion of colorectal stent
H31.5   Image guided removal of colorectal stent
H31.8   Other specified
H31.9   Unspecified

H32   **Exteriorisation of colon**
          Note: Principal H15

H32.1   Resiting of colostomy
H32.8   Other specified
H32.9   Unspecified

H33   **Excision of rectum**
          Includes: Excision of whole or part of rectum with or without part of sigmoid colon

H33.1   Abdominoperineal excision of rectum and end colostomy
H33.2   Proctectomy and anastomosis of colon to anus
H33.3   Anterior resection of rectum and anastomosis of colon to rectum using staples
          Includes: Rectosigmoidectomy and anastomosis of colon to rectum
H33.4   Anterior resection of rectum and anastomosis NEC
H33.5   Rectosigmoidectomy and closure of rectal stump and exteriorisation of bowel
          Note: Use a secondary code for type of exteriorisation of bowel (G74, H14–H15)
H33.6   Anterior resection of rectum and exteriorisation of bowel
          Note: Use a secondary code for type of exteriorisation of bowel (G74, H14–H15)
H33.7   Perineal resection of rectum HFQ
H33.8   Other specified
H33.9   Unspecified
          Includes: Rectosigmoidectomy NEC

H34   **Open extirpation of lesion of rectum**

H34.1   Open excision of lesion of rectum
H34.2   Open cauterisation of lesion of rectum
H34.3   Open cryotherapy to lesion of rectum
H34.4   Open laser destruction of lesion of rectum
H34.5   Open destruction of lesion of rectum NEC
H34.8   Other specified
H34.9   Unspecified

H35   **Fixation of rectum for prolapse**

H35.1   Anterior fixation of rectum
H35.2   Posterior fixation of rectum using prosthetic material
H35.3   Posterior fixation of rectum NEC
H35.4   Fixation of rectum using fascia lata
H35.8   Other specified
H35.9   Unspecified

H36   **Other abdominal operations for prolapse of rectum**

H36.1   Abdominal repair of levator ani muscles
           Includes: Repair of levator ani muscles NEC
                      Repair of pelvic floor muscles NEC
H36.8   Other specified
H36.9   Unspecified

H40   **Operations on rectum through anal sphincter**

H40.1   Trans-sphincteric excision of mucosa of rectum
H40.2   Trans-sphincteric excision of lesion of rectum
           Includes: Trans-sphincteric biopsy of lesion of rectum
                      Trans-sphincteric biopsy of rectum
H40.3   Trans-sphincteric destruction of lesion of rectum
H40.4   Trans-sphincteric anastomosis of colon to anus
H40.8   Other specified
H40.9   Unspecified

H41   **Other operations on rectum through anus**

H41.1   Rectosigmoidectomy and peranal anastomosis
H41.2   Peranal excision of lesion of rectum
           Includes: Peranal biopsy of lesion of rectum
                      Peranal biopsy of rectum
H41.3   Peranal destruction of lesion of rectum
H41.4   Peranal mucosal proctectomy and endoanal anastomosis
H41.5   Peranal resection of rectum using staples
           Includes: Transanal resection of rectum using staples
H41.8   Other specified
H41.9   Unspecified

H42   **Perineal operations for prolapse of rectum**
           Includes: Perineal operations for prolapse of mucosa of rectum

H42.1   Insertion of encircling suture around perianal sphincter
           Includes: Insertion of Thiersch wire around perianal sphincter
                      Insertion of suture around perianal sphincter
H42.2   Perineal plication of levator ani muscles and anal sphincters
H42.3   Insertion of supralevator sling
H42.4   Removal of encircling suture from around perianal sphincter
H42.5   Excision of mucosal prolapse of rectum NEC
H42.6   Perineal repair of prolapse of rectum NEC
H42.8   Other specified
H42.9   Unspecified

H44   **Manipulation of rectum**

H44.1   Manual removal of foreign body from rectum
H44.2   Manual reduction of prolapse of rectum
H44.3   Manual evacuation of impacted faeces from rectum
H44.4   Examination of rectum under anaesthetic
H44.5   Massage of rectum
H44.8   Other specified
H44.9   Unspecified

H46   **Other operations on rectum**

H46.1   Radiological reduction of intussusception of rectum using barium enema
H46.2   Hydrostatic reduction of intussusception of rectum
H46.3   Intubation of rectum for pressure manometry
H46.4   Intubation of rectum NEC
H46.8   Other specified
H46.9   Unspecified

H47   **Excision of anus**

H47.1   Excision of sphincter of anus
H47.8   Other specified
H47.9   Unspecified

H48   **Excision of lesion of anus**
            Includes: Perianal region

H48.1   Excision of polyp of anus
H48.2   Excision of skin tag of anus
H48.3   Excision of perianal wart
H48.8   Other specified
H48.9   Unspecified

H49   **Destruction of lesion of anus**
            Includes: Perianal region

H49.1   Cauterisation of lesion of anus
H49.2   Laser destruction of lesion of anus
H49.3   Cryotherapy to lesion of anus
H49.8   Other specified
H49.9   Unspecified

H50   **Repair of anus**
            Excludes: Other operations on the anal sphincter to control continence (H57)

H50.1   Posterior repair of anal sphincter
H50.2   Anterior repair of anal sphincter
H50.3   Cutback of covered anus
H50.4   Reanastomosis of rectum to anal canal for correction of congenital atresia of rectum
H50.8   Other specified
H50.9   Unspecified
            Includes: Anoplasty NEC

H51   **Excision of haemorrhoid**

H51.1   Haemorrhoidectomy
         Includes: Formal haemorrhoidectomy
H51.2   Partial internal sphincterotomy for haemorrhoid
H51.3   Stapled haemorrhoidectomy
H51.8   Other specified
H51.9   Unspecified

H52   **Destruction of haemorrhoid**

H52.1   Cryotherapy to haemorrhoid
H52.2   Infrared photocoagulation of haemorrhoid
H52.3   Injection of sclerosing substance into haemorrhoid
         Includes: Injection into haemorrhoid
                       Sclerotherapy to haemorrhoid
H52.4   Rubber band ligation of haemorrhoid
H52.8   Other specified
H52.9   Unspecified

H53   **Other operations on haemorrhoid**

H53.1   Evacuation of perianal haematoma
         Includes: Evacuation of thrombosed haemorrhoid
H53.2   Forced manual dilation of anus for haemorrhoid
H53.3   Manual reduction of prolapsed haemorrhoid
H53.8   Other specified
H53.9   Unspecified

H54   **Dilation of anal sphincter**

H54.1   Anorectal stretch
         Excludes: Forced manual dilation for haemorrhoid (H53.2)
H54.8   Other specified
H54.9   Unspecified

H55   **Other operations on perianal region**

H55.1   Laying open of low anal fistula
H55.2   Laying open of high anal fistula
H55.3   Laying open of anal fistula NEC
H55.4   Insertion of seton into high anal fistula and partial laying open of track HFQ
H55.5   Fistulography of anal fistula
H55.6   Probing of perineal fistula
H55.7   Repair of anal fistula using plug
H55.8   Other specified
H55.9   Unspecified

H56   **Other operations on anus**

H56.1   Biopsy of lesion of anus
         Includes: Biopsy of anus
H56.2   Lateral sphincterotomy of anus
H56.3   Incision of septum of anus
H56.4   Excision of anal fissure
H56.8   Other specified
H56.9   Unspecified

H57 **Other operations on the anal sphincter to control continence**
Excludes: Repair of anus (H50)

H57.1   Placement of artificial anal sphincter NEC
H57.2   Maintenance of artificial anal sphincter NEC
H57.3   Removal of artificial anal sphincter NEC
H57.4   Creation of graciloplasty sphincter
H57.5   Placement of dynamic graciloplasty sphincter
H57.6   Maintenance of dynamic graciloplasty sphincter
H57.7   Removal of dynamic graciloplasty sphincter
H57.8   Other specified
H57.9   Unspecified

H58 **Drainage through perineal region**

H58.1   Drainage of ischiorectal abscess
H58.2   Drainage of perianal abscess
H58.3   Drainage of perirectal abscess
H58.8   Other specified
H58.9   Unspecified

H59 **Excision of pilonidal sinus**
Includes: Pilonidal cyst
Pilonidal abscess

H59.1   Excision of pilonidal sinus and Z plasty skin flap HFQ
H59.2   Excision of pilonidal sinus and skin flap NEC
H59.3   Excision of pilonidal sinus and skin graft HFQ
H59.4   Excision of pilonidal sinus and suture HFQ
H59.8   Other specified
H59.9   Unspecified

H60 **Other operations on pilonidal sinus**
Includes: Pilonidal cyst
Pilonidal abscess

H60.1   Destruction of pilonidal sinus
H60.2   Laying open of pilonidal sinus
H60.3   Drainage of pilonidal sinus
H60.4   Injection of radiocontrast substance into pilonidal sinus
Includes: Sinography of pilonidal sinus
H60.8   Other specified
H60.9   Unspecified

H62　　**Other operations on bowel**
　　　　　Includes:　*Sigmoid colon*
　　　　　　　　　　Colon
　　　　　　　　　　Rectum

H62.1　　Laser recanalisation of bowel NEC
H62.2　　Mobilisation of bowel NEC
H62.3　　Dilation of bowel NEC
H62.4　　Intubation of bowel NEC
H62.5　　Irrigation of bowel NEC
　　　　　Includes:　*Lavage of bowel NEC*
　　　　　　　　　　Washout of bowel NEC
H62.6　　Proctoscopy
H62.8　　Other specified
H62.9　　Unspecified

H66　　**Therapeutic operations on ileoanal pouch**

H66.1　　Excision of ileoanal pouch
H66.2　　Revision of ileoanal pouch
H66.8　　Other specified
H66.9　　Unspecified

H68　　**Diagnostic endoscopic examination of enteric pouch using colonoscope**

H68.1　　Diagnostic endoscopic examination of colonic pouch and biopsy of colonic pouch using colonoscope
H68.2　　Diagnostic endoscopic examination of colonic pouch using colonoscope NEC
H68.3　　Diagnostic endoscopic examination of ileoanal pouch and biopsy of ileoanal pouch using colonoscope
H68.4　　Diagnostic endoscopic examination of ileoanal pouch using colonoscope NEC
H68.8　　Other specified
H68.9　　Unspecified

H69　　**Diagnostic endoscopic examination of enteric pouch using fibreoptic sigmoidoscope**
　　　　　Includes:　*Diagnostic examination of enteric pouch using endoscope NEC*

H69.1　　Diagnostic endoscopic examination of colonic pouch and biopsy of colonic pouch using fibreoptic sigmoidoscope
H69.2　　Diagnostic endoscopic examination of colonic pouch using fibreoptic sigmoidoscope NEC
H69.3　　Diagnostic endoscopic examination of ileoanal pouch and biopsy of ileoanal pouch using fibreoptic sigmoidoscope
H69.4　　Diagnostic endoscopic examination of ileoanal pouch using fibreoptic sigmoidoscope NEC
H69.8　　Other specified
H69.9　　Unspecified

H70　　**Diagnostic endoscopic examination of enteric pouch using rigid sigmoidoscope**

H70.1　　Diagnostic endoscopic examination of colonic pouch and biopsy of colonic pouch using rigid sigmoidoscope
H70.2　　Diagnostic endoscopic examination of colonic pouch using rigid sigmoidoscope NEC
H70.3　　Diagnostic endoscopic examination of ileoanal pouch and biopsy of ileoanal pouch using rigid sigmoidoscope
H70.4　　Diagnostic endoscopic examination of ileoanal pouch using rigid sigmoidoscope NEC
H70.8　　Other specified
H70.9　　Unspecified

CHAPTER J
OTHER ABDOMINAL ORGANS – PRINCIPALLY DIGESTIVE (CODES J01–J77)

Note: *Use a subsidiary code for minimal access approach (Y74–Y76)*

          Use a subsidiary code to identify method of image control (Y53)

          Use a subsidiary code to identify arteriotomy approach to organ under image control (Y78)

J01	**Transplantation of liver**
J01.1	Orthotopic transplantation of liver NEC
J01.2	Heterotopic transplantation of liver
	Includes: *Piggyback transplantation of liver*
	Auxillary transplantation of liver
J01.3	Replacement of previous liver transplant
J01.4	Transplantation of liver cells
J01.5	Orthotopic transplantation of whole liver
J01.8	Other specified
J01.9	Unspecified

J02	**Partial excision of liver**
J02.1	Right hemihepatectomy NEC
J02.2	Left hemihepatectomy NEC
J02.3	Resection of segment of liver
	Includes: *Resection of segments of liver*
	Resection of section of liver
J02.4	Wedge excision of liver
J02.5	Marsupialisation of lesion of liver
J02.6	Extended right hemihepatectomy
J02.7	Extended left hemihepatectomy
J02.8	Other specified
J02.9	Unspecified

J03	**Extirpation of lesion of liver**
J03.1	Excision of lesion of liver NEC
J03.2	Destruction of lesion of liver NEC
J03.3	Thermal ablation of single lesion of liver
	Includes: *Thermal ablation of lesion of liver NEC*
J03.4	Thermal ablation of multiple lesions of liver
J03.5	Excision of multiple lesions of liver
J03.8	Other specified
J03.9	Unspecified

J04	**Repair of liver**
J04.1	Removal of lacerated fragment of liver
J04.2	Repair of laceration of liver
J04.3	Packing of laceration of liver
J04.8	Other specified
J04.9	Unspecified

J05   **Incision of liver**

J05.1   Open drainage of liver
J05.2   Open removal of calculus from liver
J05.3   Open wedge biopsy of lesion of liver
          Includes: Open wedge biopsy of liver
          *   Open biopsy of lesion of liver*
          *   Open biopsy of liver*
J05.8   Other specified
J05.9   Unspecified

J06   **Other transjugular intrahepatic operations on blood vessel of liver**
                 Note: Principal J11

J06.1   Transjugular intrahepatic insertion of stent into portal vein
J06.2   Transjugular intrahepatic insertion of stent graft into portal vein
J06.8   Other specified
J06.9   Unspecified

J07   **Other open operations on liver**

J07.1   Open devascularisation of liver
J07.2   Open insertion of cannula for perfusion of liver
J07.3   Exploration of liver
J07.8   Other specified
J07.9   Unspecified

J08   **Therapeutic endoscopic operations on liver using laparoscope**
          Includes: Therapeutic endoscopic operations on liver using peritoneoscope
          *   Therapeutic endoscopic operations on liver*
          *   Gall bladder*
          Note: It is not necessary to code additionally any mention of diagnostic endoscopic examination of liver using laparoscope (J09.9)

J08.1   Endoscopic removal of calculus from liver using laparoscope
J08.2   Endoscopic insertion of cannula into gall bladder using laparoscope
J08.3   Endoscopic microwave ablation of lesion of liver using laparoscope
J08.8   Other specified
J08.9   Unspecified

J09 **Diagnostic endoscopic examination of liver using laparoscope**

Includes: *Diagnostic endoscopic examination of liver using peritoneoscope*
Diagnostic endoscopic examination of liver NEC
Gall bladder

Excludes: *Diagnostic endoscopic examination of liver using laparoscope when*
associated with general examination of the peritoneum (T43)
Endoscopic ultrasound examination of liver (J17)

J09.1 Diagnostic endoscopic examination of liver and biopsy of lesion of liver using laparoscope
Includes: *Diagnostic endoscopic examination of liver and biopsy of liver using*
laparoscope
Endoscopic biopsy of lesion of liver using laparoscope
Endoscopic biopsy of liver using laparoscope

J09.2 Laparoscopic ultrasound examination of liver and biopsy of lesion of liver
Includes: *Laparoscopic ultrasound examination of liver and biopsy of liver*
Laparoscopic ultrasonic biopsy of lesion of liver
Laparoscopic ultrasonic biopsy of liver

J09.3 Laparoscopic ultrasound examination of liver NEC
J09.8 Other specified
J09.9 Unspecified

J10 **Transluminal operations on blood vessel of liver**

Excludes: *Transjugular intrahepatic operations on blood vessel of liver (J06, J11)*
Note: **Principal category, extended at J77**
Use a subsidiary site code as necessary

J10.1 Percutaneous transluminal embolisation of hepatic artery
J10.2 Percutaneous transluminal embolisation of portal vein
J10.3 Percutaneous transluminal injection of therapeutic substance into liver
J10.4 Percutaneous transluminal angioplasty of blood vessel of liver
J10.5 Percutaneous transluminal thrombectomy of blood vessel of liver
J10.6 Percutaneous transluminal thrombolysis of blood vessel of liver
J10.7 Arteriography of hepatic artery
J10.8 Other specified
J10.9 Unspecified

J11 **Transjugular intrahepatic operations on blood vessel of liver**

Excludes: *Transluminal operations on blood vessel of liver NEC (J10, J77)*
Note: **Principal category, extended at J06**

J11.1 Transjugular intrahepatic angioplasty of portal vein
J11.2 Transjugular intrahepatic thrombectomy of portal vein
J11.3 Transjugular intrahepatic thrombolysis of portal vein
J11.4 Transjugular intrahepatic creation of portosystemic shunt
Excludes: Creation of portosystemic shunt NEC (L77.3)
J11.5 Transjugular intrahepatic venography of portal vein
J11.6 Transjugular intrahepatic pressure measurements of portal vein
J11.7 Transjugular intrahepatic pressure measurements of hepatic vein
J11.8 Other specified
J11.9 Unspecified

J12   **Other therapeutic percutaneous operations on liver**

J12.1   Percutaneous drainage of liver
J12.2   Percutaneous removal of calculus from liver
J12.3   Selective internal radiotherapy with microspheres to lesion of liver
         Note: Use an additional code to specify radiotherapy delivery (X65)
J12.4   Percutaneous radiofrequency ablation of lesion of liver
J12.5   Percutaneous thermal ablation of lesion of liver NEC
J12.6   Percutaneous chemical ablation of lesion of liver
J12.7   Percutaneous microwave ablation of lesion of liver
J12.8   Other specified
J12.9   Unspecified

J13   **Diagnostic percutaneous operations on liver**
         Excludes: Arteriography of hepatic artery (J10.7)

J13.1   Percutaneous transvascular biopsy of lesion of liver
         Includes: Percutaneous transluminal biopsy of lesion of liver
                      Percutaneous transluminal biopsy of liver
                      Transjugular biopsy of lesion of liver
                      Transjugular biopsy of liver
J13.2   Percutaneous biopsy of lesion of liver NEC
         Includes: Percutaneous biopsy of liver NEC
J13.8   Other specified
J13.9   Unspecified

J14   **Other puncture of liver**
         Excludes: Under image control (J10–J13)

J14.1   Biopsy of liver NEC
         Includes: Biopsy of lesion of liver NEC
J14.2   Aspiration of liver NEC
J14.8   Other specified
J14.9   Unspecified

J15   **Transluminal insertion of prosthesis into blood vessel of liver**
         Excludes: Transjugular intrahepatic operations on blood vessel of liver (J06, J11)
         Note: Use a subsidiary site code as necessary

J15.1   Percutaneous transluminal insertion of stent graft into hepatic artery
J15.2   Percutaneous transluminal insertion of stent into hepatic artery NEC
J15.3   Percutaneous transluminal insertion of stent graft into blood vessel of liver NEC
J15.4   Percutaneous transluminal insertion of stent into portal vein
J15.5   Percutaneous transluminal insertion of stent graft into portal vein
J15.8   Other specified
J15.9   Unspecified

J16   **Other operations on liver**

J16.1   Localised perfusion of liver
J16.2   Extracorporeal assistance to liver
J16.8   Other specified
J16.9   Unspecified

J17   **Endoscopic ultrasound examination of liver**
Excludes: Laparoscopic ultrasound examination of liver (J09)

J17.1   Endoscopic ultrasound examination of liver and biopsy of lesion of liver
Includes: Endoscopic ultrasound examination of liver and biopsy of liver
Endoscopic ultrasonic biopsy of lesion of liver
Endoscopic ultrasonic biopsy of liver

J17.8   Other specified
J17.9   Unspecified

J18   **Excision of gall bladder**
Note: Use a supplementary code for removal of lymph node (T85–T87)

J18.1   Total cholecystectomy and excision of surrounding tissue
J18.2   Total cholecystectomy and exploration of common bile duct
Includes: Cholecystectomy and exploration of common bile duct NEC
J18.3   Total cholecystectomy NEC
Includes: Cholecystectomy NEC
J18.4   Partial cholecystectomy and exploration of common bile duct
J18.5   Partial cholecystectomy NEC
J18.8   Other specified
J18.9   Unspecified

J19   **Connection of gall bladder**

J19.1   Anastomosis of gall bladder to stomach
Includes: Cholecystantrostomy
J19.2   Anastomosis of gall bladder to duodenum
J19.3   Anastomosis of gall bladder to jejunum
Includes: Cholecystojejunostomy
J19.4   Anastomosis of gall bladder to intestine NEC
J19.5   Revision of anastomosis of gall bladder
J19.6   Closure of anastomosis of gall bladder
J19.8   Other specified
J19.9   Unspecified

J20   **Repair of gall bladder**

J20.1   Closure of fistula of gall bladder
J20.2   Closure of cholecystotomy
J20.3   Repair of perforation of gall bladder
J20.8   Other specified
J20.9   Unspecified

J21   **Incision of gall bladder**

J21.1   Open removal of calculus from gall bladder
J21.2   Drainage of gall bladder
Includes: Cholecystostomy NEC
J21.3   Drainage of tissue surrounding gall bladder
J21.8   Other specified
J21.9   Unspecified

J23 Other open operations on gall bladder

J23.1 Excision of lesion of gall bladder
J23.2 Open biopsy of lesion of gall bladder
Includes: Open biopsy of gall bladder
Biopsy of lesion of gall bladder NEC
Biopsy of gall bladder NEC
J23.3 Exploration of gall bladder
J23.8 Other specified
J23.9 Unspecified

J24 Therapeutic percutaneous operations on gall bladder

J24.1 Percutaneous drainage of gall bladder
Includes: Percutaneous cholecystostomy NEC
J24.2 Percutaneous fragmentation of calculus in gall bladder
Includes: Percutaneous lithotripsy of calculus in gall bladder
J24.3 Percutaneous dissolution therapy to calculus in gall bladder
J24.8 Other specified
J24.9 Unspecified

J25 Diagnostic percutaneous operations on gall bladder

J25.1 Percutaneous biopsy of lesion of gall bladder
Includes: Percutaneous biopsy of gall bladder
J25.8 Other specified
J25.9 Unspecified

J26 Other operations on gall bladder

J26.1 Extracorporeal fragmentation of calculus in gall bladder
Includes: Extracorporeal lithotripsy of calculus in gall bladder
J26.8 Other specified
J26.9 Unspecified

J27 Excision of bile duct

J27.1 Excision of ampulla of Vater and replantation of common bile duct into duodenum
J27.2 Partial excision of bile duct and anastomosis of bile duct to duodenum
J27.3 Partial excision of bile duct and anastomosis of bile duct to jejunum
J27.4 Partial excision of bile duct and end to end anastomosis of bile duct
J27.5 Excision of extrahepatic bile ducts HFQ
Includes: Excision of extrahepatic biliary tree HFQ
J27.8 Other specified
J27.9 Unspecified

J28 Extirpation of lesion of bile duct

J28.1 Excision of lesion of bile duct
J28.2 Destruction of lesion of bile duct
J28.8 Other specified
J28.9 Unspecified

J29	**Connection of hepatic duct**
J29.1	Anastomosis of hepatic duct to transposed jejunum and insertion of tubal prosthesis HFQ
J29.2	Anastomosis of hepatic duct to jejunum NEC
J29.3	Revision of anastomosis of hepatic duct
J29.4	Open dilation of anastomosis of hepatic duct
J29.8	Other specified
J29.9	Unspecified

J30	**Connection of common bile duct**
J30.1	Anastomosis of common bile duct to duodenum
	Includes: Choledochoduodenostomy
J30.2	Anastomosis of common bile duct to transposed jejunum
J30.3	Anastomosis of common bile duct to jejunum NEC
J30.4	Revision of anastomosis of common bile duct
J30.5	Open dilation of anastomosis of common bile duct
J30.8	Other specified
J30.9	Unspecified

J31	**Open introduction of prosthesis into bile duct**
J31.1	Open insertion of tubal prosthesis into both hepatic ducts and common bile duct
J31.2	Open insertion of tubal prosthesis into one hepatic duct and common bile duct
J31.3	Open renewal of tubal prosthesis in bile duct
J31.4	Open removal of tubal prosthesis from bile duct
J31.8	Other specified
J31.9	Unspecified

J32	**Repair of bile duct**
J32.1	Reconstruction of bile duct
J32.2	Reanastomosis of bile duct
	Includes: End to end anastomosis of divided bile duct
J32.8	Other specified
J32.9	Unspecified

J33	**Incision of bile duct**
J33.1	Open removal of calculus from bile duct and drainage of bile duct
J33.2	Open removal of calculus from bile duct NEC
J33.3	Drainage of bile duct NEC
J33.8	Other specified
J33.9	Unspecified
	Includes: Exploration of bile duct
	Excludes: Exploration of bile duct when associated with excision of gall bladder (J18)

J34	**Plastic repair of sphincter of Oddi using duodenal approach**
	Includes: Plastic repair of sphincter of Oddi NEC
J34.1	Sphincteroplasty of bile duct and pancreatic duct using duodenal approach
J34.2	Sphincteroplasty of bile duct using duodenal approach NEC
J34.3	Sphincteroplasty of pancreatic duct using duodenal approach NEC
J34.8	Other specified
J34.9	Unspecified
	Includes: Sphincteroplasty of papilla of Vater using duodenal approach
	Sphincteroplasty of papilla of Vater NEC

J35   **Incision of sphincter of Oddi using duodenal approach**
Includes: *Incision of sphincter of Oddi NEC*

J35.1   Sphincterotomy of bile duct and pancreatic duct using duodenal approach
J35.2   Sphincterotomy of bile duct using duodenal approach NEC
J35.3   Sphincterotomy of pancreatic duct using duodenal approach NEC
J35.8   Other specified
J35.9   Unspecified
Includes: *Sphincterotomy of papilla of Vater using duodenal approach*
                   Sphincterotomy of papilla of Vater NEC

J36   **Other operations on ampulla of Vater using duodenal approach**
Includes: *Operations on ampulla of Vater NEC*
                   Papilla of Vater
                   Sphincter of Oddi

J36.1   Excision of ampulla of Vater using duodenal approach
J36.2   Biopsy of lesion of ampulla of Vater using duodenal approach
Includes: *Biopsy of ampulla of Vater using duodenal approach*
J36.8   Other specified
J36.9   Unspecified

J37   **Other open operations on bile duct**

J37.1   Open biopsy of lesion of bile duct
Includes: *Open biopsy of bile duct*
                   Biopsy of lesion of bile duct
                   Biopsy of bile duct
J37.2   Operative cholangiography through cystic duct
J37.3   Direct puncture operative cholangiography
Includes: *Operative cholangiography NEC*
J37.4   Operative choledochoscopy NEC
J37.8   Other specified
J37.9   Unspecified

J38   **Endoscopic incision of sphincter of Oddi**
Includes: *Endoscopic retrograde incision of sphincter of Oddi*
                   Papilla of Vater
     Note: **Use a supplementary code for concurrent diagnostic endoscopic retrograde examination of bile duct and pancreatic duct (J43)**

J38.1   Endoscopic sphincterotomy of sphincter of Oddi and removal of calculus HFQ
J38.2   Endoscopic sphincterotomy of sphincter of Oddi and insertion of tubal prosthesis into bile duct
J38.8   Other specified
J38.9   Unspecified
Includes: *Endoscopic sphincterotomy of papilla of Vater*

J39 Other therapeutic endoscopic operations on ampulla of Vater

Includes: *Therapeutic endoscopic retrograde operations on ampulla of Vater*
Papilla of Vater
Sphincter of Oddi

Note: **Use a supplementary code for concurrent diagnostic endoscopic retrograde examination of bile duct and pancreatic duct (J43)**

J39.1 Endoscopic sphincterotomy of accessory ampulla of Vater
J39.8 Other specified
J39.9 Unspecified

J40 Endoscopic retrograde placement of prosthesis in bile duct

Excludes: *When associated with endoscopic sphincterotomy of sphincter of Oddi (J38)*

Note: **Use a supplementary code for concurrent diagnostic endoscopic retrograde examination of pancreatic duct (J45)**

J40.1 Endoscopic retrograde insertion of tubal prosthesis into both hepatic ducts
J40.2 Endoscopic retrograde insertion of tubal prosthesis into bile duct NEC
J40.3 Endoscopic retrograde renewal of tubal prosthesis in bile duct NEC
J40.4 Endoscopic retrograde removal of tubal prosthesis from bile duct
Includes: *Endoscopic retrograde removal of expanding metal stent from bile duct*
J40.5 Endoscopic retrograde insertion of expanding covered metal stent into bile duct
J40.6 Endoscopic retrograde insertion of expanding metal stent into bile duct NEC
J40.7 Endoscopic retrograde renewal of expanding metal stent in bile duct
J40.8 Other specified
J40.9 Unspecified

J41 Other therapeutic endoscopic retrograde operations on bile duct

Excludes: *When associated with endoscopic sphincterotomy of sphincter of Oddi (J38)*

Note: **It is not necessary to code additionally any mention of diagnostic endoscopic examination of bile duct (J44.9)**
Use a supplementary code for concurrent diagnostic endoscopic retrograde examination of pancreatic duct (J45)

J41.1 Endoscopic retrograde extraction of calculus from bile duct
J41.2 Endoscopic dilation of bile duct NEC
Includes: *Endoscopic dilation of stricture of bile duct NEC*
J41.3 Endoscopic retrograde lithotripsy of calculus of bile duct
J41.4 Endoscopic retrograde photodynamic laser therapy of lesion of bile duct
J41.8 Other specified
J41.9 Unspecified

J42 Therapeutic endoscopic retrograde operations on pancreatic duct

Note: **It is not necessary to code additionally any mention of diagnostic endoscopic examination of pancreas (J45.9)**
Use a supplementary code for concurrent diagnostic endoscopic retrograde examination of bile duct (J44)

J42.1 Endoscopic retrograde insertion of tubal prosthesis into pancreatic duct
J42.2 Endoscopic retrograde renewal of tubal prosthesis in pancreatic duct
J42.3 Endoscopic retrograde removal of calculus from pancreatic duct
J42.4 Endoscopic retrograde drainage of lesion of pancreas
J42.5 Endoscopic retrograde dilation of pancreatic duct
J42.8 Other specified
J42.9 Unspecified

J43   **Diagnostic endoscopic retrograde examination of bile duct and pancreatic duct**
Note: *Use as a supplementary code when associated with endoscopic incision of sphincter of Oddi (J38)*

J43.1   Endoscopic retrograde cholangiopancreatography and biopsy of lesion of ampulla of Vater
Includes: *Endoscopic retrograde cholangiopancreatography and biopsy of ampulla of Vater*

J43.2   Endoscopic retrograde cholangiopancreatography and biopsy of lesion of biliary or pancreatic system NEC
Includes: *Endoscopic retrograde cholangiopancreatography and biopsy of biliary or pancreatic system NEC*
Note: *Use a subsidiary code for cytology as necessary (Y21)*
       Use a subsidiary site code as necessary

J43.3   Endoscopic retrograde cholangiopancreatography and collection of bile
J43.8   Other specified
J43.9   Unspecified
Includes: *Endoscopic retrograde cholangiopancreatography NEC*

J44   **Diagnostic endoscopic retrograde examination of bile duct**
Excludes: *When associated with diagnostic endoscopic retrograde examination of pancreatic duct (J43)*

J44.1   Endoscopic retrograde cholangiography and biopsy of lesion of bile duct
Includes: *Endoscopic retrograde cholangiography and biopsy of bile duct*
       Endoscopic retrograde biopsy of lesion of bile duct
       Endoscopic retrograde biopsy of bile duct
Note: *Use a subsidiary code for cytology as necessary (Y21)*
J44.8   Other specified
J44.9   Unspecified
Includes: *Endoscopic retrograde cholangiography NEC*

J45   **Diagnostic endoscopic retrograde examination of pancreatic duct**
Excludes: *When associated with diagnostic endoscopic retrograde examination of bile duct (J43)*

J45.1   Endoscopic retrograde pancreatography and biopsy of lesion of pancreas
Includes: *Endoscopic retrograde pancreatography and biopsy of pancreas*
       Endoscopic retrograde biopsy of lesion of pancreas
       Endoscopic retrograde biopsy of pancreas
Note: *Use a subsidiary code for cytology as necessary (Y21)*
J45.2   Endoscopic retrograde pancreatography and collection of pancreatic juice
Includes: *Endoscopic retrograde collection of pure pancreatic juice*
J45.3   Endoscopic retrograde pancreatography through accessory ampulla of Vater
J45.8   Other specified
J45.9   Unspecified
Includes: *Endoscopic retrograde pancreatography NEC*

J46   **Therapeutic percutaneous attention to connection of bile duct**
J46.1   Percutaneous dilation of anastomosis of bile duct and insertion of tubal prosthesis HFQ
J46.2   Percutaneous dilation of anastomosis of bile duct NEC
J46.8   Other specified
J46.9   Unspecified

J47   **Therapeutic percutaneous insertion of prosthesis into bile duct**

J47.1   Percutaneous insertion of tubal prosthesis into both hepatic ducts
J47.2   Percutaneous insertion of tubal prosthesis into right hepatic duct NEC
J47.3   Percutaneous insertion of tubal prosthesis into left hepatic duct NEC
J47.4   Percutaneous insertion of tubal prosthesis into hepatic duct NEC
J47.5   Percutaneous insertion of tubal prosthesis into common bile duct
J47.8   Other specified
J47.9   Unspecified

J48   **Other therapeutic percutaneous operations on bile duct**
               Note: Principal category, extended at J76

J48.1   Renewal of percutaneously inserted tubal prosthesis in bile duct
J48.2   Removal of percutaneously inserted tubal prosthesis from bile duct
J48.3   Attention to percutaneously inserted tubal prosthesis in bile duct NEC
J48.4   Percutaneous photodynamic therapy of lesion of bile duct
J48.5   Percutaneous transhepatic biliary drainage multiple
J48.6   Percutaneous transhepatic biliary drainage single
               Includes: Percutaneous transhepatic biliary drainage NEC
J48.7   Percutaneous brachytherapy of lesion of bile duct
               Note: Use an additional code to specify radiotherapy delivery (X65)
J48.8   Other specified
J48.9   Unspecified

J49   **Therapeutic operations on bile duct along T tube track**

J49.1   Endoscopic removal of calculus from bile duct along T̄ tube track
               Includes: Removal of calculus from bile duct along T tube track using choledochoscope
J49.2   Percutaneous removal of calculus from bile duct along T tube track
               Includes: Percutaneous removal of calculus from bile duct along T tube track using
                                image control
J49.8   Other specified
J49.9   Unspecified

J50   **Percutaneous examination of bile duct**

J50.1   T tube cholangiography
J50.2   Percutaneous cholangiography NEC
J50.3   Percutaneous transbiliary biopsy of lesion of bile duct
               Includes: Percutaneous transbiliary biopsy of bile duct
J50.4   Percutaneous transjejunal cholangiography
J50.5   Percutaneous transhepatic cholangiography
J50.6   Percutaneous transjejunal examination of bile duct NEC
J50.7   Percutaneous transhepatic cholangioscopy
J50.8   Other specified
J50.9   Unspecified

J51   **Laparoscopic ultrasound examination of bile duct**

J51.1   Laparoscopic ultrasound examination of bile duct and biopsy of lesion of bile duct
               Includes: Laparoscopic ultrasound examination of bile duct and biopsy of bile duct
                           Laparoscopic ultrasonic biopsy of lesion of bile duct
                           Laparoscopic ultrasonic biopsy of bile duct
J51.8   Other specified
J51.9   Unspecified

J52   **Other operations on bile duct**

J52.1   Extracorporeal lithotripsy of calculus in bile duct
J52.8   Other specified
J52.9   Unspecified

J53   **Endoscopic ultrasound examination of bile duct**

J53.1   Endoscopic ultrasound examination of bile duct and biopsy of lesion of bile duct
    Includes: Endoscopic ultrasound examination of bile duct and biopsy of bile duct
    Endoscopic ultrasonic biopsy of lesion of bile duct
    Endoscopic ultrasonic biopsy of bile duct
J53.8   Other specified
J53.9   Unspecified

J54   **Transplantation of pancreas**

J54.1   Transplantation of pancreas and duodenum
J54.2   Transplantation of whole pancreas
J54.3   Transplantation of tail of pancreas
J54.4   Transplantation of islet of Langerhans
J54.5   Renewal of transplanted pancreatic tissue
J54.8   Other specified
J54.9   Unspecified

J55   **Total excision of pancreas**

J55.1   Total pancreatectomy and excision of surrounding tissue
    Note: Use an additional code for coincidental transplantation of islet cell tissue (J54.4)
J55.2   Total pancreatectomy NEC
J55.3   Excision of transplanted pancreas
J55.8   Other specified
J55.9   Unspecified

J56   **Excision of head of pancreas**

J56.1   Pancreaticoduodenectomy and excision of surrounding tissue
J56.2   Pancreaticoduodenectomy and resection of antrum of stomach
J56.3   Pancreaticoduodenectomy NEC
J56.4   Subtotal excision of head of pancreas with preservation of duodenum and drainage HFQ
J56.8   Other specified
J56.9   Unspecified

J57   **Other partial excision of pancreas**

J57.1   Subtotal pancreatectomy
J57.2   Left pancreatectomy and drainage of pancreatic duct
J57.3   Left pancreatectomy NEC
J57.4   Excision of tail of pancreas and drainage of pancreatic duct
J57.5   Excision of tail of pancreas NEC
J57.6   Pancreatic necrosectomy
J57.8   Other specified
J57.9   Unspecified
    Includes: Pancreatectomy NEC

J58	**Extirpation of lesion of pancreas**
J58.1	Excision of lesion of islet of Langerhans
J58.2	Excision of lesion of pancreas NEC
J58.3	Destruction of lesion of pancreas
J58.8	Other specified
J58.9	Unspecified

J59	**Connection of pancreatic duct**
J59.1	Anastomosis of pancreatic duct to stomach
J59.2	Anastomosis of pancreatic duct to duodenum
J59.3	Anastomosis of pancreatic duct to transposed jejunum
J59.4	Anastomosis of pancreatic duct to jejunum NEC
J59.5	Revision of anastomosis of pancreatic duct
J59.6	Closure of anastomosis of pancreatic duct
J59.8	Other specified
J59.9	Unspecified

J60	**Other open operations on pancreatic duct**
J60.1	Drainage of pancreatic duct
J60.2	Open removal of calculus from pancreatic duct
	Includes: Removal of calculus from pancreatic duct NEC
J60.3	Insertion of T tube into pancreatic duct
J60.4	Open insertion of tubal prosthesis into pancreatic duct
	Includes: Insertion of tubal prosthesis into pancreatic duct NEC
J60.5	Open dilation of pancreatic duct
	Includes: Dilation of pancreatic duct NEC
J60.8	Other specified
J60.9	Unspecified

J61	**Open drainage of lesion of pancreas**
J61.1	Open cystogastrotomy of pancreas
J61.2	Drainage of cyst of pancreas into transposed jejunum
J61.3	Drainage of cyst of pancreas into jejunum NEC
J61.4	Drainage of cyst of pancreas NEC
J61.8	Other specified
J61.9	Unspecified

J62	**Incision of pancreas**
J62.1	Division of annular pancreas
J62.8	Other specified
J62.9	Unspecified

J63	**Open examination of pancreas**
J63.1	Open pancreatography through tail of pancreas
J63.2	Open pancreatography through papilla of Vater
J63.3	Open pancreatography NEC
J63.8	Other specified
J63.9	Unspecified

J65   **Other open operations on pancreas**

J65.1   Open biopsy of lesion of pancreas
Includes: *Open biopsy of pancreas*
Biopsy of lesion of pancreas NEC
Biopsy of pancreas NEC
J65.8   Other specified
J65.9   Unspecified

J66   **Therapeutic percutaneous operations on pancreas**

J66.1   Percutaneous drainage of lesion of pancreas and insertion of cystogastrostomy tube NEC
J66.2   Percutaneous drainage of lesion of pancreas and insertion of temporary external drain HFQ
J66.3   Percutaneous drainage of lesion of pancreas NEC
J66.4   Percutaneous aspiration of lesion of pancreas
Includes: *Needle aspiration of pancreas NEC*
J66.5   Percutaneous chemical ablation of lesion of pancreas
J66.8   Other specified
J66.9   Unspecified

J67   **Diagnostic percutaneous operations on pancreas**

J67.1   Diagnostic percutaneous aspiration of lesion of pancreas
J67.2   Percutaneous puncture of pancreatic duct and pancreatography
J67.3   Percutaneous biopsy of lesion of pancreas
Includes: *Percutaneous biopsy of pancreas*
J67.8   Other specified
J67.9   Unspecified

J68   **Other operations on pancreas**

J68.1   Extracorporeal shockwave lithotripsy of calculus of pancreas
J68.8   Other specified
J68.9   Unspecified

J69   **Total excision of spleen**

J69.1   Total excision of spleen and replantation of fragments of spleen
J69.2   Total splenectomy
J69.3   Excision of accessory spleen
J69.8   Other specified
J69.9   Unspecified
Includes: *Splenectomy NEC*

J70   **Other excision of spleen**

J70.1   Partial splenectomy
J70.2   Marsupialisation of lesion of spleen
J70.8   Other specified
J70.9   Unspecified

J72	**Other operations on spleen**
J72.1	Transplantation of spleen
J72.2	Embolisation of spleen
J72.3	Biopsy of lesion of spleen
	Includes: Biopsy of spleen
J72.4	Repair of spleen
J72.5	Banding of spleen
J72.8	Other specified
J72.9	Unspecified

J73	**Laparoscopic ultrasound examination of pancreas**
J73.1	Laparoscopic ultrasound examination of pancreas and biopsy of lesion of pancreas
	Includes: Laparoscopic ultrasound examination of pancreas and biopsy of pancreas
	Laparoscopic ultrasonic biopsy of lesion of pancreas
	Laparoscopic ultrasonic biopsy of pancreas
J73.8	Other specified
J73.9	Unspecified

J74	**Endoscopic ultrasound examination of pancreas**
J74.1	Endoscopic ultrasound examination of pancreas and biopsy of lesion of pancreas
	Includes: Endoscopic ultrasound examination of pancreas and biopsy of pancreas
	Endoscopic ultrasonic biopsy of lesion of pancreas
	Endoscopic ultrasonic biopsy of pancreas
J74.8	Other specified
J74.9	Unspecified

J76	**Therapeutic percutaneous operations on bile duct**
	Note: Principal J48
J76.1	Percutaneous transhepatic removal of calculus from bile duct
J76.2	Percutaneous balloon dilation of bile duct
J76.8	Other specified
J76.9	Unspecified

J77	**Other transluminal operations on blood vessel of liver**
	Excludes: Transjugular intrahepatic operations on blood vessel of liver (J06, J11)
	Note: Principal J10
	Use subsidiary site code as necessary
J77.1	Percutaneous transhepatic portal venous sampling
J77.8	Other specified
J77.9	Unspecified

CHAPTER K
HEART
(CODES K01–K78)

Note: *Use a subsidiary code for minimal access approach (Y74–Y76)*

        Use a subsidiary code to identify method of image control (Y53)

        Use a subsidiary code to identify cardiopulmonary bypass (Y73.1)

        Use a subsidiary code to identify arteriotomy approach to organ under image control (Y78)

K01   **Transplantation of heart and lung**

K01.1   Allotransplantation of heart and lung
K01.2   Revision of transplantation of heart and lung
K01.8   Other specified
K01.9   Unspecified

K02   **Other transplantation of heart**

K02.1   Allotransplantation of heart NEC
K02.2   Xenotransplantation of heart
K02.3   Implantation of prosthetic heart
K02.4   Piggyback transplantation of heart
K02.5   Revision of implantation of prosthetic heart
K02.6   Revision of transplantation of heart NEC
K02.8   Other specified
K02.9   Unspecified

K04   **Repair of tetralogy of Fallot**
         Includes: *Fallot-type pulmonary atresia with ventricular septal defect*
            Note: **Use a supplementary code for concurrent repair of atrioventricular septum defect (K09)**
                    Do not use secondary code for concurrent repair of defect of septum of heart (K10–K12) or construction of cardiac conduit (K18, K19)

K04.1   Repair of tetralogy of Fallot using valved right ventricular outflow conduit
K04.2   Repair of tetralogy of Fallot using right ventricular outflow conduit NEC
K04.3   Repair of tetralogy of Fallot using transannular patch
         Includes: *Repair of tetralogy of Fallot using right ventricular outflow patch*
K04.4   Revision of repair of tetralogy of Fallot
K04.5   Repair of tetralogy of Fallot with absent pulmonary valve
K04.6   Repair of Fallot-type pulmonary atresia with aortopulmonary collaterals
K04.8   Other specified
K04.9   Unspecified

K05   **Atrial inversion operations for transposition of great arteries**
            Note: **Use a supplementary code for concurrent correction of other associated abnormality**
K05.1   Reconstruction of atrium using atrial patch for transposition of great arteries
K05.2   Reconstruction of atrium using atrial wall for transposition of great arteries
K05.8   Other specified
K05.9   Unspecified

K06   **Other repair of transposition of great arteries**
            Includes: Repair of transposition of great arteries with ventricular septal defect
                          Repair of transposition of great arteries with left ventricular outflow tract
                          obstruction
                          Repair of congenitally corrected transposition of great arteries
            Note: Use a supplementary code for concurrent correction of other associated
                        abnormality

K06.1   Repositioning of transposed great arteries
        Includes: Arterial switch procedure
K06.2   Left ventricle to aorta tunnel with right ventricle to pulmonary trunk direct anastomosis
K06.3   Left ventricle to aorta tunnel with right ventricle to pulmonary artery valved conduit
K06.4   Atrial inversion and repositioning of transposed great artery
        Includes: Double switch procedure
K06.8   Other specified
K06.9   Unspecified

K07   **Correction of total anomalous pulmonary venous connection**

K07.1   Correction of total anomalous pulmonary venous connection to supracardiac vessel
K07.2   Correction of total anomalous pulmonary venous connection to coronary sinus
K07.3   Correction of total anomalous pulmonary venous connection to infradiaphragmatic vessel
K07.8   Other specified
K07.9   Unspecified

K08   **Repair of double outlet ventricle**

K08.1   Repair of double outlet right ventricle with intraventricular tunnel
K08.2   Repair of Fallot-type double outlet right ventricle
K08.3   Repair of double outlet right ventricle
K08.4   Repair of double outlet left ventricle
K08.8   Other specified
K08.9   Unspecified

K09   **Repair of defect of atrioventricular septum**
            Note: Use as a supplementary code when associated with repair of tetralogy of Fallot (K04)

K09.1   Repair of defect of atrioventricular septum using dual prosthetic patches
K09.2   Repair of defect of atrioventricular septum using prosthetic patch NEC
K09.3   Repair of defect of atrioventricular septum using tissue graft
K09.4   Repair of persistent ostium primum
K09.5   Primary repair of defect of atrioventricular septum NEC
K09.6   Revision of repair of defect of atrioventricular septum
K09.8   Other specified
K09.9   Unspecified

K10   **Repair of defect of interatrial septum**
            Excludes: When associated with repair of tetralogy of Fallot (K04)
                        Percutaneous transluminal repair of defect of interatrial septum (K13.3, K13.4)

K10.1   Repair of defect of interatrial septum using prosthetic patch
K10.2   Repair of defect of interatrial septum using pericardial patch
K10.3   Repair of defect of interatrial septum using tissue graft NEC
K10.4   Primary repair of defect of interatrial septum NEC
K10.5   Revision of repair of defect of interatrial septum
K10.8   Other specified
K10.9   Unspecified

K11   **Repair of defect of interventricular septum**

Excludes: When associated with repair of tetralogy of Fallot (K04)
Percutaneous transluminal repair of defect of interventricular septum
(K13.1, K13.2)

K11.1   Repair of defect of interventricular septum using prosthetic patch
K11.2   Repair of defect of interventricular septum using pericardial patch
K11.3   Repair of defect of interventricular septum using tissue graft NEC
K11.4   Primary repair of defect of interventricular septum NEC
K11.5   Revision of repair of defect of interventricular septum
K11.6   Repair of multiple interventricular septal defects
K11.7   Repair of interventricular septal defect using intraoperative transluminal prosthesis
K11.8   Other specified
K11.9   Unspecified

K12   **Repair of defect of unspecified septum of heart**

Excludes: When associated with repair of tetralogy of Fallot (K04)
Percutaneous transluminal repair of defect of unspecified septum
(K13.5–K13.9)

K12.1   Repair of defect of septum of heart using prosthetic patch NEC
K12.2   Repair of defect of septum of heart using pericardial patch NEC
K12.3   Repair of defect of septum of heart using tissue graft NEC
K12.4   Primary repair of defect of septum of heart NEC
K12.5   Revision of repair of septum of heart NEC
K12.8   Other specified
K12.9   Unspecified

K13   **Transluminal repair of defect of septum**

K13.1   Percutaneous transluminal repair of defect of interventricular septum using prosthesis
K13.2   Percutaneous transluminal repair of defect of interventricular septum NEC
K13.3   Percutaneous transluminal repair of defect of interatrial septum using prosthesis
K13.4   Percutaneous transluminal repair of defect of interatrial septum NEC
K13.5   Percutaneous transluminal repair of defect of unspecified septum using prosthesis
K13.8   Other specified
K13.9   Unspecified

K14   **Other open operations on septum of heart**

K14.1   Open enlargement of defect of atrial septum
K14.2   Open atrial septostomy
Includes: Open atrial septal fenestration
Atrial septostomy NEC
K14.3   Atrial septectomy
K14.4   Surgical atrial septation
K14.5   Open enlargement of defect of interventricular septum
K14.8   Other specified
K14.9   Unspecified

K15   **Closed operations on septum of heart**

K15.1   Closed enlargement of defect of atrial septum
K15.2   Closed atrial septostomy
K15.8   Other specified
K15.9   Unspecified

K16   **Other therapeutic transluminal operations on septum of heart**

K16.1   Percutaneous transluminal balloon atrial septostomy
K16.2   Percutaneous transluminal atrial septostomy NEC
K16.3   Percutaneous transluminal atrial septum fenestration closure with prosthesis
K16.4   Percutaneous transluminal atrial septum fenestration
K16.5   Percutaneous transluminal closure of patent oval foramen with prosthesis
K16.6   Percutaneous transluminal chemical mediated septal ablation
K16.8   Other specified
K16.9   Unspecified

K17   **Repair of univentricular heart**

K17.1   Total cavopulmonary connection with extracardiac inferior caval vein to pulmonary artery conduit
K17.2   Total cavopulmonary connection with lateral atrial tunnel
K17.3   Aortopulmonary reconstruction with systemic to pulmonary arterial shunt
                Includes: Primary palliation of hypoplastic left heart syndrome
K17.4   Aortopulmonary reconstruction with right ventricle to pulmonary arterial valveless conduit
                Includes: Primary palliation of hypoplastic left heart
K17.5   Biventricular repair of hypoplastic left heart syndrome
K17.6   Takedown of total cavopulmonary connection
K17.7   Conversion of atrial pulmonary anastomosis to total pulmonary connection
K17.8   Other specified
K17.9   Unspecified

K18   **Creation of valved cardiac conduit**
                Excludes: When associated with repair of tetralogy of Fallot (K04)

K18.1   Creation of valved conduit between atrium and ventricle of heart
K18.2   Creation of valved conduit between right atrium and pulmonary artery
K18.3   Creation of valved conduit between right ventricle of heart and pulmonary artery
K18.4   Creation of valved conduit between left ventricle of heart and aorta
K18.5   Revision of valved cardiac conduit
K18.6   Creation of valved conduit between left ventricle of heart and pulmonary artery
K18.7   Replacement of valved cardiac conduit
K18.8   Other specified
K18.9   Unspecified

K19   **Creation of other cardiac conduit**
                Excludes: When associated with repair of tetralogy of Fallot (K04)

K19.1   Creation of conduit between atrium and ventricle of heart NEC
K19.2   Creation of conduit between right atrium and pulmonary artery NEC
K19.3   Creation of conduit between right ventricle of heart and pulmonary artery NEC
K19.4   Creation of conduit between right ventricle of heart and vena cava
K19.5   Creation of conduit between left ventricle of heart and aorta NEC
K19.6   Revision of cardiac conduit NEC
K19.8   Other specified
K19.9   Unspecified

K20   **Refashioning of atrium**

K20.1   Correction of persistent sinus venosus
K20.2   Correction of partial anomalous pulmonary venous drainage
K20.3   Repair of cor triatriatum
K20.4   Repair of coronary sinus abnormality
K20.8   Other specified
K20.9   Unspecified

K22   **Other operations on wall of atrium**
        Excludes: Operations on coronary artery (K40–K51) or conducting system of heart
                        (K52, K57, K58)

K22.1   Excision of lesion of atrium
K22.2   Repair of atrium NEC
K22.3   Exclusion of left atrial appendage NEC
        Includes: Occlusion of left atrial appendage NEC
        Excludes: Percutaneous transluminal occlusion of left atrial appendage (K62.5)
K22.8   Other specified
K22.9   Unspecified

K23   **Other operations of wall of heart**
        Excludes: Operations on coronary artery (K40–K51) or conducting system of heart
                        (K52, K57–K58)

K23.1   Excision of lesion of wall of heart NEC
        Includes: Excision of lesion of ventricle of heart
K23.2   Biopsy of lesion of wall of heart
        Includes: Biopsy of wall of heart
                    Biopsy of lesion of heart NEC
                    Biopsy of heart NEC
K23.3   Repair of wall of heart NEC
K23.4   Revascularisation of wall of heart
        Includes: Revascularisation of heart
K23.5   Partial left ventriculectomy
K23.6   Cardiomyoplasty
K23.8   Other specified
K23.9   Unspecified

K24   **Other operations on ventricles of heart**

K24.1   Relief of right ventricular outflow tract obstruction
K24.2   Repair of double chambered right ventricle
K24.3   Repair of right ventricular aneurysm
K24.4   Repair of left ventricular aneurysm
K24.5   Relief of left ventricular outflow tract obstruction
K24.6   Myectomy of left ventricular outflow tract
K24.7   Myotomy of left ventricular outflow tract
K24.8   Other specified
K24.9   Unspecified

K25   **Plastic repair of mitral valve**

Excludes: Annuloplasty of mitral valve (K34.1)

   Note: *Use a supplementary code for concurrent multiple replacement of valves of heart (e.g. K26)*

   Use as a supplementary code when associated with bypass of coronary artery (K40–K46)

   Use a supplementary code for concurrent annuloplasty of mitral valve (K34.1)

K25.1   Allograft replacement of mitral valve
K25.2   Xenograft replacement of mitral valve
K25.3   Prosthetic replacement of mitral valve
K25.4   Replacement of mitral valve NEC
K25.5   Mitral valve repair NEC
         Includes: Mitral valvuloplasty NEC
K25.8   Other specified
K25.9   Unspecified

K26   **Plastic repair of aortic valve**

   Note: *Use as a supplementary code for concurrent multiple replacement of valves of heart (e.g. K25)*

   Use as a supplementary code when associated with bypass of coronary artery (K40–K46)

   Use a supplementary code for concurrent annuloplasty of aortic valve (K34.3)

   Use a supplementary code to identify transapical approach (Y49.4)

K26.1   Allograft replacement of aortic valve
K26.2   Xenograft replacement of aortic valve
K26.3   Prosthetic replacement of aortic valve
K26.4   Replacement of aortic valve NEC
K26.5   Aortic valve repair NEC
         Includes: Aortic valvuloplasty NEC
K26.8   Other specified
K26.9   Unspecified

K27   **Plastic repair of tricuspid valve**

   Note: *Use a supplementary code for concurrent multiple replacement of valves of heart (e.g. K28)*

   Use as a supplementary code when associated with bypass of coronary artery (K40–K46)

   Use a supplementary code for concurrent annuloplasty of tricuspid valve (K34.2)

K27.1   Allograft replacement of tricuspid valve
K27.2   Xenograft replacement of tricuspid valve
K27.3   Prosthetic replacement of tricuspid valve
K27.4   Replacement of tricuspid valve NEC
K27.5   Repositioning of tricuspid valve
K27.6   Tricuspid valve repair NEC
         Includes: Tricuspid valvuloplasty NEC
K27.8   Other specified
K27.9   Unspecified

K28   **Plastic repair of pulmonary valve**
> *Note:*   *Use as a supplementary code for concurrent multiple replacement of valves of heart (e.g. K27)*
> *Use as a supplementary code when associated with bypass of coronary artery (K40–K46)*
> *Use a supplementary code for concurrent annuloplasty of pulmonary valve (K34.3)*

K28.1   Allograft replacement of pulmonary valve
K28.2   Xenograft replacement of pulmonary valve
K28.3   Prosthetic replacement of pulmonary valve
K28.4   Replacement of pulmonary valve NEC
K28.5   Pulmonary valve repair NEC
> *Includes:*   *Pulmonary valvuloplasty NEC*

K28.8   Other specified
K28.9   Unspecified

K29   **Plastic repair of unspecified valve of heart**
> *Includes:*   *Plastic repair of other specified valve of heart*
> *Note:*   *Use as a supplementary code when associated with bypass of coronary artery (K40–K46)*
> *Use a subsidiary site code as necessary*

K29.1   Allograft replacement of valve of heart NEC
K29.2   Xenograft replacement of valve of heart NEC
K29.3   Prosthetic replacement of valve of heart NEC
K29.4   Replacement of valve of heart NEC
K29.5   Repair of valve of heart NEC
> *Includes:*   *Valvuloplasty of heart NEC*

K29.6   Truncal valve repair
> *Includes:*   *Truncal valvuloplasty*

K29.7   Replacement of truncal valve
K29.8   Other specified
K29.9   Unspecified

K30   **Revision of plastic repair of valve of heart**
> *Includes:*   *Revision of replacement of valve of heart*

K30.1   Revision of plastic repair of mitral valve
K30.2   Revision of plastic repair of aortic valve
K30.3   Revision of plastic repair of tricuspid valve
K30.4   Revision of plastic repair of pulmonary valve
K30.5   Revision of plastic repair of truncal valve
K30.8   Other specified
K30.9   Unspecified

K31   **Open incision of valve of heart**
> *Includes:*   *Incision of valve of heart NEC*

K31.1   Open mitral valvotomy
K31.2   Open aortic valvotomy
K31.3   Open tricuspid valvotomy
K31.4   Open pulmonary valvotomy
K31.5   Open truncal valvotomy
K31.8   Other specified
K31.9   Unspecified
> *Includes:*   *Valvotomy NEC*

K32   **Closed incision of valve of heart**

K32.1   Closed mitral valvotomy
K32.2   Closed aortic valvotomy
K32.3   Closed tricuspid valvotomy
K32.4   Closed pulmonary valvotomy
K32.8   Other specified
K32.9   Unspecified

K33   **Operations on aortic root**

K33.1   Aortic root replacement using pulmonary valve autograft with right ventricle to pulmonary artery valved conduit
K33.2   Aortic root replacement using pulmonary valve autograft with right ventricle to pulmonary artery valved conduit and aortoventriculoplasty
K33.3   Aortic root replacement using homograft
K33.4   Aortic root replacement using mechanical prosthesis
K33.5   Aortic root replacement NEC
K33.6   Aortoventriculoplasty with pulmonary valve autograft
K33.8   Other specified
K33.9   Unspecified

K34   **Other open operations on valve of heart**

K34.1   Annuloplasty of mitral valve
             Note: Use as a supplementary code for concurrent mitral valve repair (K25.5)
K34.2   Annuloplasty of tricuspid valve
             Note: Use as a supplementary code for concurrent tricuspid valve repair (K27.6)
K34.3   Annuloplasty of valve of heart NEC
             Note: Use as a supplementary code for concurrent aortic valve repair (K26)
             Use as a supplementary code for concurrent pulmonary valve repair (K28)
             Use as a supplementary code for concurrent valve repair NEC (K29)
K34.4   Excision of vegetations of valve of heart
             Excludes: Open excision of vegetations of heart NEC (K55.4)
             Note: Use a subsidiary site code as necessary
K34.5   Closure of tricuspid valve
K34.6   Closure of pulmonary valve
K34.8   Other specified
K34.9   Unspecified

K35   **Therapeutic transluminal operations on valve of heart**

K35.1   Percutaneous transluminal mitral valvotomy
             Includes: Percutaneous transluminal balloon valvotomy of mitral valve
K35.2   Percutaneous transluminal aortic valvotomy
             Includes: Percutaneous transluminal balloon valvotomy of aortic valve
K35.3   Percutaneous transluminal tricuspid valvotomy
             Includes: Percutaneous transluminal balloon valvotomy of tricuspid valve
K35.4   Percutaneous transluminal pulmonary valvotomy
             Includes: Percutaneous transluminal balloon valvotomy of pulmonary valve
K35.5   Percutaneous transluminal valvuloplasty
             Includes: Percutanous transluminal balloon valvuloplasty
K35.6   Percutaneous transluminal pulmonary valve perforation and dilation
K35.7   Percutaneous transluminal pulmonary valve replacement
K35.8   Other specified
K35.9   Unspecified

K36 **Excision of valve of heart**

K36.1   Tricuspid valvectomy
K36.2   Pulmonary valvectomy
K36.8   Other specified
K36.9   Unspecified

K37 **Removal of obstruction from structure adjacent to valve of heart**
Excludes: Cardiac conduit operations (K18, K19)

K37.1   Infundibulectomy of heart using patch
K37.2   Infundibulectomy of heart NEC
K37.3   Repair of subaortic stenosis
K37.4   Repair of supra-aortic stenosis
K37.5   Excision of supramitral ring
K37.6   Aortoventriculoplasty
         Excludes: Aortoventriculoplasty with aortic root replacement (K33.5)
                   Aortoventriculoplasty with pulmonary valve autograft (K33.6)
K37.8   Other specified
K37.9   Unspecified

K38 **Other operations on structure adjacent to valve of heart**

K38.1   Operations on papillary muscle
K38.2   Operations on chordae tendineae
K38.3   Operations on mitral subvalvar apparatus
K38.4   Closure of aorto-left ventricular tunnel
K38.5   Closure of aortic sinus of Valsalva fistula
K38.6   Repair of aortic sinus of Valsalva aneurysm
K38.8   Other specified
K38.9   Unspecified

K40 **Saphenous vein graft replacement of coronary artery**
Note: Use a supplementary code for concurrent repair of valve of heart (K25–K29)
Use a supplementary code for concurrent excision of lesion of ventricle of heart (K23.1) or repair of defect of interventricular septum (K11)
Use as a supplementary code for concurrent connection of thoracic artery to coronary artery (K45)

K40.1   Saphenous vein graft replacement of one coronary artery
K40.2   Saphenous vein graft replacement of two coronary arteries
K40.3   Saphenous vein graft replacement of three coronary arteries
K40.4   Saphenous vein graft replacement of four or more coronary arteries
K40.8   Other specified
K40.9   Unspecified

K41   **Other autograft replacement of coronary artery**
         Note: *Use a supplementary code for concurrent repair of valve of heart (K25–K29)*
                 Use a supplementary code for concurrent excision of lesion of ventricle of heart (K23.1) or repair of defect of interventricular septum (K11)
                 Use as a supplementary code for concurrent connection of thoracic artery to coronary artery (K45)

K41.1   Autograft replacement of one coronary artery NEC
K41.2   Autograft replacement of two coronary arteries NEC
K41.3   Autograft replacement of three coronary arteries NEC
K41.4   Autograft replacement of four or more coronary arteries NEC
K41.8   Other specified
K41.9   Unspecified

K42   **Allograft replacement of coronary artery**
         Note: *Use a supplementary code for concurrent repair of valve of heart (K25–K29)*
                 Use a supplementary code for concurrent excision of lesion of ventricle of heart (K23.1) or repair of defect of interventricular septum (K11)
                 Use as a supplementary code for concurrent connection of thoracic artery to coronary artery (K45)

K42.1   Allograft replacement of one coronary artery
K42.2   Allograft replacement of two coronary arteries
K42.3   Allograft replacement of three coronary arteries
K42.4   Allograft replacement of four or more coronary arteries
K42.8   Other specified
K42.9   Unspecified

K43   **Prosthetic replacement of coronary artery**
         Note: *Use a supplementary code for concurrent repair of valve of heart (K25–K29)*
                 Use a supplementary code for concurrent excision of lesion of ventricle of heart (K23.1) or repair of defect of interventricular septum (K11)
                 Use as a supplementary code for concurrent connection of thoracic artery to coronary artery (K45)

K43.1   Prosthetic replacement of one coronary artery
K43.2   Prosthetic replacement of two coronary arteries
K43.3   Prosthetic replacement of three coronary arteries
K43.4   Prosthetic replacement of four or more coronary arteries
K43.8   Other specified
K43.9   Unspecified

K44   **Other replacement of coronary artery**
         Includes: *Coronary artery bypass graft NEC*
         Note: *Use a supplementary code for concurrent repair of valve of heart (K25–K29)*
                 Use a supplementary code for concurrent excision of lesion of ventricle of heart (K23.1) or repair of defect of interventricular septum (K11)
                 Use as a supplementary code for concurrent connection of thoracic artery to coronary artery (K45)

K44.1   Replacement of coronary arteries using multiple methods
K44.2   Revision of replacement of coronary artery
K44.8   Other specified
K44.9   Unspecified

K45   **Connection of thoracic artery to coronary artery**
> *Note:*   *Use a supplementary code for concurrent replacement of coronary artery (K40–K44)*

K45.1   Double anastomosis of mammary arteries to coronary arteries
K45.2   Double anastomosis of thoracic arteries to coronary arteries NEC
K45.3   Anastomosis of mammary artery to left anterior descending coronary artery
K45.4   Anastomosis of mammary artery to coronary artery NEC
K45.5   Anastomosis of thoracic artery to coronary artery NEC
K45.6   Revision of connection of thoracic artery to coronary artery
K45.8   Other specified
K45.9   Unspecified

K46   **Other bypass of coronary artery**
> *Excludes:*   *Coronary artery bypass graft (K40–K44)*

K46.1   Double implantation of mammary arteries into heart
K46.2   Double implantation of thoracic arteries into heart NEC
K46.3   Implantation of mammary artery into heart NEC
K46.4   Implantation of thoracic artery into heart NEC
K46.5   Revision of implantation of thoracic artery into heart
K46.8   Other specified
K46.9   Unspecified

K47   **Repair of coronary artery**

K47.1   Endarterectomy of coronary artery
K47.2   Repair of arteriovenous fistula of coronary artery
> *Includes:*   *Percutaneous coronary fistula treatment*

K47.3   Repair of aneurysm of coronary artery
K47.4   Repair of rupture of coronary artery
K47.5   Repair of arteriovenous malformation of coronary artery
K47.8   Other specified
K47.9   Unspecified

K48   **Other open operations on coronary artery**

K48.1   Transection of muscle bridge of coronary artery
K48.2   Transposition of coronary artery NEC
> *Includes:*   *Repair of anomalous origin of coronary artery*

K48.3   Open angioplasty of coronary artery
K48.4   Exploration of coronary artery
K48.8   Other specified
K48.9   Unspecified

K49   **Transluminal balloon angioplasty of coronary artery**
> *Excludes:*   *Percutaneous transluminal balloon angioplasty and insertion of stent into coronary artery (K75)*
> *Note:*   *Use a supplementary code when associated with percutaneous atherectomy (K50.4)*

K49.1   Percutaneous transluminal balloon angioplasty of one coronary artery
> *Includes:*   *Angioplasty of coronary artery NEC*

K49.2   Percutaneous transluminal balloon angioplasty of multiple coronary arteries
K49.3   Percutaneous transluminal balloon angioplasty of bypass graft of coronary artery
K49.4   Percutaneous transluminal cutting balloon angioplasty of coronary artery
K49.8   Other specified
K49.9   Unspecified

K50 **Other therapeutic transluminal operations on coronary artery**

Excludes: Percutaneous transluminal balloon angioplasty and insertion of stent into coronary artery (K75)

K50.1   Percutaneous transluminal laser coronary angioplasty
K50.2   Percutaneous transluminal coronary thrombolysis using streptokinase
K50.3   Percutaneous transluminal injection of therapeutic substance into coronary artery NEC
K50.4   Percutaneous transluminal atherectomy of coronary artery
         Note: Use as a supplementary code for concurrent balloon angioplasty of coronary artery (K49)
K50.8   Other specified
K50.9   Unspecified

K51 **Diagnostic transluminal operations on coronary artery**

K51.1   Percutaneous transluminal angioscopy
K51.2   Intravascular ultrasound of coronary artery
K51.8   Other specified
K51.9   Unspecified

K52 **Open operations on conducting system of heart**

K52.1   Open ablation of atrioventricular node
         Includes: Ablation of atrioventricular node NEC
K52.2   Epicardial excision of rhythmogenic focus
K52.3   Endocardial excision of rhythmogenic focus
K52.4   Open division of accessory pathway within heart
K52.5   Open division of conducting system of heart NEC
K52.6   Incision of tissue in atria
K52.8   Other specified
K52.9   Unspecified

K53 **Other incision of heart**

K53.1   Inspection of valve of heart
K53.2   Exploration of heart NEC
K53.8   Other specified
K53.9   Unspecified
         Includes: Cardiotomy NEC

K54 **Open heart assist operations**

K54.1   Open implantation of ventricular assist device
K54.2   Open removal of ventricular assist device
K54.8   Other specified
K54.9   Unspecified

K55 **Other open operations on heart**

K55.1   Ligation of sinus of Valsalva
K55.2   Open chest massage of heart
K55.3   Open removal of cardiac thrombus
K55.4   Open removal of cardiac vegetations NEC
         Excludes: Open removal of vegetations of valve of heart (K34.4)
K55.5   Resection of heart tumour
K55.6   Repair of traumatic injury of heart
K55.8   Other specified
K55.9   Unspecified

K56   Transluminal heart assist operations

K56.1   Transluminal insertion of pulsation balloon into aorta
K56.2   Transluminal insertion of heart assist system NEC
K56.3   Transluminal maintenance of heart assist system
K56.4   Transluminal removal of heart assist system
K56.8   Other specified
K56.9   Unspecified

K57   Other therapeutic transluminal operations on heart
Note: Principal category, extended at K62

K57.1   Percutaneous transluminal ablation of atrioventricular node
K57.2   Percutaneous transluminal ablation of conducting system of heart NEC
K57.3   Percutaneous transluminal removal of foreign body from heart
K57.4   Percutaneous transluminal ablation of accessory pathway
K57.5   Percutaneous transluminal ablation of atrial wall NEC
K57.6   Percutaneous transluminal ablation of ventricular wall
K57.7   Percutaneous transluminal ablation for congenital heart malformation
K57.8   Other specified
K57.9   Unspecified

K58   Diagnostic transluminal operations on heart

K58.1   Percutaneous transluminal mapping of conducting system of heart NEC
K58.2   Percutaneous transluminal electrophysiological studies on conducting system of heart
K58.3   Percutaneous transluminal right ventricular biopsy
K58.4   Percutaneous transluminal left ventricular biopsy
K58.5   Transluminal intracardiac echocardiography
K58.6   Percutaneous transluminal three dimensional electroanatomic mapping of conducting system of heart
K58.8   Other specified
K58.9   Unspecified

K59   Cardioverter defibrillator introduced through the vein
Excludes: Subcutaneous cardioverter defibrillator (K72)
Evaluation of cardioverter defibrillator (X50.5)

K59.1   Implantation of cardioverter defibrillator using one electrode lead
K59.2   Implantation of cardioverter defibrillator using two electrode leads
K59.3   Resiting of lead of cardioverter defibrillator
K59.4   Renewal of cardioverter defibrillator
Includes: Maintenance of cardioverter defibrillator
K59.5   Removal of cardioverter defibrillator
K59.6   Implantation of cardioverter defibrillator using three electrode leads
K59.8   Other specified
K59.9   Unspecified

K60　　　**Cardiac pacemaker system introduced through vein**
　　　　　　Excludes: Cardioverter defibrillator introduced through the vein (K59)
　　　　　　　　　　　Subcutaneous cardioverter defibrillator (K72)

K60.1　　　Implantation of intravenous cardiac pacemaker system NEC
K60.2　　　Resiting of lead of intravenous cardiac pacemaker system
K60.3　　　Renewal of intravenous cardiac pacemaker system
　　　　　　Includes: Renewal of battery of intravenous cardiac pacemaker system
　　　　　　　　　　　Maintenance of intravenous cardiac pacemaker system NEC
K60.4　　　Removal of intravenous cardiac pacemaker system
K60.5　　　Implantation of intravenous single chamber cardiac pacemaker system
K60.6　　　Implantation of intravenous dual chamber cardiac pacemaker system
K60.7　　　Implantation of intravenous biventricular cardiac pacemaker system
K60.8　　　Other specified
K60.9　　　Unspecified

K61　　　**Other cardiac pacemaker system**
　　　　　　Includes: Epicardial implantation of cardiac pacemaker system
　　　　　　Excludes: Cardioverter defibrillator introduced through vein (K59)
　　　　　　　　　　　Subcutaneous cardioverter defibrillator (K72)

K61.1　　　Implantation of cardiac pacemaker system NEC
K61.2　　　Resiting of lead of cardiac pacemaker system NEC
K61.3　　　Renewal of cardiac pacemaker system NEC
　　　　　　Includes: Renewal of battery of cardiac pacemaker system NEC
　　　　　　　　　　　Maintenance of cardiac pacemaker system NEC
K61.4　　　Removal of cardiac pacemaker system NEC
K61.5　　　Implantation of single chamber cardiac pacemaker system
K61.6　　　Implantation of dual chamber cardiac pacemaker system
K61.7　　　Implantation of biventricular cardiac pacemaker system
K61.8　　　Other specified
K61.9　　　Unspecified

K62　　　**Therapeutic transluminal operations on heart**
　　　　　　　　Note: Principal K57

K62.1　　　Percutaneous transluminal ablation of pulmonary vein to left atrium conducting system
K62.2　　　Percutaneous transluminal ablation of atrial wall for atrial flutter
K62.3　　　Percutaneous transluminal ablation of conducting system of heart for atrial flutter NEC
K62.4　　　Percutaneous transluminal internal cardioversion NEC
　　　　　　Excludes: Implantation of cardioverter defibrillator (K59)
K62.5　　　Percutaneous transluminal occlusion of left atrial appendage
　　　　　　Includes: Percutaneous transluminal exclusion of left atrial appendage
　　　　　　Excludes: Exclusion of left atrial appendage NEC (K22.3)
K62.8　　　Other specified
K62.9　　　Unspecified

K63   **Contrast radiology of heart**
Excludes: Radionuclide angiocardiography (U10.5)
Computed tomography and magnetic resonance imaging angiography (U10.2, U10.3)

K63.1   Angiocardiography of combination of right and left side of heart
K63.2   Angiocardiography of right side of heart NEC
K63.3   Angiocardiography of left side of heart NEC
K63.4   Coronary arteriography using two catheters
K63.5   Coronary arteriography using single catheter
K63.6   Coronary arteriography NEC
K63.8   Other specified
K63.9   Unspecified

K64   **Percutaneous operations on heart**

K64.1   Percutaneous radiofrequency ablation of epicardium
K64.8   Other specified
K64.9   Unspecified

K65   **Catheterisation of heart**

K65.1   Catheterisation of combination of right and left side of heart NEC
K65.2   Catheterisation of right side of heart NEC
K65.3   Catheterisation of left side of heart NEC
K65.4   Catheterisation of left side of heart via atrial transeptal puncture
K65.8   Other specified
K65.9   Unspecified

K66   **Other operations on heart**

K66.1   Cardiotachygraphy
K66.8   Other specified
K66.9   Unspecified

K67   **Excision of pericardium**

K67.1   Excision of lesion of pericardium
K67.8   Other specified
K67.9   Unspecified

K68   **Drainage of pericardium**
Excludes: Transluminal drainage of pericardium (K77)

K68.1   Decompression of cardiac tamponade
K68.2   Pericardiocentesis NEC
K68.8   Other specified
K68.9   Unspecified

K69   **Incision of pericardium**

K69.1   Freeing of adhesions of pericardium
K69.2   Fenestration of pericardium
K69.8   Other specified
K69.9   Unspecified

K71   **Other operations on pericardium**

K71.1   Biopsy of lesion of pericardium
           Includes: Biopsy of pericardium
K71.2   Repair of pericardium
K71.3   Injection of therapeutic substance into pericardium
K71.4   Exploration of pericardium
K71.8   Other specified
K71.9   Unspecified

K72   **Other cardioverter defibrillator**
           Excludes: Cardioverter defibrillator introduced through vein (K59)
                   Evaluation of cardioverter defibrillator (X50.5)

K72.1   Implantation of subcutaneous cardioverter defibrillator
K72.2   Resiting of lead of subcutaneous cardioverter defibrillator
K72.3   Renewal of subcutaneous cardioverter defibrillator
           Includes: Renewal of battery of subcutaneous cardioverter defibrillator
                   Maintenance of subcutaneous cardioverter defibrillator
K72.4   Removal of subcutaneous cardioverter defibrillator
K72.8   Other specified
K72.9   Unspecified

K75   **Percutaneous transluminal balloon angioplasty and insertion of stent into coronary artery**
           Excludes: Transluminal balloon angioplasty of coronary artery (K49)
           Note: It is not necessary to code additionally any mention of percutaneous transluminal atherectomy of coronary artery (K50.4)

K75.1   Percutaneous transluminal balloon angioplasty and insertion of 1–2 drug-eluting stents into coronary artery
K75.2   Percutaneous transluminal balloon angioplasty and insertion of 3 or more drug-eluting stents into coronary artery
K75.3   Percutaneous transluminal balloon angioplasty and insertion of 1–2 stents into coronary artery
           Includes: Angioplasty and insertion of stent into coronary artery NEC
K75.4   Percutaneous transluminal balloon angioplasty and insertion of 3 or more stents into coronary artery NEC
K75.8   Other specified
K75.9   Unspecified

K76   **Transluminal operations on cardiac conduit**

K76.1   Percutaneous transluminal balloon dilation of cardiac conduit
K76.8   Other specified
K76.9   Unspecified

K77   **Transluminal drainage of pericardium**
           Excludes: Drainage of pericardium (K68)

K77.1   Percutaneous transluminal pericardiocentesis
K77.8   Other specified
K77.9   Unspecified

K78   **Transluminal operations on internal mammary artery side branch**

K78.1   Transluminal occlusion of left internal mammary artery side branch
K78.8   Other specified
K78.9   Unspecified

CHAPTER L
ARTERIES AND VEINS
(CODES L01–L99, O01–O05, O15, O20)

Note: *This chapter contains certain specified arteries and veins*

This specification does not extend beyond the actual named vessel

Smaller branches or tributaries of the above are to be coded to the other and unspecified vessel categories with an appropriate site code where available

Use a subsidiary code for minimal access approach (Y74–Y76)

Use a subsidiary code to identify method of image control (Y53)

Use a subsidiary code to identify cardiopulmonary bypass (Y73.1)

Use a subsidiary code to identify arteriotomy approach to organ under image control (Y78)

L01	**Open operations for combined abnormality of great vessels**
L01.1	Correction of persistent truncus arteriosus

> *Note:* *Do not code repair of defect of septum of heart separately*

L01.2	Application of band to persistent truncus arteriosus
L01.3	Repair of anomalous pulmonary artery origin from ascending aorta

Includes: *Repair of hemitruncus arteriosus*

L01.4	Closure of aortopulmonary window
L01.8	Other specified
L01.9	Unspecified

L02	**Open correction of patent ductus arteriosus**
L02.1	Division of patent ductus arteriosus
L02.2	Ligature of patent ductus arteriosus
L02.3	Closure of patent ductus arteriosus NEC
L02.4	Revision of correction of patent ductus arteriosus
L02.8	Other specified
L02.9	Unspecified

L03	**Transluminal operations on abnormality of great vessel**
L03.1	Percutaneous transluminal prosthetic occlusion of patent ductus arteriosus
L03.2	Percutaneous transluminal stent implantation into arterial duct

> *Note:* *Use a supplementary code for placement of stent (L76, L89, O20)*

L03.8	Other specified
L03.9	Unspecified

L04	**Open operations on pulmonary arterial tree**

Excludes: *Other open operations on pulmonary artery (L12)*

L04.1	Pulmonary thromboendarterectomy
L04.8	Other specified
L04.9	Unspecified

L05   **Creation of shunt to pulmonary artery from aorta using interposition tube prosthesis**

L05.1   Creation of shunt to main pulmonary artery from ascending aorta using interposition tube prosthesis

L05.2   Creation of shunt to right pulmonary artery from ascending aorta using interposition tube prosthesis

L05.3   Creation of shunt to left pulmonary artery from ascending aorta using interposition tube prosthesis

L05.4   Percutaneous transluminal balloon dilation of interposition tube prosthesis between pulmonary artery and aorta

L05.8   Other specified

L05.9   Unspecified

L06   **Other connection to pulmonary artery from aorta**

L06.1   Creation of aortopulmonary window

L06.2   Creation of anastomosis to main pulmonary artery from ascending aorta NEC

L06.3   Creation of anastomosis to right pulmonary artery from ascending aorta NEC

L06.4   Creation of anastomosis to left pulmonary artery from descending aorta NEC

L06.5   Creation of anastomosis to pulmonary artery from aorta NEC

L06.6   Revision of anastomosis to pulmonary artery from aorta

L06.7   Takedown of anastomosis to pulmonary artery from aorta

L06.8   Other specified

L06.9   Unspecified

L07   **Creation of shunt to pulmonary artery from subclavian artery using interposition tube prosthesis**

L07.1   Creation of shunt to right pulmonary artery from right subclavian artery using interposition tube prosthesis

L07.2   Creation of shunt to left pulmonary artery from left subclavian artery using interposition tube prosthesis

L07.3   Closure of prosthetic shunt to pulmonary artery from subclavian artery

L07.4   Percutaneous transluminal balloon dilation of interposition tube prosthesis between pulmonary artery and subclavian artery

L07.5   Percutaneous transluminal occlusion of interposition tube prosthesis between pulmonary artery and subclavian artery

L07.8   Other specified

L07.9   Unspecified

L08   **Other connection to pulmonary artery from subclavian artery**

L08.1   Creation of anastomosis to right pulmonary artery from right subclavian artery NEC

L08.2   Creation of anastomosis to left pulmonary artery from left subclavian artery NEC

L08.3   Creation of anastomosis to pulmonary artery from subclavian artery NEC

L08.4   Revision of anastomosis to pulmonary artery from subclavian artery

L08.6   Percutaneous transluminal balloon dilation of anastomosis between pulmonary artery and subclavian artery

L08.7   Percutaneous transluminal occlusion of anastomosis between pulmonary artery and subclavian artery

L08.8   Other specified

L08.9   Unspecified

L09 **Other connection to pulmonary artery**

L09.1   Creation of anastomosis to pulmonary artery from vena cava
L09.2   Removal of anastomosis between pulmonary artery and vena cava
L09.8   Other specified
L09.9   Unspecified

L10 **Repair of pulmonary artery**

  Note: *Use a supplementary code for concurrent operations on pulmonary valve (K28, K30–K35)*

L10.1   Repair of pulmonary artery using prosthesis
L10.2   Repair of pulmonary artery using patch
L10.3   Repair of anomalous pulmonary artery NEC
L10.4   Repair of pulmonary arterial sling
L10.8   Other specified
L10.9   Unspecified

L12 **Other open operations on pulmonary artery**

  Excludes: *Open operations on pulmonary arterial tree (L04)*

L12.1   Application of band to pulmonary artery
L12.2   Adjustment of band to pulmonary artery
L12.3   Removal of band from pulmonary artery
L12.4   Open embolectomy of pulmonary artery

  Includes: *Open thrombectomy of pulmonary artery*
   Embolectomy of pulmonary artery NEC
   Thrombectomy of pulmonary artery NEC

L12.5   Open embolisation of pulmonary artery
L12.6   Pulmonary artery ligation
L12.8   Other specified
L12.9   Unspecified

L13 **Transluminal operations on pulmonary artery**

L13.1   Percutaneous transluminal embolectomy of pulmonary artery

  Includes: *Percutaneous transluminal thrombectomy of pulmonary artery*

L13.2   Percutaneous transluminal embolisation of pulmonary artery

  Includes: *Embolisation of pulmonary artery NEC*

L13.3   Arteriography of pulmonary artery
L13.4   Percutaneous transluminal cutting balloon angioplasty of pulmonary artery
L13.5   Percutaneous transluminal balloon angioplasty of pulmonary artery NEC
L13.6   Percutaneous transluminal insertion of stent into pulmonary artery

  Note: *Use a supplementary code for placement of stent (L76, L89, O20)*

L13.8   Other specified
L13.9   Unspecified

L16   **Extra-anatomic bypass of aorta**
> *Note:*   *In categories L16–L21 reference to iliac artery (NFQ) should be understood to include:*
> *Common iliac artery;*
> *External iliac artery;*
> *Internal iliac artery.*
> *Similarly reference to femoral artery includes:*
> *Common femoral artery;*
> *Deep femoral artery;*
> *Superficial femoral artery.*

L16.1   Emergency bypass of aorta by anastomosis of axillary artery to femoral artery
L16.2   Bypass of aorta by anastomosis of axillary artery to femoral artery NEC
L16.3   Bypass of aorta by anastomosis of axillary artery to bilateral femoral arteries
          Includes: *Axillobifemoral bypass*
L16.8   Other specified
L16.9   Unspecified

L18   **Emergency replacement of aneurysmal segment of aorta**
> *Note at L16 applies*
> *Includes:*   *Emergency replacement of aneurysmal segment of aorta using prosthesis*

L18.1   Emergency replacement of aneurysmal segment of ascending aorta by anastomosis of aorta to aorta
> *Note:*   *Use a supplementary code for concurrent operations on aortic valve (K26, K30–K35)*
L18.2   Emergency replacement of aneurysmal segment of thoracic aorta by anastomosis of aorta to aorta NEC
L18.3   Emergency replacement of aneurysmal segment of suprarenal abdominal aorta by anastomosis of aorta to aorta
L18.4   Emergency replacement of aneurysmal segment of infrarenal abdominal aorta by anastomosis of aorta to aorta
L18.5   Emergency replacement of aneurysmal segment of abdominal aorta by anastomosis of aorta to aorta NEC
L18.6   Emergency replacement of aneurysmal bifurcation of aorta by anastomosis of aorta to iliac artery
L18.8   Other specified
L18.9   Unspecified

L19 **Other replacement of aneurysmal segment of aorta**
Note at L16 applies
Includes: Replacement of aneurysmal segment of aorta using prosthesis NEC

L19.1 Replacement of aneurysmal segment of ascending aorta by anastomosis of aorta to aorta NEC
Note: Use a supplementary code for concurrent operations on aortic valve (K26, K30–K35)

L19.2 Replacement of aneurysmal segment of thoracic aorta by anastomosis of aorta to aorta NEC

L19.3 Replacement of aneurysmal segment of suprarenal abdominal aorta by anastomosis of aorta to aorta NEC

L19.4 Replacement of aneurysmal segment of infrarenal abdominal aorta by anastomosis of aorta to aorta NEC

L19.5 Replacement of aneurysmal segment of abdominal aorta by anastomosis of aorta to aorta NEC

L19.6 Replacement of aneurysmal bifurcation of aorta by anastomosis of aorta to iliac artery NEC

L19.8 Other specified

L19.9 Unspecified

L20 **Other emergency bypass of segment of aorta**
Note at L16 applies
Includes: Emergency bypass of segment of aorta using prosthesis NEC
Emergency replacement of segment of aorta NEC
Emergency replacement of segment of aorta using prosthesis NEC

L20.1 Emergency bypass of segment of ascending aorta by anastomosis of aorta to aorta NEC
Note: Use a supplementary code for concurrent operations on aortic valve (K26, K30–K35)

L20.2 Emergency bypass of segment of thoracic aorta by anastomosis of aorta to aorta NEC

L20.3 Emergency bypass of segment of suprarenal abdominal aorta by anastomosis of aorta to aorta NEC

L20.4 Emergency bypass of segment of infrarenal abdominal aorta by anastomosis of aorta to aorta NEC

L20.5 Emergency bypass of segment of abdominal aorta by anastomosis of aorta to aorta NEC

L20.6 Emergency bypass of bifurcation of aorta by anastomosis of aorta to iliac artery NEC

L20.8 Other specified

L20.9 Unspecified

L21 **Other bypass of segment of aorta**
Note at L16 applies
Includes: Bypass of segment of aorta using prosthesis NEC
Replacement of segment of aorta NEC
Replacement of segment of aorta using prosthesis NEC

L21.1 Bypass of segment of ascending aorta by anastomosis of aorta to aorta NEC
Note: Use a supplementary code for concurrent operations on aortic valve (K26, K30–K35)

L21.2 Bypass of segment of thoracic aorta by anastomosis of aorta to aorta NEC

L21.3 Bypass of segment of suprarenal abdominal aorta by anastomosis of aorta to aorta NEC

L21.4 Bypass of segment of infrarenal abdominal aorta by anastomosis of aorta to aorta NEC

L21.5 Bypass of segment of abdominal aorta by anastomosis of aorta to aorta NEC

L21.6 Bypass of bifurcation of aorta by anastomosis of aorta to iliac artery NEC

L21.8 Other specified

L21.9 Unspecified

L22 **Attention to prosthesis of aorta**

L22.1 Revision of prosthesis of thoracic aorta
L22.2 Revision of prosthesis of bifurcation of aorta
L22.3 Revision of prosthesis of abdominal aorta NEC
L22.4 Removal of prosthesis from aorta
L22.8 Other specified
L22.9 Unspecified

L23 **Plastic repair of aorta**
Includes: Repair of aorta coarctation
Repair of aorta hypoplasia

L23.1 Plastic repair of aorta and end to end anastomosis of aorta
L23.2 Plastic repair of aorta using subclavian flap
L23.3 Plastic repair of aorta using patch graft
L23.4 Release of vascular ring of aorta
L23.5 Revision of plastic repair of aorta
L23.6 Plastic repair of aorta and insertion of tube graft
L23.7 Repair of interrupted aortic arch
L23.8 Other specified
L23.9 Unspecified

L25 **Other open operations on aorta**
Includes: Aortic body (L25.5)

L25.1 Endarterectomy of aorta and patch repair of aorta
L25.2 Endarterectomy of aorta NEC
L25.3 Open embolectomy of bifurcation of aorta
Includes: Open thrombectomy of bifurcation of aorta
Embolectomy of bifurcation of aorta NEC
Thrombectomy of bifurcation of aorta NEC
L25.4 Operations on aneurysm of aorta NEC
L25.5 Operations on aortic body
L25.8 Other specified
L25.9 Unspecified

L26 **Transluminal operations on aorta**
Excludes: Transluminal operations on aneurysmal segment of aorta (L28)
Note: Use a subsidiary site code as necessary

L26.1 Percutaneous transluminal balloon angioplasty of aorta
L26.2 Percutaneous transluminal angioplasty of aorta NEC
L26.3 Percutaneous transluminal embolectomy of bifurcation of aorta
Includes: Percutaneous transluminal thrombectomy of bifurcation of aorta
L26.4 Aortography
L26.5 Percutaneous transluminal insertion of stent into aorta
Note: Use a supplementary code for placement of stent (L76, L89)
L26.6 Transluminal aortic stent graft with fenestration NEC
Note: Use a supplementary code for placement of stent (O20)
L26.7 Transluminal aortic branched stent graft NEC
Note: Use a supplementary code for placement of stent (O20)
L26.8 Other specified
L26.9 Unspecified

L27   **Transluminal insertion of stent graft for aneurysmal segment of aorta**
Note: Use a supplementary code for placement of stent (O20)

L27.1   Endovascular insertion of stent graft for infrarenal abdominal aortic aneurysm
L27.2   Endovascular insertion of stent graft for suprarenal aortic aneurysm
L27.3   Endovascular insertion of stent graft for thoracic aortic aneurysm
L27.4   Endovascular insertion of stent graft for aortic dissection in any position
L27.5   Endovascular insertion of stent graft for aortic aneurysm of bifurcation NEC
L27.6   Endovascular insertion of stent graft for aorto–uniiliac aneurysm
L27.8   Other specified
L27.9   Unspecified

L28   **Transluminal operations on aneurysmal segment of aorta**
Note: Use a supplementary code for placement of stent (L76, L89)

L28.1   Endovascular insertion of stent for infrarenal abdominal aortic aneurysm
L28.2   Endovascular insertion of stent for suprarenal aortic aneurysm
L28.3   Endovascular insertion of stent for thoracic aortic aneurysm
L28.4   Endovascular insertion of stent for aortic dissection in any position
L28.5   Endovascular insertion of stent for aortic aneurysm of bifurcation NEC
L28.6   Endovascular insertion of stent for aorto–uniiliac aneurysm
L28.8   Other specified
L28.9   Unspecified

L29   **Reconstruction of carotid artery**

L29.1   Replacement of carotid artery using graft
L29.2   Intracranial bypass to carotid artery NEC
L29.3   Bypass to carotid artery NEC
L29.4   Endarterectomy of carotid artery and patch repair of carotid artery
L29.5   Endarterectomy of carotid artery NEC
L29.6   High-flow interposition extracranial to intracranial bypass from external carotid artery to middle cerebral artery
L29.7   Bypass of carotid artery by anastomosis of superficial temporal artery to middle cerebral artery
L29.8   Other specified
L29.9   Unspecified

L30   **Other open operations on carotid artery**
Includes: Carotid body (L30.5)

L30.1   Repair of carotid artery NEC
L30.2   Ligation of carotid artery
L30.3   Open embolectomy of carotid artery
Includes: Open thrombectomy of carotid artery
Embolectomy of carotid artery NEC
Thrombectomy of carotid artery NEC
L30.4   Operations on aneurysm of carotid artery
L30.5   Operations on carotid body
L30.8   Other specified
L30.9   Unspecified

L31   **Transluminal operations on carotid artery**

L31.1   Percutaneous transluminal angioplasty of carotid artery
L31.2   Arteriography of carotid artery
L31.3   Endovascular repair of carotid artery
L31.4   Percutaneous transluminal insertion of stent into carotid artery
        Note: Use a supplementary code for placement of stent (L76, L89, O20)
L31.8   Other specified
L31.9   Unspecified

L33   **Operations on aneurysm of cerebral artery**
       Includes: Artery of circle of Willis

L33.1   Excision of aneurysm of cerebral artery
L33.2   Clipping of aneurysm of cerebral artery
L33.3   Ligation of aneurysm of cerebral artery NEC
L33.4   Obliteration of aneurysm of cerebral artery NEC
L33.8   Other specified
L33.9   Unspecified

L34   **Other open operations on cerebral artery**
       Includes: Artery of circle of Willis

L34.1   Reconstruction of cerebral artery
L34.2   Anastomosis of cerebral artery
L34.3   Open embolectomy of cerebral artery
       Includes: Open thrombectomy of cerebral artery
                    Embolectomy of cerebral artery NEC
                    Thrombectomy of cerebral artery NEC
L34.4   Open embolisation of cerebral artery
L34.8   Other specified
L34.9   Unspecified

L35   **Transluminal operations on cerebral artery**
       Includes: Artery of circle of Willis

L35.1   Percutaneous transluminal embolisation of cerebral artery
       Includes: Embolisation of cerebral artery NEC
L35.2   Arteriography of cerebral artery
L35.3   Percutaneous transluminal insertion of stent into cerebral artery
        Note: Use a supplementary code for placement of stent (L76, L89, O20)
L35.8   Other specified
L35.9   Unspecified

L37   **Reconstruction of subclavian artery**
       Includes: Axillary artery
                    Brachial artery
                    Vertebral artery

L37.1   Bypass of subclavian artery NEC
L37.2   Endarterectomy of vertebral artery
L37.3   Endarterectomy of subclavian artery and patch repair of subclavian artery
L37.4   Endarterectomy of subclavian artery NEC
L37.8   Other specified
L37.9   Unspecified

L38 **Other open operations on subclavian artery**
Includes: Axillary artery
Brachial artery
Vertebral artery

L38.1 Repair of subclavian artery NEC
L38.2 Ligation of subclavian artery
L38.3 Open embolectomy of subclavian artery
Includes: Open thrombectomy of subclavian artery
Embolectomy of subclavian artery NEC
Thrombectomy of subclavian artery NEC
L38.4 Operations on aneurysm of subclavian artery
L38.8 Other specified
L38.9 Unspecified

L39 **Transluminal operations on subclavian artery**
Includes: Axillary artery
Brachial artery
Vertebral artery

L39.1 Percutaneous transluminal angioplasty of subclavian artery
L39.2 Percutaneous transluminal embolectomy of subclavian artery
Includes: Percutaneous transluminal thrombectomy of subclavian artery
L39.3 Percutaneous transluminal embolisation of subclavian artery
Includes: Embolisation of subclavian artery NEC
L39.4 Arteriography of subclavian artery
L39.5 Percutaneous transluminal insertion of stent into subclavian artery
Note: **Use a supplementary code for placement of stent (L76, L89, O20)**
L39.8 Other specified
L39.9 Unspecified

L41 **Reconstruction of renal artery**

L41.1 Plastic repair of renal artery and end to end anastomosis of renal artery
L41.2 Bypass of renal artery
L41.3 Replantation of renal artery
L41.4 Endarterectomy of renal artery
L41.5 Translocation of branch of renal artery
L41.6 Patch angioplasty of renal artery
L41.8 Other specified
L41.9 Unspecified

L42 **Other open operations on renal artery**

L42.1 Open embolectomy of renal artery
Includes: Open thrombectomy of renal artery
Embolectomy of renal artery NEC
Thrombectomy of renal artery NEC
L42.2 Open embolisation of renal artery
L42.3 Ligation of renal artery
L42.4 Operations on aneurysm of renal artery
L42.8 Other specified
L42.9 Unspecified

L43   **Transluminal operations on renal artery**

L43.1   Percutaneous transluminal angioplasty of renal artery

L43.2   Percutaneous transluminal embolectomy of renal artery

             Includes: Percutaneous transluminal thrombectomy of renal artery

L43.3   Percutaneous transluminal embolisation of renal artery

             Includes: Embolisation of renal artery NEC

L43.4   Arteriography of renal artery

L43.5   Percutaneous transluminal insertion of stent into renal artery

             Note: Use a supplementary code for placement of stent (L76, L89, O20)

L43.6   Percutaneous transluminal radiofrequency denervation of renal artery

L43.8   Other specified

L43.9   Unspecified

L45   **Reconstruction of other visceral branch of abdominal aorta**

             Includes: Coeliac artery

                       Superior mesenteric artery

                       Inferior mesenteric artery

                       Suprarenal artery

L45.1   Bypass of visceral branch of abdominal aorta NEC

L45.2   Replantation of visceral branch of abdominal aorta NEC

L45.3   Endarterectomy of visceral branch of abdominal aorta and patch repair of visceral branch of abdominal aorta NEC

L45.4   Endarterectomy of visceral branch of abdominal aorta NEC

L45.8   Other specified

L45.9   Unspecified

L46   **Other open operations on other visceral branch of abdominal aorta**

             Includes: Coeliac artery

                       Superior mesenteric artery

                       Inferior mesenteric artery

                       Suprarenal artery

L46.1   Open embolectomy of visceral branch of abdominal aorta NEC

             Includes: Open thrombectomy of visceral branch of abdominal aorta NEC

                       Embolectomy of visceral branch of abdominal aorta NEC

                       Thrombectomy of visceral branch of abdominal aorta NEC

L46.2   Open embolisation of visceral branch of abdominal aorta NEC

L46.3   Ligation of visceral branch of abdominal aorta NEC

L46.4   Operations on aneurysm of visceral branch of abdominal aorta NEC

L46.8   Other specified

L46.9   Unspecified

L47 **Transluminal operations on other visceral branch of abdominal aorta**
Includes: *Coeliac artery*
Superior mesenteric artery
Inferior mesenteric artery
Suprarenal artery

L47.1 Percutaneous transluminal angioplasty of visceral branch of abdominal aorta NEC
L47.2 Percutaneous transluminal embolisation of visceral branch of abdominal aorta NEC
Includes: *Embolisation of visceral branch of abdominal aorta NEC*
L47.3 Arteriography of visceral branch of abdominal aorta NEC
L47.4 Percutaneous transluminal insertion of stent into visceral branch of abdominal aorta NEC
Note: **Use a supplementary code for placement of stent (L76, L89, O20)**
L47.8 Other specified
L47.9 Unspecified

L48 **Emergency replacement of aneurysmal iliac artery**
Includes: *Emergency replacement of aneurysmal iliac artery using prosthesis*
Note: **In categories L48–L54 reference to iliac artery (NFQ) should be understood**
to include:
Common iliac artery;
External iliac artery;
Internal iliac artery.
Similarly reference to femoral artery includes:
Common femoral artery;
Deep femoral artery;
Superficial femoral artery.

L48.1 Emergency replacement of aneurysmal common iliac artery by anastomosis of aorta to common iliac artery
L48.2 Emergency replacement of aneurysmal iliac artery by anastomosis of aorta to external iliac artery
Includes: *Emergency replacement of aneurysmal iliac artery by anastomosis of aorta to internal iliac artery*
L48.3 Emergency replacement of aneurysmal artery of leg by anastomosis of aorta to common femoral artery
L48.4 Emergency replacement of aneurysmal artery of leg by anastomosis of aorta to superficial femoral artery
Includes: *Emergency replacement of aneurysmal artery of leg by anastomosis of aorta to deep femoral artery*
Emergency replacement of aneurysmal artery of leg by anastomosis of aorta to popliteal artery
L48.5 Emergency replacement of aneurysmal iliac artery by anastomosis of iliac artery to iliac artery
L48.6 Emergency replacement of aneurysmal artery of leg by anastomosis of iliac artery to femoral artery
Includes: *Emergency replacement of aneurysmal artery of leg by anastomosis of iliac artery to popliteal artery*
L48.8 Other specified
L48.9 Unspecified

L49   **Other replacement of aneurysmal iliac artery**
Note at L48 applies
Includes: Replacement of aneurysmal iliac artery using prosthesis NEC

L49.1   Replacement of aneurysmal common iliac artery by anastomosis of aorta to common iliac artery NEC

L49.2   Replacement of aneurysmal iliac artery by anastomosis of aorta to external iliac artery NEC
Includes: Replacement of aneurysmal iliac artery by anastomosis of aorta to internal iliac artery NEC

L49.3   Replacement of aneurysmal artery of leg by anastomosis of aorta to common femoral artery NEC

L49.4   Replacement of aneurysmal artery of leg by anastomosis of aorta to superficial femoral artery NEC
Includes: Replacement of aneurysmal artery of leg by anastomosis of aorta to deep femoral artery NEC
Replacement of aneurysmal artery of leg by anastomosis of aorta to popliteal artery NEC

L49.5   Replacement of aneurysmal iliac artery by anastomosis of iliac artery to iliac artery NEC

L49.6   Replacement of aneurysmal artery of leg by anastomosis of iliac artery to femoral artery NEC
Includes: Replacement of aneurysmal artery of leg by anastomosis of iliac artery to popliteal artery NEC

L49.8   Other specified
L49.9   Unspecified

L50   **Other emergency bypass of iliac artery**
Note at L48 applies
Includes: Emergency bypass of iliac artery using prosthesis NEC
Emergency replacement of iliac artery NEC
Emergency replacement of iliac artery using prosthesis NEC

L50.1   Emergency bypass of common iliac artery by anastomosis of aorta to common iliac artery NEC

L50.2   Emergency bypass of iliac artery by anastomosis of aorta to external iliac artery NEC
Includes: Emergency bypass of iliac artery by anastomosis of aorta to internal iliac artery NEC

L50.3   Emergency bypass of artery of leg by anastomosis of aorta to common femoral artery NEC

L50.4   Emergency bypass of artery of leg by anastomosis of aorta to deep femoral artery NEC
Includes: Emergency bypass of artery of leg by anastomosis of aorta to superficial femoral artery NEC
Emergency bypass of artery of leg by anastomosis of aorta to popliteal artery NEC

L50.5   Emergency bypass of iliac artery by anastomosis of iliac artery to iliac artery NEC
L50.6   Emergency bypass of artery of leg by anastomosis of iliac artery to femoral artery NEC
Includes: Emergency bypass of artery of leg by anastomosis of iliac artery to popliteal artery NEC

L50.8   Other specified
Includes: Emergency aortoiliac anastomosis NEC
Emergency aortofemoral anastomosis NEC
Emergency iliofemoral anastomosis NEC

L50.9   Unspecified

L51 **Other bypass of iliac artery**
Note at L48 applies
Includes: *Bypass of iliac artery using prosthesis NEC*
Replacement of iliac artery NEC
Replacement of iliac artery using prosthesis NEC

L51.1 Bypass of common iliac artery by anastomosis of aorta to common iliac artery NEC
L51.2 Bypass of iliac artery by anastomosis of aorta to external iliac artery NEC
Includes: *Bypass of iliac artery by anastomosis of aorta to internal iliac artery NEC*
L51.3 Bypass of artery of leg by anastomosis of aorta to common femoral artery NEC
L51.4 Bypass of artery of leg by anastomosis of aorta to deep femoral artery NEC
Includes: *Bypass of artery of leg by anastomosis of aorta to superficial femoral*
artery NEC
Bypass of artery of leg by anastomosis of aorta to popliteal artery NEC
L51.5 Bypass of iliac artery by anastomosis of iliac artery to iliac artery NEC
L51.6 Bypass of artery of leg by anastomosis of iliac artery to femoral artery NEC
Includes: *Bypass of artery of leg by anastomosis of iliac artery to popliteal artery NEC*
L51.8 Other specified
Includes: *Aortoiliac anastomosis NEC*
Aortofemoral anastomosis NEC
Iliofemoral anastomosis NEC
L51.9 Unspecified

L52 **Reconstruction of iliac artery**
Note at L48 applies

L52.1 Endarterectomy of iliac artery and patch repair of iliac artery
L52.2 Endarterectomy of iliac artery NEC
L52.8 Other specified
L52.9 Unspecified

L53 **Other open operations on iliac artery**
Note at L48 applies

L53.1 Repair of iliac artery NEC
L53.2 Open embolectomy of iliac artery
Includes: *Open thrombectomy of iliac artery*
Embolectomy of iliac artery NEC
Thrombectomy of iliac artery NEC
L53.3 Operations on aneurysm of iliac artery NEC
L53.8 Other specified
L53.9 Unspecified

L54 **Transluminal operations on iliac artery**
Note at L48 applies

L54.1 Percutaneous transluminal angioplasty of iliac artery
L54.2 Percutaneous transluminal embolectomy of iliac artery
Includes: *Percutaneous transluminal thrombectomy of iliac artery*
L54.3 Arteriography of iliac artery
L54.4 Percutaneous transluminal insertion of stent into iliac artery
Note: ***Use a supplementary code for placement of stent (L76, L89, O20)***
L54.8 Other specified
L54.9 Unspecified

L56 **Emergency replacement of aneurysmal femoral artery**

Excludes: *When associated with connection from aorta or iliac artery (L48)*

> *Note:* ***In categories L56–L65 reference to iliac artery (NFQ) should be understood to include:***
> ***Common iliac artery;***
> ***External iliac artery;***
> ***Internal iliac artery.***
> ***Similarly reference to femoral artery includes:***
> ***Common femoral artery;***
> ***Deep femoral artery;***
> ***Superficial femoral artery.***

L56.1 Emergency replacement of aneurysmal femoral artery by anastomosis of femoral artery to femoral artery

Includes: *Emergency replacement of aneurysmal femoral artery by anastomosis of femoral artery to femoral artery using prosthesis*

L56.2 Emergency replacement of aneurysmal femoral artery by anastomosis of femoral artery to popliteal artery using prosthesis

L56.3 Emergency replacement of aneurysmal femoral artery by anastomosis of femoral artery to popliteal artery using vein graft

Includes: *Emergency replacement of aneurysmal femoral artery by anastomosis of femoral artery to popliteal artery NEC*

L56.4 Emergency replacement of aneurysmal femoral artery by anastomosis of femoral artery to tibial artery using prosthesis

Includes: *Popliteal artery*

L56.5 Emergency replacement of aneurysmal femoral artery by anastomosis of femoral artery to tibial artery using vein graft

Includes: *Emergency replacement of aneurysmal femoral artery by anastomosis of femoral artery to tibial artery NEC*
Popliteal artery

L56.6 Emergency replacement of aneurysmal femoral artery by anastomosis of femoral artery to peroneal artery using prosthesis

Includes: *Popliteal artery*

L56.7 Emergency replacement of aneurysmal femoral artery by anastomosis of femoral artery to peroneal artery using vein graft

Includes: *Emergency replacement of aneurysmal femoral artery by anastomosis of femoral artery to peroneal artery NEC*
Popliteal artery

L56.8 Other specified

L56.9 Unspecified

L57 **Other replacement of aneurysmal femoral artery**
Note at L56 applies
Excludes: When associated with connection from aorta or iliac artery (L49)

L57.1 Replacement of aneurysmal femoral artery by anastomosis of femoral artery to femoral artery NEC
Includes: Replacement of aneurysmal femoral artery by anastomosis of femoral artery to femoral artery using prosthesis NEC

L57.2 Replacement of aneurysmal femoral artery by anastomosis of femoral artery to popliteal artery using prosthesis NEC

L57.3 Replacement of aneurysmal femoral artery by anastomosis of femoral artery to popliteal artery using vein graft NEC
Includes: Replacement of aneurysmal femoral artery by anastomosis of femoral artery to popliteal artery NEC

L57.4 Replacement of aneurysmal femoral artery by anastomosis of femoral artery to tibial artery using prosthesis NEC
Includes: Popliteal artery

L57.5 Replacement of aneurysmal femoral artery by anastomosis of femoral artery to tibial artery using vein graft NEC
Includes: Replacement of aneurysmal femoral artery by anastomosis of femoral artery to tibial artery NEC
Popliteal artery

L57.6 Replacement of aneurysmal femoral artery by anastomosis of femoral artery to peroneal artery using prosthesis NEC
Includes: Popliteal artery

L57.7 Replacement of aneurysmal femoral artery by anastomosis of femoral artery to peroneal artery using vein graft NEC
Includes: Replacement of aneurysmal femoral artery by anastomosis of femoral artery to peroneal artery NEC
Popliteal artery

L57.8 Other specified
L57.9 Unspecified

L58   **Other emergency bypass of femoral artery**
Note at L56 applies
Includes: Emergency replacement of femoral artery NEC
Excludes: When associated with connection from aorta or iliac artery (L50)

L58.1   Emergency bypass of femoral artery by anastomosis of femoral artery to femoral artery NEC
Includes: Emergency bypass of femoral artery by anastomosis of femoral artery to femoral artery using prosthesis NEC

L58.2   Emergency bypass of femoral artery by anastomosis of femoral artery to popliteal artery using prosthesis NEC

L58.3   Emergency bypass of femoral artery by anastomosis of femoral artery to popliteal artery using vein graft NEC
Includes: Emergency bypass of femoral artery by anastomosis of femoral artery to popliteal artery NEC

L58.4   Emergency bypass of femoral artery by anastomosis of femoral artery to tibial artery using prosthesis NEC
Includes: Popliteal artery

L58.5   Emergency bypass of femoral artery by anastomosis of femoral artery to tibial artery using vein graft NEC
Includes: Emergency bypass of femoral artery by anastomosis of femoral artery to tibial artery NEC
Popliteal artery

L58.6   Emergency bypass of femoral artery by anastomosis of femoral artery to peroneal artery using prosthesis NEC
Includes: Popliteal artery

L58.7   Emergency bypass of femoral artery by anastomosis of femoral artery to peroneal artery using vein graft NEC
Includes: Emergency bypass of femoral artery by anastomosis of femoral artery to peroneal artery NEC
Popliteal artery

L58.8   Other specified

L58.9   Unspecified

L59   **Other bypass of femoral artery**
Note at L56 applies
Includes: *Replacement of femoral artery NEC*
Excludes: *When associated with connection from aorta or iliac artery (L51)*

L59.1   Bypass of femoral artery by anastomosis of femoral artery to femoral artery NEC
Includes: *Bypass of femoral artery by anastomosis of femoral artery to femoral artery using prosthesis NEC*

L59.2   Bypass of femoral artery by anastomosis of femoral artery to popliteal artery using prosthesis NEC

L59.3   Bypass of femoral artery by anastomosis of femoral artery to popliteal artery using vein graft NEC
Includes: *Bypass of femoral artery by anastomosis of femoral artery to popliteal artery NEC*

L59.4   Bypass of femoral artery by anastomosis of femoral artery to tibial artery using prosthesis NEC
Includes: *Popliteal artery*

L59.5   Bypass of femoral artery by anastomosis of femoral artery to tibial artery using vein graft NEC
Includes: *Bypass of femoral artery by anastomosis of femoral artery to tibial artery NEC*
          Popliteal artery

L59.6   Bypass of femoral artery by anastomosis of femoral artery to peroneal artery using prosthesis NEC
Includes: *Popliteal artery*

L59.7   Bypass of femoral artery by anastomosis of femoral artery to peroneal artery using vein graft NEC
Includes: *Bypass of femoral artery by anastomosis of femoral artery to peroneal artery NEC*
          Popliteal artery

L59.8   Other specified
L59.9   Unspecified

L60   **Reconstruction of femoral artery**
Note at L56 applies
Includes: *Popliteal artery*

L60.1   Endarterectomy of femoral artery and patch repair of femoral artery
L60.2   Endarterectomy of femoral artery NEC
L60.3   Profundoplasty of femoral artery and patch repair of deep femoral artery
L60.4   Profundoplasty of femoral artery NEC
L60.8   Other specified
L60.9   Unspecified

L62   **Other open operations on femoral artery**
Note at L56 applies
Includes: *Popliteal artery*

L62.1   Repair of femoral artery NEC
L62.2   Open embolectomy of femoral artery
Includes: *Open thrombectomy of femoral artery*
          Embolectomy of femoral artery NEC
          Thrombectomy of femoral artery NEC
L62.3   Ligation of aneurysm of popliteal artery
L62.4   Operations on aneurysm of femoral artery NEC
L62.8   Other specified
L62.9   Unspecified

L63 **Transluminal operations on femoral artery**
Note at L56 applies
Includes: Popliteal artery

L63.1 Percutaneous transluminal angioplasty of femoral artery
Includes: Percutaneous transluminal balloon angioplasty of femoral artery
L63.2 Percutaneous transluminal embolectomy of femoral artery
Includes: Percutaneous transluminal thrombectomy of femoral artery
L63.3 Percutaneous transluminal embolisation of femoral artery
Includes: Embolisation of femoral artery NEC
L63.4 Arteriography of femoral artery
L63.5 Percutaneous transluminal insertion of stent into femoral artery
Note: Use a supplementary code for placement of stent (L76, L89, O20)
L63.8 Other specified
L63.9 Unspecified

L65 **Revision of reconstruction of artery**
Note at L56 applies

L65.1 Revision of reconstruction involving aorta
L65.2 Revision of reconstruction involving iliac artery
L65.3 Revision of reconstruction involving femoral artery
L65.8 Other specified
L65.9 Unspecified

L66 **Other therapeutic transluminal operations on artery**
Note: Principal L71

L66.1 Percutaneous transluminal arterial thrombolysis and reconstruction
Includes: Percutaneous transluminal thrombolysis with angioplasty of artery
Percutaneous transluminal thrombolysis with placement of stent into artery
Note: Use a supplementary code for placement of stent (L76, L89, O20)
L66.2 Percutaneous transluminal stent reconstruction of artery
Note: Use a supplementary code for placement of stent (L76, L89, O20)
L66.3 Percutaneous transluminal occlusion of artery
L66.4 Percutaneous transluminal balloon test occlusion of artery
L66.5 Percutaneous transluminal balloon angioplasty of artery
Includes: Percutaneous transluminal cutting balloon angioplasty of artery
L66.7 Percutaneous transluminal placement of peripheral stent in artery
Note: Use a supplementary code for placement of stent (L76, L89, O20)
L66.8 Other specified
L66.9 Unspecified

L67 **Excision of other artery**
Includes: Unspecified artery
Note: These codes should not normally be used when more specific site codes may be identified (L01–L65)

L67.1 Biopsy of artery NEC
L67.8 Other specified
L67.9 Unspecified

L68   **Repair of other artery**
Note at L67 applies
Includes: Unspecified artery

L68.1   Endarterectomy and patch repair of artery NEC
L68.2   Endarterectomy NEC
L68.3   Repair of artery using prosthesis NEC
L68.4   Repair of artery using vein graft NEC
Includes: Repair of artery using graft NEC
L68.8   Other specified
L68.9   Unspecified

L69   **Operations on major systemic to pulmonary collateral arteries**

L69.1   Major systemic to pulmonary collateral artery occlusion
L69.2   Pulmonary unifocalisation
L69.3   Percutaneous transluminal embolisation of major systemic to pulmonary collateral artery
L69.4   Percutaneous transluminal balloon angioplasty of major systemic to pulmonary collateral artery
L69.5   Percutaneous transluminal insertion of stent into major systemic to pulmonary collateral artery
Note: Use a supplementary code for placement of stent (L76, L89, O20)
L69.8   Other specified
L69.9   Unspecified

L70   **Other open operations on other artery**
Note at L67 applies
Includes: Unspecified artery

L70.1   Open embolectomy of artery NEC
Includes: Open thrombectomy of artery NEC
Embolectomy of artery NEC
Thrombectomy of artery NEC
L70.2   Open embolisation of artery NEC
L70.3   Ligation of artery NEC
L70.4   Open cannulation of artery
L70.5   Operations on aneurysm of artery NEC
L70.8   Other specified
L70.9   Unspecified

L71   **Therapeutic transluminal operations on other artery**
Note at L67 applies
Includes: Unspecified artery
Note: Principal category, extended at L66

L71.1   Percutaneous transluminal angioplasty of artery
L71.2   Percutaneous transluminal embolectomy of artery
Includes: Percutaneous transluminal thrombectomy of artery
L71.3   Percutaneous transluminal embolisation of artery
Includes: Percutaneous transluminal chemoembolisation of artery
L71.4   Percutaneous transluminal cannulation of artery
L71.5   Percutaneous transluminal dilation of artery
L71.6   Percutaneous transluminal thrombolysis of artery
Includes: Percutaneous transluminal Streptokinase thrombolysis of artery
Excludes: Percutaneous transluminal thrombolysis of artery and reconstruction (L66.1)
L71.7   Percutaneous transluminal atherectomy
L71.8   Other specified
L71.9   Unspecified

L72   **Diagnostic transluminal operations on other artery**
Note at L67 applies
Includes: *Unspecified artery*

L72.1	Arteriography NEC
L72.2	Monitoring of arterial pressure
L72.3	Percutaneous transluminal angioscopy NEC
L72.5	Stimulated arteriography of pancreas
L72.6	Intravascular ultrasound of artery NEC
L72.8	Other specified
L72.9	Unspecified

L73   **Mechanical embolic protection of blood vessel**
Excludes: *Endovascular placement of metallic stent with mechanical embolic protection (L76.7)*

L73.1	Mechanical embolic protection NEC
L73.2	Mechanical embolic protection of artery
L73.3	Mechanical embolic protection of vein
L73.8	Other specified
L73.9	Unspecified

L74   **Arteriovenous shunt**

L74.1	Insertion of arteriovenous prosthesis
L74.2	Creation of arteriovenous fistula NEC
L74.3	Attention to arteriovenous shunt
L74.4	Banding of arteriovenous fistula
L74.5	Thrombectomy of arteriovenous fistula
	Includes: *Thrombectomy of synthetic graft*
L74.6	Creation of graft fistula for dialysis
L74.7	Injection of radiocontrast substance into arteriovenous fistula
	Includes: *Fistulography of arteriovenous fistula*
L74.8	Other specified
L74.9	Unspecified

L75   **Other arteriovenous operations**
Excludes: *Operations on dural arteriovenous fistula (O05)*

L75.1	Excision of congenital arteriovenous malformation
	Includes: *Ligation of congenital arteriovenous malformation*
L75.2	Repair of acquired arteriovenous fistula
	Includes: *Ligation of acquired arteriovenous fistula*
L75.3	Embolisation of arteriovenous abnormality NEC
L75.4	Percutaneous transluminal embolisation of arteriovenous malformation NEC
L75.5	Percutaneous transluminal venous embolisation of arteriovenous malformation
L75.6	Percutaneous transluminal arterial and venous embolisation of arteriovenous malformation
L75.8	Other specified
L75.9	Unspecified

L76   **Endovascular placement of stent**
> *Note: Principal category, extended at L89*
> *Codes in this category are not intended as primary codes. They may be used in a supplementary position with codes from Chapter L*

L76.1   Endovascular placement of one metallic stent
L76.2   Endovascular placement of one plastic stent
L76.3   Endovascular placement of two metallic stents
L76.4   Endovascular placement of two plastic stents
L76.5   Endovascular placement of three or more metallic stents
L76.6   Endovascular placement of three or more plastic stents
L76.7   Endovascular placement of metallic stent with mechanical embolic protection
> *Excludes: Mechanical embolic protection of blood vessel NEC (L73)*

L76.8   Other specified
L76.9   Unspecified

L77   **Connection of vena cava or branch of vena cava**

L77.1   Creation of portocaval shunt
L77.2   Creation of mesocaval shunt
L77.3   Creation of portosystemic shunt NEC
> *Excludes: Transjugular intrahepatic creation of portosystemic shunt (J11.4)*

L77.4   Creation of distal splenorenal shunt
L77.5   Creation of proximal splenorenal shunt
L77.8   Other specified
L77.9   Unspecified

L79   **Other operations on vena cava**

L79.1   Insertion of filter into vena cava
L79.2   Plication of vena cava
L79.3   Insertion of stent into vena cava NEC
> *Note: Use a supplementary code for placement of stent (L76, L89, O20)*

L79.4   Attention to filter into vena cava NEC
L79.5   Removal of filter in vena cava
L79.6   Repair of anomalous caval vein connection
L79.7   Excision of lesion of vena cava
L79.8   Other specified
L79.9   Unspecified

L80   **Operations on individual pulmonary veins**
> *Excludes: Percutaneous transluminal ablation of pulmonary vein to left atrium conducting system (K62.1)*

L80.1   Repair of pulmonary vein stenosis
L80.2   Percutaneous transluminal balloon angioplasty of pulmonary vein
L80.3   Percutaneous transluminal cutting balloon angioplasty of pulmonary vein
L80.4   Percutaneous transluminal insertion of stent into pulmonary vein
> *Note: Use a supplementary code for placement of stent (L76, L89, O20)*

L80.8   Other specified
L80.9   Unspecified

L81   **Other bypass operations on vein**

L81.1   Creation of peritovenous shunt
L81.2   Bypass operations for priapism
L81.8   Other specified
L81.9   Unspecified

L82   **Repair of valve of vein**

L82.1   Transposition of valve of vein
L82.2   Interposition of valve of vein
L82.8   Other specified
L82.9   Unspecified

L83   **Other operations for venous insufficiency**

L83.1   Crossover graft of saphenous vein
L83.2   Subfascial ligation of perforating vein of leg
L83.8   Other specified
L83.9   Unspecified

L84   **Combined operations on varicose vein of leg**

L84.1   Combined operations on primary long saphenous vein
L84.2   Combined operations on primary short saphenous vein
L84.3   Combined operations on primary long and short saphenous vein
L84.4   Combined operations on recurrent long saphenous vein
L84.5   Combined operations on recurrent short saphenous vein
L84.6   Combined operations on recurrent long and short saphenous vein
L84.8   Other specified
L84.9   Unspecified

L85   **Ligation of varicose vein of leg**
              Excludes: Combined operations on varicose vein of leg (L84)

L85.1   Ligation of long saphenous vein
L85.2   Ligation of short saphenous vein
L85.3   Ligation of recurrent varicose vein of leg
L85.8   Other specified
L85.9   Unspecified

L86   **Injection into varicose vein of leg**

L86.1   Injection of sclerosing substance into varicose vein of leg NEC
L86.2   Ultrasound guided foam sclerotherapy for varicose vein of leg
L86.8   Other specified
L86.9   Unspecified

L87   **Other operations on varicose vein of leg**
              Excludes: Combined operations on varicose vein of leg (L84)

L87.1   Stripping of long saphenous vein
L87.2   Stripping of short saphenous vein
L87.3   Stripping of varicose vein of leg NEC
L87.4   Avulsion of varicose vein of leg
L87.5   Local excision of varicose vein of leg
L87.6   Incision of varicose vein of leg
L87.7   Transilluminated powered phlebectomy of varicose vein of leg
L87.8   Other specified
L87.9   Unspecified

L88   **Transluminal operations on varicose vein of leg**

L88.1   Percutaneous transluminal laser ablation of long saphenous vein
L88.2   Radiofrequency ablation of varicose vein of leg
L88.3   Percutaneous transluminal laser ablation of varicose vein of leg NEC
L88.8   Other specified
L88.9   Unspecified

L89   **Other endovascular placement of stent**

> *Note: Principal L76*
> *Codes in this category are not intended as primary codes. They may be used in a supplementary position with codes from Chapter L*

L89.1   Endovascular placement of two drug-eluting stents
L89.2   Endovascular placement of two coated stents
L89.3   Endovascular placement of three or more drug-eluting stents
L89.4   Endovascular placement of three or more coated stents
L89.5   Endovascular placement of one drug-eluting stent
L89.6   Endovascular placement of one coated stent
L89.8   Other specified
L89.9   Unspecified

L90   **Open removal of thrombus from vein**

L90.1   Open thrombectomy of vein of upper limb
L90.2   Open thrombectomy of vein of lower limb
L90.3   Open thrombectomy of renal vein
L90.8   Other specified
L90.9   Unspecified

L91   **Other vein related operations**

L91.1   Open insertion of central venous catheter
L91.2   Insertion of central venous catheter NEC
> *Includes: Insertion of non-tunnelled venous catheter*
> *Excludes: Percutaneous transluminal insertion of subcutaneous port (L94.3)*
> *Percutaneous transluminal peripheral insertion of central catheter (L99.7)*
> *Insertion of umbilical venous catheter (O15.2)*
> *Insertion of umbilical arterial catheter (O15.3)*
L91.3   Attention to central venous catheter NEC
> *Includes: Linogram of central venous catheter*
L91.4   Removal of central venous catheter
L91.5   Insertion of tunnelled venous catheter
L91.6   Cannulation of vein NEC
L91.8   Other specified
L91.9   Unspecified

L92   **Unblocking of access catheter**

L92.1   Fibrin sheath stripping of access catheter
L92.2   Wire brushing of access catheter
L92.3   Thrombolysis of access catheter
L92.8   Other specified
L92.9   Unspecified

L93   **Other open operations on vein**
          Excludes: Operations on varicocele (N19)

L93.1   Excision of vein NEC
          Includes: Biopsy of vein
L93.2   Incision of vein NEC
L93.3   Ligation of vein NEC
L93.4   Open cannulation of vein
L93.5   Vein graft
          Note: Use as a supplementary code when associated with concurrent microvascular free tissue transfer of flap of muscle (T76.1)
L93.6   Excision of lesion of vein NEC
L93.8   Other specified
L93.9   Unspecified

L94   **Therapeutic transluminal operations on vein**
          Note: Principal category, extended at L99

L94.1   Percutaneous transluminal embolisation of vein
          Includes: Percutaneous transluminal chemoembolisation of vein
L94.2   Percutaneous transluminal cannulation of vein
L94.3   Percutaneous transluminal insertion of subcutaneous port
L94.4   Percutaneous transluminal replacement of subcutaneous port
L94.5   Percutaneous transluminal insertion of stent into vein NEC
          Note: Use a supplementary code for placement of stent (L76, L89, O20)
L94.6   Percutaneous transluminal venoplasty
L94.7   Percutaneous transluminal balloon angioplasty of vein NEC
          Includes: Percutaneous transluminal cutting balloon angioplasty of vein
          Excludes: Percutaneous transluminal angioplasty of vein NEC (L99.1)
L94.8   Other specified
L94.9   Unspecified

L95   **Diagnostic transluminal operations on vein**

L95.1   Venography
L95.2   Monitoring of venous pressure NEC
L95.8   Other specified
L95.9   Unspecified

L96   **Percutaneous removal of thrombus from vein**

L96.1   Percutaneous mechanical thromboembolectomy
L96.2   Percutaneous aspiration thromboembolectomy
L96.8   Other specified
L96.9   Unspecified

L97   **Other operations on blood vessel**
          Note: Principal category, extended at O15

L97.1   Revascularisation for impotence
L97.2   Peroperative angioplasty
L97.3   Isolated limb perfusion
L97.4   Operations on artery NEC
L97.5   Operations on vein NEC
L97.6   Insertion of vascular closure device
L97.7   Thrombin injection for pseudoaneurysm
L97.8   Other specified
L97.9   Unspecified

L98   **Operations on microvascular vessel**

L98.1   Microvascular vessel anastomosis
L98.2   Microvascular lymphatic vessel anastomosis
L98.3   Microvascular lymphatico-venous anastomosis
L98.4   Anastomosis of vessel using microvascular anastomotic device
L98.5   Revision of microvascular vessel anastomosis
L98.6   Placement of doppler ultrasound probe into microvascular vessel anastomosis
L98.8   Other specified
L98.9   Unspecified

L99   **Other therapeutic transluminal operations on vein**
             Note: Principal L94

L99.1   Percutaneous transluminal angioplasty of vein NEC
             Excludes: Percutaneous transluminal balloon angioplasty of vein (L94.7)
                         Percutaneous transluminal cutting balloon angioplasty of vein (L94.7)
L99.2   Percutaneous transluminal stent reconstruction of vein
             Note: Use a supplementary code for placement of stent (L76, L89, O20)
L99.3   Percutaneous transluminal venous thrombolysis with reconstruction
             Includes: Percutaneous transluminal thrombolysis with angioplasty of vein NEC
                         Percutaneous transluminal thrombolysis with placement of stent into
                         vein NEC
             Note: Use a supplementary code for placement of stent (L76, L89, O20)
L99.4   Percutaneous transluminal venous thrombolysis NEC
L99.5   Percutaneous transluminal occlusion of vein NEC
L99.6   Percutaneous transluminal balloon test occlusion of vein
L99.7   Percutaneous transluminal peripheral insertion of central catheter
L99.8   Other specified
L99.9   Unspecified

O01   **Transluminal coil embolisation of aneurysm of artery**
             Excludes: Transluminal balloon assisted coil embolisation of aneurysm of artery (O02)
                         Transluminal stent assisted coil embolisation of aneurysm of artery (O03)
             Note: Use a subsidiary site code as necessary

O01.1   Percutaneous transluminal coil embolisation of small aneurysm of artery
O01.2   Percutaneous transluminal coil embolisation of medium aneurysm of artery
O01.3   Percutaneous transluminal coil embolisation of large aneurysm of artery
O01.4   Percutaneous transluminal coil embolisation of giant aneurysm of artery
O01.8   Other specified
O01.9   Unspecified

O02   **Transluminal balloon assisted coil embolisation of aneurysm of artery**
             Excludes: Transluminal coil embolisation of aneurysm of artery (O01)
                         Transluminal stent assisted coil embolisation of aneurysm of artery (O03)
             Note: Use a subsidiary site code as necessary

O02.1   Percutaneous transluminal balloon assisted coil embolisation of three or more aneurysms
             of artery
O02.2   Percutaneous transluminal balloon assisted coil embolisation of two aneurysms of artery
O02.3   Percutaneous transluminal balloon assisted coil embolisation of single aneurysm of artery
O02.8   Other specified
O02.9   Unspecified

O03   **Transluminal stent assisted coil embolisation of aneurysm of artery**
Excludes: *Transluminal coil embolisation of aneurysm of artery (O01)*
                 Transluminal balloon assisted coil embolisation of aneurysm of artery (O02)
       Note: **Use a subsidiary site code as necessary**

O03.1   Percutaneous transluminal stent assisted coil embolisation of three or more aneurysms of artery
O03.2   Percutaneous transluminal stent assisted coil embolisation of two aneurysms of artery
O03.3   Percutaneous transluminal stent assisted coil embolisation of single aneurysm of artery
O03.8   Other specified
O03.9   Unspecified

O04   **Other transluminal embolisation of aneurysm of artery**
       Note: **Use a subsidiary site code as necessary**

O04.1   Percutaneous transluminal liquid polymer embolisation of aneurysm of artery
O04.2   Percutaneous transluminal stent assisted liquid polymer embolisation of aneurysm of artery
O04.8   Other specified
O04.9   Unspecified

O05   **Operations on dural arteriovenous fistula**

O05.1   Percutaneous transluminal arterial and venous embolisation of dural arteriovenous fistula
O05.2   Percutaneous transluminal arterial embolisation of dural arteriovenous fistula
O05.3   Percutaneous transluminal venous embolisation of dural arteriovenous fistula
O05.8   Other specified
O05.9   Unspecified

O15   **Operations on blood vessel**
       Note: **Principal L97**

O15.1   Duplex ultrasound guided compression of pseudoaneurysm
O15.2   Insertion of umbilical venous catheter
O15.3   Insertion of umbilical arterial catheter
O15.8   Other specified
O15.9   Unspecified

O20   **Endovascular placement of stent graft**
       Note: **Codes in this category are not intended as primary codes. They may be used in a supplementary position with codes from Chapter L**

O20.1   Endovascular placement of one branched stent graft
O20.2   Endovascular placement of one fenestrated stent graft
O20.3   Endovascular placement of one stent graft NEC
O20.4   Endovascular placement of two stent grafts
O20.5   Endovascular placement of three or more stent grafts
O20.8   Other specified
O20.9   Unspecified

CHAPTER M
URINARY
(CODES M01–M86)

Includes: *PROSTATE*
Excludes: *PENIS (except URETHRAL ORIFICE)*   *(Chapter N)*
           OPERATIONS FOR DISORDERS OF SEX DEVELOPMENT   *(Chapter X)*
           OPERATIONS FOR SEXUAL TRANSFORMATION   *(Chapter X)*
      Note: **Use a subsidiary code for minimal access approach (Y74–Y76)**
               Use a subsidiary code to identify method of image control (Y53)

M01   **Transplantation of kidney**

M01.1   Autotransplantation of kidney
M01.2   Allotransplantation of kidney from live donor
               Note: **Use a subsidiary code to identify donor status (Y99)**
M01.3   Allotransplantation of kidney from cadaver NEC
M01.4   Allotransplantation of kidney from cadaver heart beating
M01.5   Allotransplantation of kidney from cadaver heart non-beating
M01.8   Other specified
M01.9   Unspecified

M02   **Total excision of kidney**

M02.1   Nephrectomy and excision of perirenal tissue
            Includes: *Nephroureterectomy and excision of perirenal tissue*
M02.2   Nephroureterectomy NEC
M02.3   Bilateral nephrectomy
M02.4   Excision of half of horseshoe kidney
M02.5   Nephrectomy NEC
M02.6   Excision of rejected transplanted kidney
M02.7   Excision of transplanted kidney NEC
M02.8   Other specified
M02.9   Unspecified

M03   **Partial excision of kidney**

M03.1   Heminephrectomy of duplex kidney
M03.2   Division of isthmus of horseshoe kidney
M03.8   Other specified
M03.9   Unspecified
            Includes: *Partial nephrectomy NEC*

M04   **Open extirpation of lesion of kidney**

M04.1   Deroofing of cyst of kidney
M04.2   Open excision of lesion of kidney NEC
M04.3   Open destruction of lesion of kidney
M04.8   Other specified
M04.9   Unspecified

M05   **Open repair of kidney**

M05.1   Open pyeloplasty
M05.2   Open revision of pyeloplasty
M05.3   Nephropexy
M05.4   Plication of kidney
               Note: **Use an additional code for coincidental translocation of branch of renal artery (L41.5)**
M05.5   Repair of laceration of kidney
M05.8   Other specified
M05.9   Unspecified

M06	**Incision of kidney**

M06   **Incision of kidney**
         Includes: Pelvis of kidney

M06.1   Open removal of calculus from kidney
         Includes: Nephrolithotomy
                     Pyelolithotomy
         Excludes: Percutaneous nephrolithotomy (M16.4)

M06.2   Drainage of kidney NEC
         Includes: Nephrostomy NEC
                     Insertion of nephrostomy tube NEC
         Excludes: Percutaneous insertion of nephrostomy tube (M13.6)

M06.3   Closure of nephrostomy
M06.4   Attention to nephrostomy tube NEC
M06.8   Other specified
M06.9   Unspecified

M08   **Other open operations on kidney**
         Includes: Pelvis of kidney

M08.1   Open biopsy of lesion of kidney
         Includes: Open biopsy of kidney
M08.2   Open denervation of kidney
M08.3   Exploration of kidney
M08.4   Exploration of transplanted kidney
M08.8   Other specified
M08.9   Unspecified

M09   **Therapeutic endoscopic operations on calculus of kidney**
         Includes: Nephroscopic percutaneous lithotripsy of calculus of kidney
                     Percutaneous lithotripsy of calculus of kidney NEC
         Note: It is not necessary to code additionally any mention of diagnostic endoscopic examination of kidney (M11.9)

M09.1   Endoscopic ultrasound fragmentation of calculus of kidney
M09.2   Endoscopic electrohydraulic shockwave fragmentation of calculus of kidney
M09.3   Endoscopic laser fragmentation of calculus of kidney
M09.4   Endoscopic extraction of calculus of kidney NEC
M09.8   Other specified
M09.9   Unspecified

M10   **Other therapeutic endoscopic operations on kidney**
         Note: It is not necessary to code additionally any mention of diagnostic endoscopic examination of kidney (M11.9)

M10.1   Endoscopic extirpation of lesion of kidney NEC
         Includes: Enucleation of lesion of kidney
M10.2   Endoscopic pyeloplasty
M10.3   Endoscopic deroofing of multiple cysts of kidney
M10.4   Endoscopic cryoablation of lesion of kidney
M10.5   Endoscopic endoluminal balloon rupture of stenosis of pelviureteric junction of kidney
M10.8   Other specified
M10.9   Unspecified

M11 **Diagnostic endoscopic examination of kidney**

M11.1   Diagnostic endoscopic examination of kidney and biopsy of lesion of kidney NEC
       Includes: *Diagnostic endoscopic examination of kidney and biopsy of kidney NEC*
                       Endoscopic biopsy of lesion of kidney NEC
                       Endoscopic biopsy of kidney NEC

M11.2   Diagnostic endoscopic retrograde examination of kidney and biopsy of lesion of kidney
       Includes: *Diagnostic endoscopic retrograde examination of kidney and biopsy of kidney*
                       Endoscopic retrograde biopsy of lesion of kidney
                       Endoscopic retrograde biopsy of kidney

M11.3   Diagnostic endoscopic retrograde examination of kidney NEC
       Includes: *Ureterorenoscopy NEC*

M11.8   Other specified

M11.9   Unspecified
       Includes: *Nephroscopy NEC*

M12 **Percutaneous studies of upper urinary tract**

M12.1   Percutaneous pyeloureterodynamics
M12.8   Other specified
M12.9   Unspecified

M13 **Percutaneous puncture of kidney**
       Includes: *Pelvis of kidney*

M13.1   Percutaneous needle biopsy of lesion of kidney
       Includes: *Percutaneous needle biopsy of kidney*
                       Biopsy of lesion of kidney NEC
                       Biopsy of kidney NEC

M13.2   Percutaneous drainage of kidney
M13.3   Percutaneous aspiration of kidney NEC
M13.4   Percutaneous injection of therapeutic substance into kidney
M13.5   Percutaneous injection of radiocontrast substance into kidney
       Includes: *Antegrade pyelography*
M13.6   Percutaneous insertion of nephrostomy tube
M13.7   Percutaneous radiofrequency ablation of lesion of kidney
M13.8   Other specified
M13.9   Unspecified

M14 **Extracorporeal fragmentation of calculus of kidney**

M14.1   Extracorporeal shock wave lithotripsy of calculus of kidney
M14.8   Other specified
M14.9   Unspecified

M15 **Operations on kidney along nephrostomy tube track**

M15.1   Nephrostomography
M15.8   Other specified
M15.9   Unspecified

M16   **Other operations on kidney**
            Excludes: Renal dialysis (X40.1)

M16.1   Irrigation of kidney
M16.2   Maintenance of drainage tube of kidney
            Includes: Maintenance of nephrostomy tube
M16.4   Percutaneous nephrolithotomy NEC
M16.5   Removal of nephrostomy tube
M16.8   Other specified
M16.9   Unspecified

M17   **Interventions associated with transplantation of kidney**

M17.1   Live kidney donor screening
M17.2   Pre-transplantation of kidney work-up – recipient
M17.3   Pre-transplantation of kidney work-up – live donor
M17.4   Post-transplantation of kidney examination – recipient
M17.5   Post-transplantation of kidney examination – live donor
M17.8   Other specified
M17.9   Unspecified

M18   **Excision of ureter**

M18.1   Total ureterectomy
            Includes: Ureterectomy NEC
M18.2   Excision of segment of ureter
M18.3   Secondary ureterectomy
M18.4   Excision of duplex ureter
M18.8   Other specified
M18.9   Unspecified

M19   **Urinary diversion**

M19.1   Construction of ileal conduit
            Note: Use as a supplementary code when associated with concurrent total excision of bladder (M34)
M19.2   Creation of urinary diversion to intestine NEC
            Note: Use as a supplementary code when associated with concurrent total excision of bladder (M34)
M19.3   Revision of urinary diversion
            Includes: Revision of ileal conduit
            Urinary undiversion
M19.4   Cutaneous ureterostomy NEC
M19.5   Revision of ureterostomy stoma
M19.6   Percutaneous tunnelled kidney to bladder bypass using prosthesis
M19.8   Other specified
M19.9   Unspecified

M20   **Replantation of ureter**

M20.1   Bilateral replantation of ureter
M20.2   Unilateral replantation of ureter
M20.3   Replantation of ureter after urinary diversion
M20.8   Other specified
M20.9   Unspecified

M21 Other connection of ureter

M21.1	Direct anastomosis of ureter to bladder
M21.2	Anastomosis of ureter to bladder using flap of bladder
M21.3	Ileal replacement of ureter
M21.4	Colonic replacement of ureter
M21.5	Revision of anastomosis of ureter NEC
M21.6	Ureteroureterostomy
M21.8	Other specified
M21.9	Unspecified

M22 Repair of ureter

M22.1	Suture of ureter
M22.2	Removal of ligature from ureter
M22.3	Closure of ureteric fistula
M22.8	Other specified
M22.9	Unspecified

M23 Incision of ureter

M23.1	Open ureterolithotomy
M23.8	Other specified
M23.9	Unspecified

M25 Other open operations on ureter

M25.1	Excision of ureterocele
M25.2	Open excision of lesion of ureter NEC
M25.3	Ureterolysis
M25.4	Open biopsy of lesion of ureter
	Includes: Open biopsy of ureter
M25.5	Open exploration of ureter
M25.8	Other specified
M25.9	Unspecified

M26 Therapeutic nephroscopic operations on ureter

Note: It is not necessary to code additionally any mention of diagnostic endoscopic examination of ureter (M30.9)

M26.1	Nephroscopic laser fragmentation of calculus of ureter
M26.2	Nephroscopic fragmentation of calculus of ureter NEC
M26.3	Nephroscopic extraction of calculus of ureter
M26.4	Nephroscopic insertion of tubal prosthesis into ureter
M26.8	Other specified
M26.9	Unspecified

M27   **Therapeutic ureteroscopic operations on ureter**
             Note: *It is not necessary to code additionally any mention of diagnostic endoscopic*
                       examination of ureter (M30.9)

M27.1   Ureteroscopic laser fragmentation of calculus of ureter
M27.2   Ureteroscopic fragmentation of calculus of ureter NEC
M27.3   Ureteroscopic extraction of calculus of ureter
M27.4   Ureteroscopic insertion of ureteric stent
         Includes: *Ureteroscopic insertion of ureteric stent using guide catheter*
M27.5   Ureteroscopic removal of ureteric stent
         Includes: *Ureteroscopic removal of ureteric stent using guide catheter*
                       Ureteroscopic removal of ureteric stent using snare
M27.6   Ureteroscopic endoluminal balloon rupture of stenosis of ureter
M27.7   Ureteroscopic dilation of ureter
M27.8   Other specified
M27.9   Unspecified

M28   **Other endoscopic removal of calculus from ureter**
             Includes: *Cystoscopic removal of calculus from ureter*
             Note: *It is not necessary to code additionally any mention of diagnostic endoscopic*
                       examination of ureter (M30.9)

M28.1   Endoscopic laser fragmentation of calculus of ureter NEC
M28.2   Endoscopic fragmentation of calculus of ureter NEC
M28.3   Endoscopic extraction of calculus of ureter NEC
M28.4   Endoscopic catheter drainage of calculus of ureter
M28.5   Endoscopic drainage of calculus of ureter by dilation of ureter
M28.8   Other specified
M28.9   Unspecified

M29   **Other therapeutic endoscopic operations on ureter**
             Includes: *Therapeutic cystoscopic operations on ureter NEC*
             Note: *It is not necessary to code additionally any mention of diagnostic endoscopic*
                       examination of ureter (M30.9)

M29.1   Endoscopic extirpation of lesion of ureter
M29.2   Endoscopic insertion of tubal prosthesis into ureter NEC
         Excludes: Ureteroscopic insertion of ureteric stent (M27.4)
M29.3   Endoscopic removal of tubal prosthesis from ureter
         Excludes: Ureteroscopic removal of ureteric stent (M27.5)
M29.4   Endoscopic dilation of ureter
         Excludes: Ureteroscopic dilation of ureter (M27.7)
M29.5   Endoscopic renewal of tubal prosthesis into ureter
         Excludes: Ureteroscopic renewal of ureteric stent (M27)
M29.8   Other specified
M29.9   Unspecified

M30   **Diagnostic endoscopic examination of ureter**
           *Note: Use as a supplementary code when associated with diagnostic endoscopic
           examination of bladder (M45)*

M30.1   Endoscopic retrograde pyelography
M30.2   Endoscopic catheterisation of ureter
M30.3   Endoscopic ureteric urine sampling
M30.4   Nephroscopic ureteroscopy
M30.5   Diagnostic endoscopic examination of ureter and biopsy of lesion of ureter NEC
           *Includes: Diagnostic endoscopic examination of ureter and biopsy of ureter NEC
           Endoscopic biopsy of lesion of ureter NEC
           Endoscopic biopsy of ureter NEC
           Biopsy of lesion of ureter NEC
           Biopsy of ureter NEC*
M30.6   Diagnostic endoscopic examination of ureter and biopsy of lesion of ureter using rigid
           ureteroscope
           *Includes: Diagnostic endoscopic examination of ureter and biopsy of ureter using rigid
           ureteroscope
           Endoscopic biopsy of lesion of ureter using rigid ureteroscope
           Endoscopic biopsy of ureter using rigid ureteroscope*
M30.8   Other specified
M30.9   Unspecified
           Includes: Ureteroscopy NEC

M31   **Extracorporeal fragmentation of calculus of ureter**

M31.1   Extracorporeal shockwave lithotripsy of calculus of ureter
M31.8   Other specified
M31.9   Unspecified

M32   **Operations on ureteric orifice**
           *Note: It is not necessary to code additionally any mention of diagnostic endoscopic
           examination of ureter (M30.9)*

M32.1   Endoscopic extirpation of lesion of ureteric orifice
M32.2   Endoscopic meatotomy of ureteric orifice
M32.3   Endoscopic injection of inert substance around ureteric orifice
M32.4   Endoscopic dilation of ureteric orifice
M32.5   Endoscopic incision of ureterocele
M32.6   Endoscopic transurethral resection of ureteric orifice
M32.8   Other specified
M32.9   Unspecified

M33   **Percutaneous ureteric stent procedures**

M33.1   Percutaneous insertion of metallic stent into ureter
M33.2   Percutaneous insertion of plastic stent into ureter
M33.3   Percutaneous replacement of metallic stent into ureter
M33.4   Percutaneous replacement of plastic stent into ureter
M33.5   Percutaneous insertion of ureteric stent into ureter NEC
M33.6   Percutaneous removal of ureteric stent from ureter NEC
M33.8   Other specified
M33.9   Unspecified

M34   **Total excision of bladder**
   Note: Use a supplementary code for concurrent construction of ileal conduit (M19.1)

M34.1   Cystoprostatectomy
M34.2   Cystourethrectomy
M34.3   Cystectomy NEC
M34.4   Simple cystectomy
M34.8   Other specified
M34.9   Unspecified

M35   **Partial excision of bladder**

M35.1   Diverticulectomy of bladder
M35.8   Other specified
M35.9   Unspecified
   Includes: Partial cystectomy NEC

M36   **Enlargement of bladder**

M36.1   Caecocystoplasty
M36.2   Ileocystoplasty
M36.3   Colocystoplasty
M36.8   Other specified
M36.9   Unspecified

M37   **Other repair of bladder**
   Excludes: Reconstruction of neck of male bladder NEC (M64.6)
   Reconstruction of neck of female bladder NEC (M54.2)

M37.1   Cystourethroplasty
M37.2   Repair of vesicocolic fistula
M37.3   Repair of rupture of bladder
M37.4   Closure of exstrophy
M37.5   Repair of fistula of bladder NEC
M37.8   Other specified
M37.9   Unspecified

M38   **Open drainage of bladder**

M38.1   Perineal urethrostomy and drainage of bladder
M38.2   Cystostomy and insertion of suprapubic tube into bladder
M38.3   Cystostomy NEC
M38.8   Other specified
M38.9   Unspecified

M39   **Other open operations on contents of bladder**

M39.1   Open removal of calculus from bladder
M39.2   Open removal of foreign body from bladder
M39.8   Other specified
M39.9   Unspecified

M41　　　　**Other open operations on bladder**

M41.1　　　Open extirpation of lesion of bladder
M41.2　　　Creation of vesicovaginal fistula
M41.3　　　Open transection of bladder
M41.4　　　Open biopsy of lesion of bladder
　　　　　　　Includes:　Open biopsy of bladder
M41.5　　　Exploration of bladder
M41.6　　　Detrusor myotomy
M41.8　　　Other specified
M41.9　　　Unspecified

M42　　　　**Endoscopic extirpation of lesion of bladder**
　　　　　　　Note:　It is not necessary to code additionally any mention of diagnostic endoscopic
　　　　　　　　　　　examination of bladder (M45.5, M45.9)

M42.1　　　Endoscopic resection of lesion of bladder
M42.2　　　Endoscopic cauterisation of lesion of bladder
M42.3　　　Endoscopic destruction of lesion of bladder NEC
M42.8　　　Other specified
M42.9　　　Unspecified

M43　　　　**Endoscopic operations to increase capacity of bladder**
　　　　　　　Note:　It is not necessary to code additionally any mention of diagnostic endoscopic
　　　　　　　　　　　examination of bladder (M45.5, M45.9)

M43.1　　　Endoscopic transection of bladder
M43.2　　　Endoscopic hydrostatic distension of bladder
M43.3　　　Endoscopic overdistension of bladder NEC
M43.4　　　Endoscopic injection of neurolytic substance into nerve of bladder
M43.8　　　Other specified
M43.9　　　Unspecified

M44　　　　**Other therapeutic endoscopic operations on bladder**
　　　　　　　Note:　It is not necessary to code additionally any mention of diagnostic endoscopic
　　　　　　　　　　　examination of bladder (M45.5, M45.9)

M44.1　　　Endoscopic lithopaxy
M44.2　　　Endoscopic extraction of calculus of bladder NEC
M44.3　　　Endoscopic removal of foreign body from bladder
M44.4　　　Endoscopic removal of blood clot from bladder
M44.8　　　Other specified
M44.9　　　Unspecified

M45   **Diagnostic endoscopic examination of bladder**
Includes: *Prostate (M45.2)*
        Note: ***Use a supplementary code for diagnostic endoscopic examination of ureter (M30)***

M45.1   Diagnostic endoscopic examination of bladder and biopsy of lesion of bladder NEC
        Includes: *Diagnostic endoscopic examination of bladder and biopsy of bladder NEC*
                   Endoscopic biopsy of lesion of bladder NEC
                   Endoscopic biopsy of bladder NEC
                   Biopsy of lesion of bladder NEC
                   Biopsy of bladder NEC

M45.2   Diagnostic endoscopic examination of bladder and biopsy of lesion of prostate NEC
        Includes: *Diagnostic endoscopic examination of bladder and biopsy of prostate NEC*
                   Endoscopic biopsy of lesion of prostate NEC
                   Endoscopic biopsy of prostate NEC

M45.3   Diagnostic endoscopic examination of bladder and biopsy of lesion of bladder using rigid cystoscope
        Includes: *Diagnostic endoscopic examination of bladder and biopsy of bladder using rigid cystoscope*
                   Endoscopic biopsy of lesion of bladder using rigid cystoscope
                   Endoscopic biopsy of bladder using rigid cystoscope

M45.4   Diagnostic endoscopic examination of bladder and biopsy of lesion of prostate using rigid cystoscope
        Includes: *Diagnostic endoscopic examination of bladder and biopsy of prostate using rigid endoscope*
                   Endoscopic biopsy of lesion of prostate using rigid cystoscope
                   Endoscopic biopsy of prostate using rigid cystoscope

M45.5   Diagnostic endoscopic examination of bladder using rigid cystoscope
        Includes: *Rigid cystourethroscopy*
                   Rigid cystoscopy

M45.8   Other specified
M45.9   Unspecified
        Includes: *Cystourethroscopy NEC*
                   Cystoscopy NEC

M47   **Urethral catheterisation of bladder**
        Excludes: *Voiding cystourethrogram (U12.1)*
                   Micturating cystography (M49.6)

M47.1   Urethral irrigation of bladder
        Includes: *Urethral lavage of bladder*
M47.2   Change of urethral catheter into bladder
M47.3   Removal of urethral catheter from bladder
M47.4   Urodynamic studies using catheter
        Excludes: *Urodynamics NEC (U26.4)*
                   Urodynamic studies using suprapubic tube (M48.2)
M47.5   Maintenance of urethral catheter in bladder
M47.8   Other specified
M47.9   Unspecified

M48   **Operations on bladder**
> *Note:*   *Principal M49*

M48.1   Suprapubic aspiration of bladder
M48.2   Urodynamic studies using suprapubic tube
> *Excludes: Urodynamics NEC (U26.4)*
>   *Urodynamic studies using catheter (M47.4)*
M48.8   Other specified
M48.9   Unspecified

M49   **Other operations on bladder**
> *Note:*   *Principal category, extended at M48*

M49.1   Closure of cystostomy
M49.2   Change of suprapubic tube into bladder
M49.3   Removal of suprapubic tube from bladder
M49.4   Introduction of therapeutic substance into bladder
> *Includes: Instillation of therapeutic substance into bladder*
M49.5   Injection of therapeutic substance into bladder wall
M49.6   Micturating cystography
> *Excludes: Nuclear cystography (U12.7)*
M49.7   High intensity focused ultrasound of bladder
M49.8   Other specified
M49.9   Unspecified

M51   **Combined abdominal and vaginal operations to support outlet of female bladder**

M51.1   Abdominoperineal suspension of urethra
> *Includes: Abdominovaginal suspension of urethra*
M51.2   Endoscopic suspension of neck of bladder
M51.8   Other specified
M51.9   Unspecified

M52   **Abdominal operations to support outlet of female bladder**

M52.1   Suprapubic sling operation
M52.2   Retropubic suspension of neck of bladder
M52.3   Colposuspension of neck of bladder
M52.4   Urethrolysis
M52.8   Other specified
M52.9   Unspecified

M53   **Vaginal operations to support outlet of female bladder**

M53.1   Vaginal buttressing of urethra
M53.2   Introduction of biethium bean through vagina
M53.3   Introduction of tension-free vaginal tape
M53.4   Total removal of tension-free vaginal tape
M53.5   Partial removal of tension-free vaginal tape
M53.6   Introduction of transobturator tape
M53.7   Removal of transobturator tape
M53.8   Other specified
M53.9   Unspecified

M54   **Open operations on outlet of female bladder**
           Note: Principal M55

M54.1   Creation of urethrovaginal fistula
M54.2   Reconstruction of neck of female bladder NEC
M54.3   Removal of artificial urinary sphincter from outlet of female bladder
M54.8   Other specified
M54.9   Unspecified

M55   **Other open operations on outlet of female bladder**
           Note: Principal category, extended at M54

M55.1   Open resection of outlet of female bladder
M55.2   Implantation of artificial urinary sphincter into outlet of female bladder
M55.3   Insertion of prosthetic collar around outlet of female bladder
M55.4   Maintenance of prosthetic collar around outlet of female bladder
M55.5   Removal of prosthetic collar from around outlet of female bladder
M55.6   Insertion of retropubic device for female stress urinary incontinence NEC
         Includes: Insertion of female adjustable continence therapy balloon
M55.7   Removal of female retropubic device NEC
         Includes: Removal of female adjustable continence therapy balloon
M55.8   Other specified
M55.9   Unspecified

M56   **Therapeutic endoscopic operations on outlet of female bladder**
           Note: It is not necessary to code additionally any mention of diagnostic endoscopic
           examination of bladder (M45.5, M45.9)

M56.1   Endoscopic resection of outlet of female bladder
M56.2   Endoscopic incision of outlet of female bladder
M56.3   Endoscopic injection of inert substance into outlet of female bladder
M56.8   Other specified
M56.9   Unspecified

M58   **Other operations on outlet of female bladder**

M58.1   Closed urethrotomy of outlet of female bladder
M58.2   Dilation of outlet of female bladder
M58.8   Other specified
M58.9   Unspecified

M60   **Open operations on outlet of male bladder**
           Note: Principal M64

M60.1   Insertion of male retropubic continence device NEC
         Includes: Insertion of male adjustable continence therapy balloon
M60.2   Removal of male retropubic device NEC
         Includes: Removal of male adjustable continence therapy balloon
M60.3   Removal of artificial urinary sphincter from outlet of male bladder
M60.8   Other specified
M60.9   Unspecified

M61	**Open excision of prostate**
	Excludes: Cystoprostatectomy (M34.1)
M61.1	Total excision of prostate and capsule of prostate
M61.2	Retropubic prostatectomy
M61.3	Transvesical prostatectomy
M61.4	Perineal prostatectomy
M61.8	Other specified
M61.9	Unspecified
	Includes: Prostatectomy NEC

M62	**Other open operations on prostate**
M62.1	Open extirpation of lesion of prostate
M62.2	Open biopsy of lesion of prostate
	Includes: Open biopsy of prostate
M62.3	Prostatotomy
M62.4	Repair of rectoprostatic fistula
M62.8	Other specified
M62.9	Unspecified

M64	**Other open operations on outlet of male bladder**
	Note: Principal category, extended at M60
M64.1	Open resection of outlet of male bladder
M64.2	Implantation of artificial urinary sphincter into outlet of male bladder
M64.3	Insertion of prosthetic collar around outlet of male bladder
M64.4	Maintenance of prosthetic collar around outlet of male bladder
M64.5	Removal of prosthetic collar from around outlet of male bladder
M64.6	Reconstruction of neck of male bladder NEC
M64.7	Introduction of transobturator sling
M64.8	Other specified
M64.9	Unspecified

M65	**Endoscopic resection of outlet of male bladder**
	Includes: Endoscopic resection of lesion of outlet of male bladder
	Transurethral resection of prostate
	*Note: **It is not necessary to code additionally any mention of diagnostic endoscopic examination of bladder (M45.5, M45.9)***
	Use a subsidiary code for robotic assisted minimal access approach to body cavity (Y76.5)
M65.1	Endoscopic resection of prostate using electrotome
M65.2	Endoscopic resection of prostate using punch
M65.3	Endoscopic resection of prostate NEC
M65.4	Endoscopic resection of prostate using laser
M65.5	Endoscopic resection of prostate using vapotrode
M65.8	Other specified
M65.9	Unspecified

M66   **Other therapeutic endoscopic operations on outlet of male bladder**
> *Note:*   *It is not necessary to code additionally any mention of diagnostic endoscopic examination of bladder (M45.5, M45.9)*

M66.1   Endoscopic sphincterotomy of external sphincter of male bladder
M66.2   Endoscopic incision of outlet of male bladder NEC
M66.3   Endoscopic injection of inert substance into outlet of male bladder
M66.8   Other specified
M66.9   Unspecified

M67   **Other therapeutic endoscopic operations on prostate**
> *Note:*   *It is not necessary to code additionally any mention of diagnostic endoscopic examination of bladder (M45.5, M45.9)*

M67.1   Endoscopic cryotherapy to lesion of prostate
M67.2   Endoscopic destruction of lesion of prostate NEC
M67.3   Endoscopic drainage of prostate
M67.4   Endoscopic removal of calculus from prostate
M67.5   Endoscopic microwave destruction of lesion of prostate
M67.6   Endoscopic radiofrequency ablation of lesion of prostate
> *Excludes:*   *Transurethral radiofrequency needle ablation prostate (M70.7)*

M67.8   Other specified
M67.9   Unspecified

M68   **Endoscopic insertion of prosthesis into prostate**
> *Note:*   *It is not necessary to code additionally any mention of diagnostic endoscopic examination of bladder (M45.5, M45.9)*

M68.1   Endoscopic insertion of prostatic stent
M68.2   Endoscopic removal of prostatic stent
M68.8   Other specified
M68.9   Unspecified

M70   **Other operations on outlet of male bladder**
> *Note:*   *Principal category, extended at M71*

M70.1   Aspiration of prostate NEC
M70.2   Perineal needle biopsy of prostate
> *Includes:*   *Needle biopsy of prostate NEC*
>   *Biopsy of prostate NEC*

M70.3   Rectal needle biopsy of prostate
M70.4   Balloon dilation of prostate
M70.5   Massage of prostate
M70.6   Radioactive seed implantation into prostate
> *Note:*   *Use an additional code to specify radiotherapy delivery (X65)*

M70.7   Transurethral radiofrequency needle ablation of prostate
> *Excludes:*   *Endoscopic radiofrequency ablation of lesion of prostate (M67.6)*

M70.8   Other specified
M70.9   Unspecified

M71   **Other operations on prostate**
          Note: Principal M70

M71.1   High intensity focused ultrasound of prostate
M71.2   Implantation of radioactive substance into prostate
          Note: Use an additional code to specify radiotherapy delivery (X65)
M71.8   Other specified
M71.9   Unspecified

M72   **Excision of urethra**

M72.1   Partial urethrectomy
M72.2   Urethrectomy NEC
M72.3   Excision of lesion of urethra NEC
M72.4   Secondary urethrectomy
M72.8   Other specified
M72.9   Unspecified

M73   **Repair of urethra**

M73.1   Repair of hypospadias
M73.2   Repair of epispadias
M73.3   Closure of fistula of urethra
M73.4   Reconstruction of urethra
M73.5   Pull through of urethra
M73.6   Urethroplasty NEC
M73.7   Repair of rupture of urethra NEC
M73.8   Other specified
M73.9   Unspecified

M75   **Other open operations on urethra**

M75.1   Open biopsy of lesion of urethra
          Includes: Open biopsy of urethra
M75.2   Insertion of prosthesis for compression of bulb of male urethra
M75.3   External urethrotomy
          Note: Do not use as approach code (Y52.2)
M75.4   Open extraction of calculus from urethra
M75.8   Other specified
M75.9   Unspecified

M76   **Therapeutic endoscopic operations on urethra**
          Note: It is not necessary to code additionally any mention of examination of urethra (M77.9)

M76.1   Endoscopic extirpation of lesion of urethra
M76.2   Endoscopic removal of foreign body from urethra
M76.3   Optical urethrotomy
M76.4   Endoscopic dilation of urethra
M76.5   Endoscopic destruction of urethral valves
M76.6   Endoscopic insertion of urethral stent
M76.7   Endoscopic removal of urethral stent
M76.8   Other specified
M76.9   Unspecified

M77　　Diagnostic endoscopic examination of urethra

M77.1　　Diagnostic endoscopic examination of urethra and biopsy of lesion of urethra
　　　　　Includes:　Diagnostic endoscopic examination of urethra and biopsy of urethra
　　　　　　　　　　Endoscopic biopsy of lesion of urethra
　　　　　　　　　　Endoscopic biopsy of urethra
　　　　　　　　　　Biopsy of lesion of urethra NEC
　　　　　　　　　　Biopsy of urethra NEC
M77.8　　Other specified
M77.9　　Unspecified
　　　　　Includes:　Urethroscopy NEC

M79　　Other operations on urethra

M79.1　　Bouginage of urethra
M79.2　　Dilation of urethra NEC
M79.3　　Calibration of urethra
M79.4　　Internal urethrotomy NEC
M79.5　　Urethrography ascending and descending
M79.6　　Urethrography ascending NEC
M79.7　　Urethrography descending NEC
M79.8　　Other specified
M79.9　　Unspecified

M81　　Operations on urethral orifice

M81.1　　Extirpation of lesion of meatus of urethra
M81.2　　Meatoplasty of urethra
M81.3　　External meatotomy of urethral orifice
M81.4　　Dilation of meatus of urethra
M81.8　　Other specified
M81.9　　Unspecified

M83　　Other operations on urinary tract

M83.1　　Drainage of paravesical abscess
M83.2　　Exploration of retropubic space
M83.3　　Removal of foreign body from urinary tract NEC
M83.8　　Other specified
M83.9　　Unspecified

M85　　Diagnostic endoscopic examination of urinary diversion

M85.1　　Endoscopic examination of intestinal conduit
M85.8　　Other specified
M85.9　　Unspecified

M86　　Therapeutic endoscopic operations on urinary diversion

M86.1　　Endoscopic extraction of calculus of urinary diversion
M86.8　　Other specified
M86.9　　Unspecified

CHAPTER N
MALE GENITAL ORGANS
(CODES N01–N35)

Excludes:	PROSTATE	(Chapter M)
	URETHRAL ORIFICE	(Chapter M)
	OPERATIONS FOR MALE SEXUAL TRANSFORMATION	(Chapter X)
	OPERATIONS FOR DISORDERS OF SEX DEVELOPMENT	(Chapter X)

Note: **Use a subsidiary code for minimal access approach (Y74–Y76)**

Use a subsidiary code to identify method of image control (Y53)

N01   **Extirpation of scrotum**

Includes: *Skin of scrotum*

    Note: **Codes from Chapter S may be used to enhance these codes**

N01.1   Excision of scrotum
N01.2   Excision of lesion of scrotum
N01.3   Destruction of lesion of scrotum
N01.8   Other specified
N01.9   Unspecified

N03   **Other operations on scrotum**

     Note at N01 applies

Includes: *Skin of scrotum*

Excludes: *Dermatological non-operative interventions involving the scrotum (N35.1)*

N03.1   Biopsy of lesion of scrotum

Includes: *Biopsy of scrotum*

N03.2   Drainage of scrotum
N03.3   Suture of scrotum
N03.4   Exploration of scrotum
N03.5   Removal of foreign body from scrotum
N03.6   Reconstruction of scrotum
N03.8   Other specified
N03.9   Unspecified

N05   **Bilateral excision of testes**

N05.1   Bilateral subcapsular orchidectomy
N05.2   Bilateral orchidectomy NEC
N05.3   Bilateral inguinal orchidectomy

Includes: *Bilateral inguinal orchidectomy and excision of spermatic cord*

N05.8   Other specified
N05.9   Unspecified

Includes: *Male castration*

N06   **Other excision of testis**

N06.1   Subcapsular orchidectomy NEC
N06.2   Excision of aberrant testis
N06.3   Orchidectomy NEC
N06.4   Excision of testicular appendage
N06.5   Division of cremaster
N06.6   Inguinal orchidectomy NEC
          Includes: Inguinal orchidectomy and excision of spermatic cord NEC
N06.8   Other specified
N06.9   Unspecified

N07   **Extirpation of lesion of testis**

N07.1   Excision of lesion of testis
          Includes: Excision of hydatid of Morgagni of testis
N07.2   Destruction of lesion of testis
N07.8   Other specified
N07.9   Unspecified

N08   **Bilateral placement of testes in scrotum**

N08.1   Bilateral microvascular transfer of testes to scrotum
N08.2   One stage bilateral orchidopexy NEC
N08.3   First stage bilateral orchidopexy
N08.4   Second stage bilateral orchidopexy
N08.8   Other specified
N08.9   Unspecified

N09   **Other placement of testis in scrotum**

N09.1   Microvascular transfer of testis to scrotum NEC
N09.2   One stage orchidopexy NEC
N09.3   First stage orchidopexy NEC
N09.4   Second stage orchidopexy NEC
N09.8   Other specified
N09.9   Unspecified

N10   **Prosthesis of testis**

N10.1   Insertion of prosthetic replacement for testis
N10.2   Removal of prosthetic replacement for testis
N10.8   Other specified
N10.9   Unspecified

N11   **Operations on hydrocele sac**
          Excludes: Correction of hydrocele of infancy (T19.3)

N11.1   Excision of hydrocele sac
N11.2   Plication of hydrocele sac
N11.3   Eversion of hydrocele sac
N11.4   Drainage of hydrocele sac
N11.5   Aspiration of hydrocele sac
          Includes: Tapping of hydrocele sac
N11.6   Injection sclerotherapy to hydrocele sac
N11.8   Other specified
N11.9   Unspecified

N13   **Other operations on testis**
            Excludes: Testicular sperm extraction (N34.6)

N13.1   Drainage of testis
N13.2   Fixation of testis
            Includes: Tether of testis
N13.3   Reduction of torsion of testis
N13.4   Biopsy of testis
            Includes: Biopsy of lesion of testis
N13.5   Exploration of testis
N13.6   Removal of foreign body from testis
N13.7   Repair of rupture of testis
N13.8   Other specified
N13.9   Unspecified

N15   **Operations on epididymis**

N15.1   Bilateral epididymectomy
N15.2   Unilateral epididymectomy
N15.3   Excision of lesion of epididymis
            Includes: Excision of hydatid of Morgagni of epididymis
N15.4   Drainage of epididymis
N15.5   Biopsy of lesion of epididymis
            Includes: Biopsy of epididymis
N15.6   Aspiration of lesion of epididymis
            Excludes: Microsurgical epididymal sperm aspiration (N34.4)
                        Percutaneous epldldymal sperm aspiration (N34.5)
N15.7   Epididymovasostomy
N15.8   Other specified
N15.9   Unspecified
            Includes: Epididymectomy NEC

N17   **Excision of vas deferens**

N17.1   Bilateral vasectomy
            Includes: Vasectomy NEC
N17.2   Ligation of vas deferens NEC
N17.8   Other specified
N17.9   Unspecified

N18   **Repair of spermatic cord**

N18.1   Reversal of bilateral vasectomy
N18.2   Suture of vas deferens NEC
N18.8   Other specified
N18.9   Unspecified

N19   **Operations on varicocele**

N19.1   Ligation of varicocele
N19.2   Embolisation of varicocele
N19.8   Other specified
N19.9   Unspecified

N20   **Other operations on spermatic cord**

N20.1   Excision of lesion of spermatic cord
            Includes: Excision of hydatid of Morgagni of spermatic cord
N20.2   Biopsy of spermatic cord
            Includes: Biopsy of lesion of spermatic cord
N20.3   Drainage of spermatic cord
N20.4   Vasotomy
N20.5   Vasography
N20.8   Other specified
N20.9   Unspecified

N22   **Operations on seminal vesicle**

N22.1   Excision of seminal vesicle
N22.2   Incision of seminal vesicle
N22.3   Seminal vesiculography
N22.4   Transrectal needle biopsy of seminal vesicle
N22.5   Resection of ejaculatory duct
N22.8   Other specified
N22.9   Unspecified

N24   **Operations on male perineum**
            Includes: Skin of male perineum (N24.1, N24.2)
            Excludes: Dermatological non-operative interventions involving the male perineum (N35.3)
               Note: Codes from Chapter S may be used to enhance these codes

N24.1   Excision of sweat gland bearing skin of male perineum
N24.2   Operations on skin of male perineum NEC
N24.3   Excision of male periurethral tissue NEC
N24.4   Incision of male periurethral tissue
N24.8   Other specified
N24.9   Unspecified

N26   **Amputation of penis**

N26.1   Total amputation of penis
N26.2   Partial amputation of penis
N26.8   Other specified
N26.9   Unspecified

N27   **Extirpation of lesion of penis**
            Includes: Skin of penis
               Note: Codes from Chapter S may be used to enhance these codes

N27.1   Excision of lesion of penis
N27.2   Cauterisation of lesion of penis
N27.3   Destruction of lesion of penis NEC
N27.4   Extracorporeal shockwave lithotripsy to lesion of penis
            Includes: Shockwave treatment for Peyronie's disease
N27.8   Other specified
N27.9   Unspecified

N28   **Plastic operations on penis**
            Note at N27 applies
            Includes: Skin of penis

N28.1   Construction of penis
N28.2   Reconstruction of penis
N28.3   Plication of corpora of penis
N28.4   Frenuloplasty of penis
N28.5   Correction of chordee of penis
N28.6   Repair of fracture of penis
N28.7   Graft to penis
            Note: Use a supplementary code for concurrent incision of penis (N32.3)
N28.8   Other specified
N28.9   Unspecified

N29   **Prosthesis of penis**

N29.1   Implantation of prosthesis into penis
N29.2   Attention to prosthesis in penis
N29.8   Other specified
N29.9   Unspecified

N30   **Operations on prepuce**
            Includes: Skin of prepuce
            Note: Codes from Chapter S may be used to enhance these codes

N30.1   Prepuceplasty
N30.2   Freeing of adhesions of prepuce
N30.3   Circumcision
N30.4   Dorsal slit of prepuce
            Includes: Lateral slit of prepuce
N30.5   Stretching of prepuce
N30.6   Manual reduction of prepuce
N30.8   Other specified
N30.9   Unspecified

N32   **Other operations on penis**
            Note at N27 applies
            Includes: Skin of penis
            Excludes: Dermatological non-operative interventions involving the penis (N35.2)

N32.1   Biopsy of lesion of penis
            Includes: Biopsy of penis
N32.2   Drainage of penis
N32.3   Incision of penis NEC
            Includes: Incision of penis for Peyronie's disease
            ***Note: Use as a supplementary code when associated with concurrent graft to
                        penis (N28.7)***
N32.4   Injection of therapeutic substance into penis
            Includes: Penile injection to produce erection
            *   Penile injection to deflate priapism*
N32.5   Removal of constricting object from penis
N32.6   Operations on penis for erectile dysfunction NEC
            Excludes: Injection of therapeutic substance into penis for erectile dysfunction (N32.4)
N32.8   Other specified
N32.9   Unspecified

N34 **Other operations on male genital tract**
Excludes: Non-operative interventions to male genitalia (N35)

N34.1   Fertility investigation of male NEC
N34.2   Collection of sperm NEC
N34.3   Male colposcopy
N34.4   Microsurgical epididymal sperm aspiration
N34.5   Percutaneous epididymal sperm aspiration
N34.6   Testicular sperm extraction
N34.8   Other specified
N34.9   Unspecified

N35 **Non-operative interventions to male genitalia**

N35.1   Dermatological non-operative interventions involving the scrotum
N35.2   Dermatological non-operative interventions involving the penis
N35.3   Dermatological non-operative interventions involving the male perineum
N35.8   Other specified
N35.9   Unspecified

CHAPTER P
LOWER FEMALE GENITAL TRACT
(CODES P01–P32)

Excludes: *GYNAECOLOGICAL OPERATIONS ON FEMALE URETHRA*
AND BLADDER   *(Chapter M)*
OBSTETRIC OPERATIONS   *(Chapter R)*
OPERATIONS FOR FEMALE SEXUAL TRANSFORMATION   *(Chapter X)*
OPERATIONS FOR DISORDERS OF SEX DEVELOPMENT   *(Chapter X)*

Note: **Obstetric operations are normally carried out in relation to delivery at or near term or in**
pregnancy expected to go to term
They do not include abortion or termination of pregnancy
Use a subsidiary code for minimal access approach (Y74–Y76)
Use a subsidiary code to identify method of image control (Y53)

P01   **Operations on clitoris**

P01.1   Clitoridectomy
P01.2   Reduction of clitoris
P01.8   Other specified
P01.9   Unspecified

P03   **Operations on Bartholin gland**
             Includes: Bartholin duct (P03.5)

P03.1   Excision of Bartholin gland
P03.2   Marsupialisation of Bartholin gland
P03.3   Excision of lesion of Bartholin gland
P03.4   Drainage of Bartholin gland
P03.5   Operations on Bartholin duct
P03.8   Other specified
P03.9   Unspecified

P05   **Excision of vulva**
             Includes: Skin of vulva
             Note: Codes from Chapter S may be used to enhance these codes

P05.1   Total excision of vulva
P05.2   Partial excision of vulva
P05.3   Marsupialisation of lesion of vulva
P05.4   Excision of lesion of vulva NEC
P05.5   Excision of excess labial tissue
P05.6   Reduction labia minor
P05.7   Reduction labia major
P05.8   Other specified
P05.9   Unspecified
             Includes: Vulvectomy NEC

P06   **Extirpation of lesion of vulva**
Note at P05 applies
Includes: Skin of vulva

P06.1   Laser destruction of lesion of vulva
P06.2   Cryosurgery to lesion of vulva
P06.3   Cauterisation of lesion of vulva
P06.4   Implantation of radioactive substance into vulva
Note: Use an additional code to specify radiotherapy delivery (X65)
P06.8   Other specified
P06.9   Unspecified

P07   **Repair of vulva**
Note at P05 applies
Includes: Skin of vulva

P07.1   Plastic repair of vulva
P07.2   Deinfibulation of vulva
Excludes: Deinfibulation of vulva to facilitate delivery (R27.2)
P07.8   Other specified
P07.9   Unspecified

P09   **Other operations on vulva**
Note at P05 applies
Includes: Skin of vulva

P09.1   Biopsy of lesion of vulva
Includes: Biopsy of vulva
P09.2   Drainage of lesion of vulva
P09.3   Evacuation of haematoma from vulva
P09.8   Other specified
P09.9   Unspecified

P11   **Extirpation of lesion of female perineum**
Includes: Skin of female perineum
Note: Codes from Chapter S may be used to enhance these codes

P11.1   Excision of lesion of female perineum
P11.2   Laser destruction of lesion of female perineum
P11.3   Cauterisation of lesion of female perineum
P11.4   Destruction of lesion of female perineum NEC
P11.8   Other specified
P11.9   Unspecified

P13	**Other operations on female perineum**
	Note at P11 applies
	Includes: Skin of female perineum

P13.1	Drainage of female perineum
	Includes: Drainage of lesion of female perineum
P13.2	Female perineorrhaphy
	Excludes: Colpoperineorrhaphy (P25.5)
P13.3	Female perineoplasty
P13.4	Closure of fistula of female perineum
P13.5	Female perineotomy NEC
P13.6	Operations on female periurethral tissue NEC
P13.7	Excision of sweat gland bearing skin of female perineum
P13.8	Other specified
P13.9	Unspecified

| P14 | **Incision of introitus of vagina** |

P14.1	Posterior episiotomy and division of levator ani muscle
P14.2	Posterior episiotomy NEC
P14.3	Anterior episiotomy
P14.8	Other specified
P14.9	Unspecified
	Includes: Episiotomy NEC

| P15 | **Other operations on introitus of vagina** |

P15.1	Hymenectomy
P15.2	Excision of hymenal tag
P15.3	Repair of hymen
P15.4	Incision of hymen
	Includes: Hymenotomy
P15.5	Stretching of hymen
P15.8	Other specified
P15.9	Unspecified

| P17 | **Excision of vagina** |

P17.1	Total colpectomy
P17.2	Partial colpectomy
P17.3	Marsupialisation of lesion of vagina
P17.8	Other specified
P17.9	Unspecified

| P18 | **Other obliteration of vagina** |

P18.1	Complete colpocleisis
P18.2	Partial colpocleisis
P18.8	Other specified
P18.9	Unspecified

P19   **Excision of band of vagina**

P19.1   Laser excision of septum of vagina
P19.2   Excision of septum of vagina NEC
P19.3   Excision of transverse septum high
P19.4   Excision of transverse septum low
P19.5   Excision of transverse septum vertical
P19.8   Other specified
P19.9   Unspecified

P20   **Extirpation of lesion of vagina**

P20.1   Excision of lesion of vagina
P20.2   Laser destruction of lesion of vagina
P20.3   Cauterisation of lesion of vagina
P20.4   Cryotherapy to lesion of vagina
P20.5   Implantation of radioactive substance into vagina
        Note: *Use an additional code to specify radiotherapy delivery (X65)*
P20.8   Other specified
P20.9   Unspecified

P21   **Plastic operations on vagina**
        Note: *Principal category, extended at P32*

P21.1   Construction of vagina
P21.2   Reconstruction of vagina NEC
P21.3   Vaginoplasty NEC
P21.4   Vaginoplasty in presence of uterus for absent vagina
P21.5   Vaginoplasty using olive
P21.8   Other specified
P21.9   Unspecified

P22   **Repair of prolapse of vagina and amputation of cervix uteri**

P22.1   Anterior and posterior colporrhaphy and amputation of cervix uteri
P22.2   Anterior colporrhaphy and amputation of cervix uteri NEC
P22.3   Posterior colporrhaphy and amputation of cervix uteri NEC
P22.8   Other specified
P22.9   Unspecified
        Includes: *Colporrhaphy and amputation of cervix uteri NEC*

P23   **Other repair of prolapse of vagina**
        Note: *Use a supplementary code for concurrent excision of uterus (Q08)*

P23.1   Anterior and posterior colporrhaphy NEC
P23.2   Anterior colporrhaphy NEC
P23.3   Posterior colporrhaphy NEC
P23.4   Repair of enterocele NEC
P23.5   Paravaginal repair
P23.6   Anterior colporrhaphy with mesh reinforcement
P23.7   Posterior colporrhaphy with mesh reinforcement
P23.8   Other specified
P23.9   Unspecified
        Includes: *Colporrhaphy NEC*

P24	**Repair of vault of vagina**
	Excludes: *Operations to support female bladder (M51–M55)*
P24.1	Repair of vault of vagina using combined abdominal and vaginal approach
P24.2	Sacrocolpopexy
P24.3	Repair of vault of vagina using abdominal approach NEC
P24.4	Repair of vault of vagina using vaginal approach NEC
P24.5	Repair of vault of vagina with mesh using abdominal approach
P24.6	Repair of vault of vagina with mesh using vaginal approach
P24.7	Sacrospinous fixation of vagina
P24.8	Other specified
P24.9	Unspecified
	Includes: *Suspension of vagina NEC*

P25	**Other repair of vagina**
P25.1	Repair of vesicovaginal fistula
P25.2	Repair of urethrovaginal fistula
P25.3	Repair of rectovaginal fistula
P25.4	Repair of uterovaginal fistula
P25.5	Suture of vagina
	Includes: *Colpoperineorrhaphy*
P25.8	Other specified
P25.9	Unspecified

P26	**Introduction of supporting pessary into vagina**
	Excludes: *Insertion of abortifacient pessary (Q14)*
P26.1	Insertion of Hodge pessary into vagina
P26.2	Insertion of ring pessary into vagina
P26.3	Removal of supporting pessary from vagina
P26.4	Renewal of supporting pessary in vagina
P26.8	Other specified
P26.9	Unspecified

P27	**Exploration of vagina**
P27.1	Evacuation of haematoma from vagina
P27.2	Toilet to vagina
P27.3	Colposcopy of vagina
	Excludes: *Colposcopy of cervix (Q55.4)*
P27.8	Other specified
P27.9	Unspecified

P29	**Other operations on vagina**
P29.1	Freeing of adhesions of vagina
P29.2	Colpotomy NEC
P29.3	Biopsy of lesion of vagina
	Includes: *Biopsy of vagina*
P29.4	Removal of foreign body from vagina
P29.5	Dilation of vagina
	Includes: *Dilator therapy of vagina*
P29.8	Other specified
P29.9	Unspecified

P31   **Operations on pouch of Douglas**

P31.1   Culdoplasty
P31.2   Drainage of pouch of Douglas
P31.3   Aspiration of pouch of Douglas
P31.4   Culdotomy NEC
P31.5   Removal of intrauterine contraceptive device from pouch of Douglas
P31.6   Removal of foreign body from pouch of Douglas NEC
P31.8   Other specified
P31.9   Unspecified

P32   **Other plastic operations on vagina**
              Note: *Principal P21*

P32.1   Reconstruction of vagina using bowel interposition
P32.2   Reconstruction of vagina using pelvic peritoneal graft
P32.3   Reconstruction of vagina with urethral dissection
P32.4   Vaginoplasty using rotational skin flaps
P32.5   Vaginoplasty using tissue expanders
P32.6   Vaginoplasty using a mould and skin graft
P32.7   Vaginoplasty using a mould NEC
P32.8   Other specified
P32.9   Unspecified

CHAPTER Q
UPPER FEMALE GENITAL TRACT
(CODES Q01–Q56)

Includes:	*UTERUS*	
	FALLOPIAN TUBE	
	OVARY	
	LIGAMENT OF UTERUS	
Excludes:	*OBSTETRIC OPERATIONS*	*(Chapter R)*
	OPERATIONS FOR FEMALE SEXUAL TRANSFORMATION	*(Chapter X)*
	OPERATIONS FOR DISORDERS OF SEX DEVELOPMENT	*(Chapter X)*

Note: **Obstetric operations are normally carried out in relation to delivery at or near or in pregnancy expected to go to term**

They do not include abortion or termination of pregnancy

Use a subsidiary code for minimal access approach (Y74–Y76)

Use a subsidiary code to identify method of image control (Y53)

Q01   Excision of cervix uteri

Q01.1   Amputation of cervix uteri
               Excludes: When associated with repair of prolapse of vagina (P22)
Q01.2   Wedge excision of cervix uteri and suture HFQ
Q01.3   Excision of lesion of cervix uteri
Q01.4   Large loop excision of transformation zone
Q01.8   Other specified
Q01.9   Unspecified

Q02   Destruction of lesion of cervix uteri

Q02.1   Avulsion of lesion of cervix uteri
Q02.2   Laser destruction of lesion of cervix uteri
Q02.3   Cauterisation of lesion of cervix uteri
Q02.4   Cryotherapy to lesion of cervix uteri
Q02.8   Other specified
Q02.9   Unspecified

Q03   Biopsy of cervix uteri
               Includes: Biopsy of lesion of cervix uteri

Q03.1   Knife cone biopsy of cervix uteri
Q03.2   Laser cone biopsy of cervix uteri
Q03.3   Cone biopsy of cervix uteri NEC
Q03.4   Punch biopsy of cervix uteri
Q03.5   Ring biopsy of cervix uteri
Q03.8   Other specified
Q03.9   Unspecified

Q05   Other operations on cervix uteri

Q05.1   Repair of cervix uteri NEC
               Includes: Cerclage of cervix of non-gravid uterus
               Excludes: Cerclage of cervix of gravid uterus (R12.1)
Q05.2   Dilation of cervix uteri
               *Excludes: When associated with curettage of uterus (Q10.1) or other evacuation of
                                 uterus (Q11.1, Q11.2)*
Q05.8   Other specified
Q05.9   Unspecified

Q07   **Abdominal excision of uterus**
       Note: *Use a supplementary code for concurrent excision of ovary and/or fallopian tube (Q22–Q24)*

Q07.1   Abdominal hysterocolpectomy and excision of periuterine tissue
Q07.2   Abdominal hysterectomy and excision of periuterine tissue NEC
Q07.3   Abdominal hysterocolpectomy NEC
Q07.4   Total abdominal hysterectomy NEC
            Includes: *Hysterectomy NEC*
Q07.5   Subtotal abdominal hysterectomy
Q07.6   Excision of accessory uterus
            Excludes: *Excision of Mullerian duct remnant (X16.1)*
                         Excision of uterine horn (X16.1)
                         Excision of rudimentary uterus (X16.1)
Q07.8   Other specified
Q07.9   Unspecified

Q08   **Vaginal excision of uterus**
       Note: *Use as a supplementary code when associated with concurrent repair of prolapse of vagina (P23)*
                Use a supplementary code for concurrent excision of ovary and/or fallopian tube (Q22–Q24)

Q08.1   Vaginal hysterocolpectomy and excision of periuterine tissue
Q08.2   Vaginal hysterectomy and excision of periuterine tissue NEC
Q08.3   Vaginal hysterocolpectomy NEC
Q08.8   Other specified
Q08.9   Unspecified
            Includes: *Vaginal hysterectomy NEC*

Q09   **Other open operations on uterus**

Q09.1   Open removal of products of conception from uterus
            Note: *Use a subsidiary code to identify gestational age (Y95)*
Q09.2   Open myomectomy
Q09.3   Open excision of lesion of uterus NEC
            Includes: *Excision of lesion of uterus NEC*
Q09.4   Open biopsy of lesion of uterus
            Includes: *Open biopsy of uterus*
Q09.5   Metroplasty
Q09.6   Incision of uterus NEC
            Includes: *Hysterotomy NEC*
Q09.8   Other specified
Q09.9   Unspecified

Q10   **Curettage of uterus**

Q10.1   Dilation of cervix uteri and curettage of products of conception from uterus
            Note: *Use a subsidiary code to identify gestational age (Y95)*
Q10.2   Curettage of products of conception from uterus NEC
             Note: *Use a subsidiary code to identify gestational age (Y95)*
Q10.3   Dilation of cervix uteri and curettage of uterus NEC
Q10.8   Other specified
Q10.9   Unspecified

Q11   **Other evacuation of contents of uterus**
                Note: Use a subsidiary code to identify gestational age (Y95)

Q11.1   Vacuum aspiration of products of conception from uterus NEC
                Includes: Dilation of cervix uteri and vacuum aspiration of products of conception from
                                 uterus NEC
Q11.2   Dilation of cervix uteri and evacuation of products of conception from uterus NEC
Q11.3   Evacuation of products of conception from uterus NEC
Q11.4   Extraction of menses
Q11.5   Vacuum aspiration of products of conception from uterus using rigid cannula
Q11.6   Vacuum aspiration of products of conception from uterus using flexible cannula
Q11.8   Other specified
Q11.9   Unspecified

Q12   **Intrauterine contraceptive device**

Q12.1   Introduction of intrauterine contraceptive device
Q12.2   Replacement of intrauterine contraceptive device
Q12.3   Removal of displaced intrauterine contraceptive device NEC
                Excludes: Removal of displaced intrauterine contraceptive device from pouch of
                                   Douglas (P31.5)
Q12.4   Removal of intrauterine contraceptive device NEC
Q12.8   Other specified
Q12.9   Unspecified

Q13   **Introduction of gametes into uterine cavity**
                Includes: Introduction of embryo into uterine cavity
                Note: Principal category, extended at Q21

Q13.1   Transfer of embryo to uterus NEC
                Includes: In vitro fertilisation
                                 Implantation of fertilised egg into uterus
                Note: Use a subsidiary code to identify method of in vitro fertilisation (Y96)
Q13.2   Intracervical artificial insemination
Q13.3   Intrauterine artificial insemination
                Includes: Artificial insemination NEC
Q13.4   Intrauterine insemination with superovulation using partner sperm
Q13.5   Intrauterine insemination with superovulation using donor sperm
Q13.6   Intrauterine insemination without superovulation using partner sperm
Q13.7   Intrauterine insemination without superovulation using donor sperm
Q13.8   Other specified
Q13.9   Unspecified

Q14   **Introduction of abortifacient into uterine cavity**
                Note: Use a subsidiary code to identify gestational age (Y95)

Q14.1   Intra-amniotic injection of prostaglandin
Q14.2   Intra-amniotic injection of abortifacient NEC
Q14.3   Extra-amniotic injection of prostaglandin
Q14.4   Extra-amniotic injection of abortifacient NEC
Q14.5   Insertion of prostaglandin pessary
Q14.6   Insertion of abortifacient pessary NEC
Q14.8   Other specified
Q14.9   Unspecified

Q15   **Introduction of other substance into uterine cavity**

Q15.1   Introduction of radioactive substance into uterine cavity
          Note: *Use an additional code to specify radiotherapy delivery (X65)*
Q15.2   Introduction of therapeutic substance into uterine cavity NEC
Q15.3   Injection into uterine cavity NEC
Q15.4   Removal of therapeutic substance from uterine cavity
Q15.8   Other specified
Q15.9   Unspecified

Q16   **Other vaginal operations on uterus**

Q16.1   Vaginal excision of lesion of uterus
Q16.2   Balloon ablation of endometrium
Q16.3   Microwave ablation of endometrium NEC
          Excludes: Endoscopic microwave ablation of endometrium (Q17.6)
Q16.4   Free circulating saline ablation of endometrium
Q16.5   Radiofrequency ablation of endometrium
Q16.6   Photodynamic ablation of endometrium
Q16.8   Other specified
Q16.9   Unspecified

Q17   **Therapeutic endoscopic operations on uterus**
          Note: *It is not necessary to code additionally any mention of diagnostic endoscopic*
                  examination of uterus (Q18.9)

Q17.1   Endoscopic resection of lesion of uterus
          Includes: Endoscopic resection of uterus
Q17.2   Endoscopic cauterisation of lesion of uterus
          Includes: Endoscopic cauterisation of uterus
Q17.3   Endoscopic cryotherapy to lesion of uterus
          Includes: Endoscopic cryotherapy of uterus
Q17.4   Endoscopic destruction of lesion of uterus NEC
          Includes: Endoscopic destruction of uterus NEC
Q17.5   Endoscopic metroplasty
Q17.6   Endoscopic microwave ablation of endometrium
          Excludes: Microwave ablation of endometrium NEC (Q16.3)
Q17.7   Endoscopic balloon ablation of endometrium
Q17.8   Other specified
Q17.9   Unspecified

Q18   **Diagnostic endoscopic examination of uterus**

Q18.1   Diagnostic endoscopic examination of uterus and biopsy of lesion of uterus
          Includes: Diagnostic endoscopic examination of uterus and biopsy of uterus
                      Endoscopic biopsy of lesion of uterus
                      Endoscopic biopsy of uterus
Q18.8   Other specified
Q18.9   Unspecified
          Includes: Hysteroscopy NEC

Q19   **Plastic operations on uterus**

Q19.1   Connection of uterus to vagina
          Includes: Uterovaginal anastomosis
Q19.8   Other specified
Q19.9   Unspecified

Q20   **Other operations on uterus**

Q20.1   Freeing of adhesions of uterus
Q20.2   Biopsy of lesion of uterus NEC
               Includes: Biopsy of uterus NEC
Q20.3   Manual manipulation of uterus
               Excludes: Manual manipulation of gravid uterus (R12.3) or delivered uterus (R30)
Q20.4   Vaginofixation of uterus
Q20.5   Exploration of uterus NEC
Q20.6   Focused ultrasound to lesion of uterus
Q20.8   Other specified
Q20.9   Unspecified

Q21   **Other introduction of gametes into uterine cavity**
               Includes: Introduction of embryo into uterine cavity
                   Note: Principal Q13

Q21.1   Transmyometrial transfer of embryo to uterus
                   Note: Use a subsidiary code to identify method of in vitro fertilisation (Y96)
                   It is not necessary to code additionally any mention of transvaginal ultrasound
                   scan (Q55.5)
Q21.8   Other specified
Q21.9   Unspecified

Q22   **Bilateral excision of adnexa of uterus**
                   Note: Use as a supplementary code when associated with concurrent excision of
                   uterus (Q07, Q08)

Q22.1   Bilateral salpingoophorectomy
Q22.2   Bilateral salpingectomy NEC
Q22.3   Bilateral oophorectomy NEC
Q22.8   Other specified
Q22.9   Unspecified

Q23   **Unilateral excision of adnexa of uterus**
                   Note: Use as a supplementary code when associated with concurrent excision of
                   uterus (Q07, Q08)

Q23.1   Unilateral salpingoophorectomy NEC
Q23.2   Salpingoophorectomy of remaining solitary fallopian tube and ovary
Q23.3   Unilateral salpingectomy NEC
                   Note: Use a subsidiary code to identify gestational age (Y95)
Q23.4   Salpingectomy of remaining solitary fallopian tube NEC
                   Note: Use a subsidiary code to identify gestational age (Y95)
Q23.5   Unilateral oophorectomy NEC
Q23.6   Oophorectomy of remaining solitary ovary NEC
Q23.8   Other specified
Q23.9   Unspecified

Q24   **Other excision of adnexa of uterus**
> *Note:*   *Use as a supplementary code when associated with concurrent excision of uterus (Q07, Q08)*

Q24.1   Salpingoophorectomy NEC
Q24.2   Salpingectomy NEC
> *Note:*   *Use a subsidiary code to identify gestational age (Y95)*

Q24.3   Oophorectomy NEC
Q24.8   Other specified
Q24.9   Unspecified

Q25   **Partial excision of fallopian tube**
> *Excludes:*   *When associated with sterilisation (Q27, Q28)*
> > *Note:*   *Use a subsidiary code to identify gestational age (Y95)*

Q25.1   Excision of lesion of fallopian tube
Q25.8   Other specified
Q25.9   Unspecified
> *Includes:*   *Partial salpingectomy NEC*

Q26   **Placement of prosthesis in fallopian tube**

Q26.1   Insertion of tubal prosthesis into fallopian tube
Q26.2   Revision of tubal prosthesis in fallopian tube
Q26.3   Removal of tubal prosthesis from fallopian tube
Q26.8   Other specified
Q26.9   Unspecified

Q27   **Open bilateral occlusion of fallopian tubes**

Q27.1   Open bilateral ligation of fallopian tubes
Q27.2   Open bilateral clipping of fallopian tubes
> *Includes:*   *Open bilateral ringing of fallopian tubes*

Q27.8   Other specified
Q27.9   Unspecified

Q28   **Other open occlusion of fallopian tube**

Q28.1   Open ligation of remaining solitary fallopian tube
Q28.2   Open ligation of fallopian tube NEC
Q28.3   Open clipping of remaining solitary fallopian tube
> *Includes:*   *Open ringing of remaining solitary fallopian tube*

Q28.4   Open clipping of fallopian tube NEC
> *Includes:*   *Open ringing of fallopian tube NEC*

Q28.8   Other specified
Q28.9   Unspecified

Q29   **Open reversal of female sterilisation**

Q29.1   Reanastomosis of fallopian tube NEC
Q29.2   Open removal of clip from fallopian tube NEC
> *Includes:*   *Open removal of ring from fallopian tube NEC*

Q29.8   Other specified
Q29.9   Unspecified

Q30 Other repair of fallopian tube

Q30.1	Reconstruction of fallopian tube
Q30.2	Replantation of fallopian tube
Q30.3	Anastomosis of fallopian tube NEC
Q30.4	Salpingostomy
Q30.5	Suture of fallopian tube
Q30.8	Other specified
Q30.9	Unspecified

Q31 Incision of fallopian tube

Q31.1	Removal of products of conception from fallopian tube
	Note: Use a subsidiary code to identify gestational age (Y95)
Q31.2	Drainage of fallopian tube
Q31.8	Other specified
Q31.9	Unspecified
	Includes: Salpingotomy NEC

Q32 Operations on fimbria

Q32.1	Excision of fimbria
Q32.2	Burying of fimbria in wall of uterus
Q32.3	Excision of hydatid of Morgagni
Q32.8	Other specified
Q32.9	Unspecified

Q34 Other open operations on fallopian tube

Q34.1	Open freeing of adhesions of fallopian tube
Q34.2	Open biopsy of fallopian tube
	Includes: Open biopsy of lesion of fallopian tube
Q34.3	Open dilation of fallopian tube
Q34.4	Exploration of fallopian tube
Q34.8	Other specified
Q34.9	Unspecified

Q35 Endoscopic bilateral occlusion of fallopian tubes

Note: It is not necessary to code additionally any mention of diagnostic endoscopic examination of fallopian tube (Q39.9)

Q35.1	Endoscopic bilateral cauterisation of fallopian tubes
Q35.2	Endoscopic bilateral clipping of fallopian tubes
Q35.3	Endoscopic bilateral ringing of fallopian tubes
Q35.4	Endoscopic bilateral placement of intrafallopian implants
	Includes: Hysteroscopic placement of intrafallopian implants
Q35.8	Other specified
Q35.9	Unspecified

Q36 **Other endoscopic occlusion of fallopian tube**
> *Note:* *It is not necessary to code additionally any mention of diagnostic endoscopic examination of fallopian tube (Q39.9)*

Q36.1 Endoscopic occlusion of remaining solitary fallopian tube
Q36.2 Endoscopic placement of intrafallopian implant into remaining solitary fallopian tube
> *Includes:* *Hysteroscopic placement of intrafallopian implant into remaining solitary fallopian tube*

Q36.8 Other specified
Q36.9 Unspecified

Q37 **Endoscopic reversal of female sterilisation**
> *Note:* *It is not necessary to code additionally any mention of diagnostic endoscopic examination of fallopian tube (Q39.9)*

Q37.1 Endoscopic removal of clip from fallopian tube
Q37.8 Other specified
Q37.9 Unspecified

Q38 **Other therapeutic endoscopic operations on fallopian tube**
> *Note:* *It is not necessary to code additionally any mention of endoscopic examination of fallopian tube (Q39.9)*

Q38.1 Endoscopic freeing of adhesions of fallopian tube
Q38.2 Endoscopic injection into fallopian tube
Q38.3 Endoscopic intrafallopian transfer of gametes
> *Note:* *Use a subsidiary code to identify method of in vitro fertilisation (Y96)*

Q38.8 Other specified
Q38.9 Unspecified

Q39 **Diagnostic endoscopic examination of fallopian tube**

Q39.1 Diagnostic endoscopic examination of fallopian tube and biopsy of lesion of fallopian tube
> *Includes:* *Diagnostic endoscopic examination of fallopian tube and biopsy of fallopian tube*
> *Endoscopic biopsy of lesion of fallopian tube*
> *Endoscopic biopsy of fallopian tube*
> *Biopsy of lesion of fallopian tube NEC*
> *Biopsy of fallopian tube NEC*

Q39.8 Other specified
Q39.9 Unspecified
> *Includes:* *Laparoscopy of fallopian tube NEC*
> *Falloposcopy NEC*

Q41 Other operations on fallopian tube

Q41.1 Salpingography
Includes: Hysterosalpingography
Q41.2 Hydrotubation of fallopian tube
Q41.3 Dye test of fallopian tube
Note: Use an additional code to identify laparoscopy of fallopian tube (Q39.9) or gynaecological laparoscopy (T43.9)
Q41.4 Insufflation of fallopian tube
Q41.5 Operations to ensure patency of fallopian tube NEC
Includes: Dilation of fallopian tube NEC
Q41.6 Recanalisation of fallopian tube
Q41.7 Aspiration of fallopian tube
Q41.8 Other specified
Q41.9 Unspecified

Q43 Partial excision of ovary

Q43.1 Excision of wedge of ovary
Q43.2 Excision of lesion of ovary
Q43.3 Marsupialisation of lesion of ovary
Q43.8 Other specified
Q43.9 Unspecified

Q44 Open destruction of lesion of ovary

Q44.1 Open cauterisation of lesion of ovary
Q44.8 Other specified
Q44.9 Unspecified

Q45 Repair of ovary

Q45.1 Replantation of ovary
Q45.2 Fixation of ovary NEC
Q45.3 Suture of ovary
Q45.4 Suture of rupture of corpus luteum
Q45.8 Other specified
Q45.9 Unspecified

Q47 Other open operations on ovary

Q47.1 Transposition of ovary
Q47.2 Open freeing of adhesions of ovary
Q47.3 Open biopsy of lesion of ovary
Includes: Open biopsy of ovary
Q47.4 Open drainage of cyst of ovary
Q47.8 Other specified
Q47.9 Unspecified

Q48 Oocyte recovery

Q48.1 Endoscopic transurethral ultrasound directed oocyte recovery
Q48.2 Endoscopic transvesical oocyte recovery
Q48.3 Laparoscopic oocyte recovery
Includes: Endoscopic oocyte recovery NEC
Q48.4 Transvaginal oocyte recovery
Q48.8 Other specified
Q48.9 Unspecified

Q49   **Therapeutic endoscopic operations on ovary**
      Note: It is not necessary to code additionally any mention of diagnostic endoscopic examination of ovary (Q50.9)

Q49.1   Endoscopic extirpation of lesion of ovary NEC
Q49.2   Endoscopic freeing of adhesions of ovary
Q49.3   Endoscopic drainage of cyst of ovary
Q49.4   Endoscopic drilling of ovary
Q49.8   Other specified
Q49.9   Unspecified

Q50   **Diagnostic endoscopic examination of ovary**

Q50.1   Diagnostic endoscopic examination of ovary and biopsy of lesion of ovary
      Includes: Diagnostic endoscopic examination of ovary and biopsy of ovary
            Endoscopic biopsy of lesion of ovary
            Endoscopic biopsy of ovary
            Biopsy of lesion of ovary NEC
            Biopsy of ovary NEC
Q50.8   Other specified
Q50.9   Unspecified
      Includes: Laparoscopy of ovary NEC

Q51   **Other operations on ovary**

Q51.1   Transvaginal ultrasound guided aspiration of ovarian cyst
Q51.8   Other specified
Q51.9   Unspecified

Q52   **Operations on broad ligament of uterus**

Q52.1   Excision of lesion of broad ligament of uterus
Q52.2   Destruction of lesion of broad ligament of uterus
Q52.3   Shortening of broad ligament of uterus
Q52.8   Other specified
Q52.9   Unspecified

Q54   **Operations on other ligament of uterus**

Q54.1   Suspension of uterus NEC
Q54.2   Plication of round ligament of uterus
Q54.3   Division of uteropelvic ligament
Q54.4   Suspension of uterus using mesh NEC
Q54.5   Sacrohysteropexy
Q54.6   Infracoccygeal hysteropexy
Q54.8   Other specified
Q54.9   Unspecified

Q55   **Other examination of female genital tract**

Q55.1   Examination of female genital tract under anaesthetic and Papanicolau smear
            Includes: Examination of female genital tract under anaesthetic and cervical smear
Q55.2   Examination of female genital tract under anaesthetic NEC
Q55.3   Papanicolau smear NEC
            Includes: Cervical smear NEC
Q55.4   Colposcopy of cervix
            Includes: Colposcopy NEC
            Excludes: Colposcopy limited to vagina (P27.3)
Q55.5   Transvaginal ultrasound examination of female genital tract
            Includes: Examination vagina ultrasound
Q55.6   Genital swab
            Includes: High vaginal swab
Q55.8   Other specified
Q55.9   Unspecified
            Includes: Gynaecological examination under anaesthetic

Q56   **Other operations on female genital tract**

Q56.1   Fertility investigation of female NEC
            Excludes: Patency operations on fallopian tube (Q41)
Q56.2   Fertiloscopy
Q56.8   Other specified
Q56.9   Unspecified

CHAPTER R
FEMALE GENITAL TRACT ASSOCIATED WITH PREGNANCY, CHILDBIRTH AND PUERPERIUM
(CODES R01–R43)

Excludes:	*OPERATIONS ASSOCIATED WITH PREGNANCY*	
	WITH ABORTIVE OUTCOME	*(Chapter Q)*
Note:	*Use a subsidiary code for minimal access approach (Y74–Y76)*	
	Use a subsidiary code to identify method of image control (Y53)	

R01   **Therapeutic endoscopic operations on fetus**
            Note: *Use a subsidiary code to identify gestational age (Y95)*
                       It is not necessary to code additionally any mention of diagnostic endoscopic examination of fetus (R02.9)

R01.1   Fetoscopic blood transfusion of fetus
R01.2   Fetoscopic insertion of tracheal plug for congenital diaphragmatic hernia
R01.8   Other specified
R01.9   Unspecified

R02   **Diagnostic endoscopic examination of fetus**
            Note: *Use a subsidiary code to identify gestational age (Y95)*

R02.1   Fetoscopic examination of fetus and fetoscopic biopsy of fetus
            Includes: *Fetoscopic biopsy of fetus NEC*
R02.2   Fetoscopic examination of fetus and fetoscopic sampling of fetal blood
            Includes: *Fetoscopic sampling of fetal blood NEC*
R02.8   Other specified
R02.9   Unspecified
            Includes: *Fetoscopy NEC*

R03   **Category retired – refer to introduction**

R04   **Therapeutic percutaneous operations on fetus**
            Note: *Use a subsidiary code to identify gestational age (Y95)*

R04.1   Percutaneous insertion of fetal vesicoamniotic shunt
R04.2   Percutaneous insertion of fetal pleuroamniotic shunt
R04.3   Percutaneous blood transfusion of fetus
R04.4   Percutaneous insertion of fetal pleural drain
R04.5   Percutaneous insertion of fetal bladder drain
R04.6   Percutaneous insertion of fetal tracheal plug for congenital diaphragmatic hernia
R04.7   Percutaneous laser ablation of lesion of fetus
R04.8   Other specified
R04.9   Unspecified

R05   **Diagnostic percutaneous examination of fetus**
            Includes: *Placenta*
            Note: *Use a subsidiary code to identify gestational age (Y95)*

R05.1   Percutaneous biopsy of fetus
R05.2   Percutaneous sampling of fetal blood
R05.3   Percutaneous sampling of chorionic villus
R05.8   Other specified
R05.9   Unspecified

R06   **Destruction of fetus**
> *Note: Use a subsidiary code to identify gestational age (Y95)*

R06.1   Selective feticide
R06.2   Feticide NEC
R06.8   Other specified
R06.9   Unspecified

R07   **Therapeutic endoscopic operations for twin to twin transfusion syndrome**
> *Note: Use a subsidiary code to identify gestational age (Y95)*

R07.1   Endoscopic laser ablation of placental arteriovenous anastomosis
R07.2   Endoscopic serial drainage of amniotic fluid for twin to twin transfusion syndrome
R07.8   Other specified
R07.9   Unspecified

R08   **Therapeutic percutaneous operations for twin to twin transfusion syndrome**
> *Note: Use a subsidiary code to identify gestational age (Y95)*

R08.1   Percutaneous laser ablation of placental arteriovenous anastomosis
R08.2   Percutaneous serial drainage of amniotic fluid for twin to twin transfusion syndrome
R08.8   Other specified
R08.9   Unspecified

R10   **Other operations on amniotic cavity**
> *Note: Use a subsidiary code to identify gestational age (Y95)*

R10.1   Drainage of amniotic cavity
R10.2   Diagnostic amniocentesis
         Includes: Amniocentesis NEC
R10.3   Amnioscopy
R10.4   Sampling of chorionic villus NEC
         Includes: Sampling of chorionic villus using vaginal approach
R10.5   Biopsy of placenta NEC
R10.8   Other specified
R10.9   Unspecified

R12   **Operations on gravid uterus**
> *Note: Use a subsidiary code to identify gestational age (Y95)*

R12.1   Cerclage of cervix of gravid uterus
R12.2   Removal of cerclage from cervix of gravid uterus
R12.3   Repositioning of retroverted gravid uterus
R12.4   External cephalic version
R12.8   Other specified
R12.9   Unspecified

R14   **Surgical induction of labour**
         Includes: Surgical augmentation of labour
> *Note: Use as a supplementary code when associated with delivery (R17–R25)*

R14.1   Forewater rupture of amniotic membrane
R14.2   Hindwater rupture of amniotic membrane
R14.8   Other specified
R14.9   Unspecified

R15	**Other induction of labour**

Includes: *Other augmentation of labour*
    Note: **Use as a supplementary code when associated with delivery (R17–R25)**

R15.1	Medical induction of labour

Includes: *Induction of labour using prostaglandins*
              Induction of labour using oxytocin
              Induction of labour using misoprostol

R15.8	Other specified
R15.9	Unspecified

R17	**Elective caesarean delivery**

R17.1	Elective upper uterine segment caesarean delivery
R17.2	Elective lower uterine segment caesarean delivery
R17.8	Other specified
R17.9	Unspecified

R18	**Other caesarean delivery**

Includes: *Emergency caesarean delivery*
Excludes: *Caesarean hysterectomy (R25.1)*

R18.1	Upper uterine segment caesarean delivery NEC
R18.2	Lower uterine segment caesarean delivery NEC
R18.8	Other specified
R18.9	Unspecified

R19	**Breech extraction delivery**

R19.1	Breech extraction delivery with version
R19.8	Other specified
R19.9	Unspecified

R20	**Other breech delivery**

R20.1	Spontaneous breech delivery
R20.2	Assisted breech delivery
R20.8	Other specified
R20.9	Unspecified

R21	**Forceps cephalic delivery**

R21.1	High forceps cephalic delivery with rotation
R21.2	High forceps cephalic delivery NEC
R21.3	Mid forceps cephalic delivery with rotation
R21.4	Mid forceps cephalic delivery NEC
R21.5	Low forceps cephalic delivery
R21.8	Other specified
R21.9	Unspecified

R22	**Vacuum delivery**

R22.1	High vacuum delivery
R22.2	Low vacuum delivery
R22.3	Vacuum delivery before full dilation of cervix
R22.8	Other specified
R22.9	Unspecified

R23 **Cephalic vaginal delivery with abnormal presentation of head at delivery without instrument**

R23.1 Manipulative cephalic vaginal delivery with abnormal presentation of head at delivery without instrument

R23.2 Non-manipulative cephalic vaginal delivery with abnormal presentation of head at delivery without instrument

R23.8 Other specified

R23.9 Unspecified

R24 **Normal delivery**

R24.9 All

R25 **Other methods of delivery**

R25.1 Caesarean hysterectomy

R25.2 Destructive operation to facilitate delivery

R25.8 Other specified

R25.9 Unspecified

R27 **Other operations to facilitate delivery**

R27.1 Episiotomy to facilitate delivery

R27.2 Deinfibulation of vulva to facilitate delivery

R27.8 Other specified

R27.9 Unspecified

R28 **Instrumental removal of products of conception from delivered uterus**
Excludes: After termination of pregnancy (Q10, Q11)

R28.1 Curettage of delivered uterus

R28.8 Other specified

R28.9 Unspecified

R29 **Manual removal of products of conception from delivered uterus**
Excludes: Expression of placenta (R30.2)

R29.1 Manual removal of placenta from delivered uterus

R29.8 Other specified

R29.9 Unspecified

R30 **Other operations on delivered uterus**

R30.1 Repositioning of inverted delivered uterus

R30.2 Expression of placenta

R30.3 Instrumental exploration of delivered uterus NEC

R30.4 Manual exploration of delivered uterus NEC
Includes: Exploration of delivered uterus NEC

R30.8 Other specified

R30.9 Unspecified

R32	**Repair of obstetric laceration**

Includes: Immediate and non-immediate repair of obstetric laceration

R32.1	Repair of obstetric laceration of uterus or cervix uteri
R32.2	Repair of obstetric laceration of perineum and sphincter of anus

Includes: Repair of third degree obstetric tear

R32.3	Repair of obstetric laceration of vagina and floor of pelvis

Includes: Repair of second degree obstetric tear

R32.4	Repair of minor obstetric laceration

Includes: Repair of first degree obstetric tear

R32.5	Repair of obstetric laceration of perineum and sphincter and mucosa of anus

Includes: Repair of fourth degree obstetric tear

R32.8	Other specified
R32.9	Unspecified

R34	**Other obstetric operations**
R34.8	Other specified
R34.9	Unspecified

R36	**Routine obstetric scan**

Note: Use a subsidiary code to identify gestational age (Y95)

R36.1	Dating scan
R36.2	Viability scan
R36.3	Mid trimester scan
R36.8	Other specified
R36.9	Unspecified

R37	**Non-routine obstetric scan for fetal observations**

Note: Use a subsidiary code to identify gestational age (Y95)

R37.1	Biophysical profile
R37.2	Detailed structural scan

Excludes: Nuchal translucency scan NEC (R37.4)

R37.3	Fetal biometry

Includes: Growth scan NEC

R37.4	Nuchal translucency scan

Excludes: Nuchal translucency scan performed as part of a detailed structural scan (R37.2)

R37.5	Fetal ascites scan
R37.6	Rhesus detailed scan
R37.8	Other specified
R37.9	Unspecified

R38	**Other non-routine obstetric scan**

Note: Use a subsidiary code to identify gestational age (Y95)

R38.1	Placental localisation scan
R38.2	Liquor volume scan
R38.8	Other specified
R38.9	Unspecified

R40 **Other maternal physiological assessments**
         Note: Use a subsidiary code to identify gestational age (Y95)

R40.1   Maternal cervical assessment
R40.2   Cervical length scanning at 24 weeks
R40.8   Other specified
R40.9   Unspecified

R42 **Obstetric doppler ultrasound**
         Note: Use a subsidiary code to identify gestational age (Y95)

R42.1   Doppler ultrasound scan of umbilical artery
R42.2   Doppler ultrasound scan of uterine artery
R42.3   Doppler ultrasound scan of middle cerebral artery of fetus
R42.8   Other specified
R42.9   Unspecified

R43 **Ultrasound monitoring**
         Note: Use a subsidiary code to identify gestational age (Y95)

R43.1   Ultrasound monitoring of luteal phase
R43.2   Ultrasound monitoring of early pregnancy
R43.8   Other specified
R43.9   Unspecified

CHAPTER S
SKIN
(CODES S01–S70)

Excludes: *SKIN TESTS* *(U27, U28, U40)*

Note: *Use a subsidiary code for minimal access approach (Y74–Y76)*

Use a subsidiary code to identify method of image control (Y53)

Codes from this chapter are not to be used as primary codes for following skin sites:

SKIN SITE	CHAPTER	CODE
NIPPLE	B	B35 B36
EYEBROW	C	C10
LIP	F	F01–F06

and for skin of following sites:

SITE	CHAPTER	CODE
CANTHUS	C	C11
EYELID	C	C12 C17 C19 C22
EXTERNAL EAR	D	D02–D06
EXTERNAL NOSE	E	E09
SCROTUM	N	N01–N03
MALE PERINEUM	N	N24
PENIS	N	N27–N28 N32
Includes: Prepuce	N	N30
VULVA	P	P05–P09
FEMALE PERINEUM	P	P11–P13
UMBILICUS	T	T29

Codes from this chapter may, however, be used to enhance these codes where necessary

---

S01   **Plastic excision of skin of head or neck**
    Includes: Subcutaneous tissue of head or neck

S01.1   Facelift and tightening of platysma
S01.2   Facelift NEC
S01.3   Submental lipectomy
S01.4   Browlift NEC
S01.5   Direct browlift
S01.6   Internal browlift
S01.8   Other specified
S01.9   Unspecified

S02   **Plastic excision of skin of abdominal wall**
    Includes: Subcutaneous tissue of abdominal wall
    Excludes: Plastic excision of skin of umbilicus (T29.6)

S02.1   Abdominoplasty
S02.2   Abdominolipectomy
S02.8   Other specified
S02.9   Unspecified

S03   **Plastic excision of skin of other site**
    Includes: Subcutaneous tissue NEC

S03.1   Buttock lift
S03.2   Thigh lift
S03.3   Excision of redundant skin or fat of arm
S03.8   Other specified
S03.9   Unspecified

S04   **Other excision of skin**

S04.1   Excision of sweat gland bearing skin of axilla
S04.2   Excision of sweat gland bearing skin of groin
S04.3   Excision of sweat gland bearing skin NEC
           *Excludes: Excision of sweat gland bearing skin of male perineum (N24.1) or female
                   perineum (P13.7)*
S04.8   Other specified
S04.9   Unspecified

S05   **Microscopically controlled excision of lesion of skin**
           Includes: Subcutaneous tissue

S05.1   Microscopically controlled excision of lesion of skin of head or neck using fresh tissue
           technique
S05.2   Microscopically controlled excision of lesion of skin using fresh tissue technique NEC
S05.3   Microscopically controlled excision of lesion of skin of head or neck using chemosurgical
           technique
S05.4   Microscopically controlled excision of lesion of skin using chemosurgical technique NEC
S05.5   Microscopically controlled excision of lesion of skin of head or neck NEC
S05.8   Other specified
S05.9   Unspecified

S06   **Other excision of lesion of skin**
           Includes: Subcutaneous tissue

S06.1   Marsupialisation of lesion of skin of head or neck
S06.2   Marsupialisation of lesion of skin NEC
S06.3   Shave excision of lesion of skin of head or neck
S06.4   Shave excision of lesion of skin NEC
S06.5   Excision of lesion of skin of head or neck NEC
S06.6   Re-excision of skin margins of head or neck
           Includes: Wider excision of skin margins of head or neck
S06.7   Re-excision of skin margins NEC
           Includes: Wider excision of skin margins NEC
S06.8   Other specified
S06.9   Unspecified

S07   **Photodynamic therapy of skin**

S07.1   Photodynamic therapy of skin of whole body
S07.8   Other specified
S07.9   Unspecified

S08   **Curettage of lesion of skin**
           Includes: Subcutaneous tissue

S08.1   Curettage and cauterisation of lesion of skin of head or neck
S08.2   Curettage and cauterisation of lesion of skin NEC
S08.3   Curettage of lesion of skin of head or neck NEC
S08.8   Other specified
S08.9   Unspecified

S09   **Photodestruction of lesion of skin**
           Includes: Subcutaneous tissue

S09.1   Laser destruction of lesion of skin of head or neck
S09.2   Laser destruction of lesion of skin NEC
S09.3   Photodestruction of lesion of skin of head or neck NEC
S09.4   Infrared photocoagulation of lesion of skin of head or neck
S09.5   Infrared photocoagulation of lesion of skin NEC
S09.8   Other specified
S09.9   Unspecified

S10   **Other destruction of lesion of skin of head or neck**
           Includes: Subcutaneous tissue

S10.1   Cauterisation of lesion of skin of head or neck NEC
S10.2   Cryotherapy to lesion of skin of head or neck
S10.3   Chemical peeling of lesion of skin of head or neck
S10.4   Electrolysis to lesion of skin of head or neck
S10.5   Electrodessication of lesion of skin of head or neck
S10.8   Other specified
S10.9   Unspecified

S11   **Other destruction of lesion of skin of other site**
           Includes: Subcutaneous tissue

S11.1   Cauterisation of lesion of skin NEC
S11.2   Cryotherapy to lesion of skin NEC
S11.3   Chemical peeling of lesion of skin NEC
S11.4   Electrolysis to lesion of skin NEC
S11.5   Electrodessication of lesion of skin NEC
S11.8   Other specified
S11.9   Unspecified

S12   **Phototherapy to skin**

S12.1   Ultraviolet A light therapy to skin
S12.2   Ultraviolet B light therapy to skin
S12.3   Combined photochemotherapy and ultraviolet A light therapy to skin
S12.4   Combined photochemotherapy and ultraviolet B light therapy to skin
S12.8   Other specified
S12.9   Unspecified

S13   **Punch biopsy of skin**

S13.1   Punch biopsy of lesion of skin of head or neck
S13.2   Punch biopsy of lesion of skin NEC
S13.8   Other specified
S13.9   Unspecified

S14   **Shave biopsy of skin**

S14.1   Shave biopsy of lesion of skin of head or neck
S14.2   Shave biopsy of lesion of skin NEC
S14.3   Shaved deep ellipse biopsy of lesion of skin of head or neck
S14.4   Shaved deep ellipse biopsy of lesion of skin NEC
S14.8   Other specified
S14.9   Unspecified

S15   **Other biopsy of skin**
Includes: Subcutaneous tissue

S15.1   Biopsy of lesion of skin of head or neck NEC
S15.2   Biopsy of lesion of skin NEC
S15.8   Other specified
S15.9   Unspecified

S17   **Distant flap of skin and muscle**

S17.1   Distant myocutaneous subcutaneous pedicle flap to head or neck
S17.2   Distant myocutaneous subcutaneous pedicle flap NEC
S17.3   Distant myocutaneous flap to head or neck NEC
S17.8   Other specified
S17.9   Unspecified
Includes: Distant myocutaneous flap NEC

S18   **Distant flap of skin and fascia**

S18.1   Distant fasciocutaneous subcutaneous pedicle flap to head or neck
S18.2   Distant fasciocutaneous subcutaneous pedicle flap NEC
S18.3   Distant fasciocutaneous flap to head or neck NEC
S18.8   Other specified
S18.9   Unspecified
Includes: Distant fasciocutaneous flap NEC

S19   **Distant pedicle flap of skin**

S19.1   Distant tube pedicle flap of skin to head or neck
S19.2   Distant tube pedicle flap of skin NEC
S19.8   Other specified
S19.9   Unspecified

S20   **Other distant flap of skin**

S20.1   Axial pattern distant flap of skin to head or neck
S20.2   Axial pattern distant flap of skin NEC
S20.3   Random pattern distant flap of skin to head or neck
S20.4   Random pattern distant flap of skin NEC
S20.5   Distant flap of skin to head or neck NEC
S20.8   Other specified
S20.9   Unspecified

S21   **Hair bearing flap of skin**
Excludes: Hair bearing flap of skin to eyebrow (C10.2)

S21.1   Hair bearing flap of skin to scalp for male pattern baldness
S21.2   Hair bearing flap of skin to scalp NEC
S21.3   Hair bearing flap of skin to nasolabial area
S21.4   Hair bearing flap of skin to chin area
S21.8   Other specified
S21.9   Unspecified

S22   **Sensory flap of skin**

S22.1   Neurovascular island sensory flap of skin to head or neck
S22.2   Neurovascular island sensory flap of skin NEC
S22.3   Local sensory flap of skin to head or neck
S22.4   Local sensory flap of skin NEC
S22.8   Other specified
S22.9   Unspecified

S23   **Flap operations to relax contracture of skin**

S23.1   Z plasty to head or neck
S23.2   Z plasty NEC
S23.3   W plasty to head or neck
S23.4   W plasty NEC
S23.8   Other specified
S23.9   Unspecified

S24   **Local flap of skin and muscle**
              Includes: Myocutaneous flap NEC

S24.1   Local myocutaneous subcutaneous pedicle flap to head or neck
S24.2   Local myocutaneous subcutaneous pedicle flap NEC
S24.3   Local myocutaneous flap to head or neck NEC
S24.8   Other specified
S24.9   Unspecified
              Includes: Local myocutaneous flap NEC

S25   **Local flap of skin and fascia**
              Includes: Fasciocutaneous flap NEC

S25.1   Local fasciocutaneous subcutaneous pedicle flap to head or neck
S25.2   Local fasciocutaneous subcutaneous pedicle flap NEC
S25.3   Local fasciocutaneous flap to head or neck NEC
S25.8   Other specified
S25.9   Unspecified
              Includes: Local fasciocutaneous flap NEC

S26   **Local subcutaneous pedicle flap of skin**
              Includes: Subcutaneous pedicle flap of skin NEC

S26.1   Axial pattern local subcutaneous pedicle flap of skin to head or neck
S26.2   Axial pattern local subcutaneous pedicle flap of skin NEC
S26.3   Random pattern local subcutaneous pedicle flap of skin to head or neck
S26.4   Random pattern local subcutaneous pedicle flap of skin NEC
S26.5   Local subcutaneous pedicle flap of skin to head or neck NEC
S26.8   Other specified
S26.9   Unspecified

S27   **Other local flap of skin**
             Includes: Flap of skin NEC

S27.1   Axial pattern local flap of skin to head or neck NEC
S27.2   Axial pattern local flap of skin NEC
S27.3   Random pattern local flap of skin to head or neck NEC
S27.4   Random pattern local flap of skin NEC
S27.5   Local flap of skin to head or neck NEC
S27.8   Other specified
S27.9   Unspecified

S28   **Flap of mucosa**

S28.1   Tongue flap
S28.8   Other specified
S28.9   Unspecified

S30   **Other operations on flap of skin to head or neck**

S30.1   Delay of flap of skin to head or neck
S30.2   Transfer of flap of skin to head or neck
S30.3   Revision of flap of skin to head or neck
S30.4   Final inset of flap of skin to head or neck
S30.5   Thinning of flap of skin to head or neck
S30.6   Removal of flap of skin to head or neck
S30.8   Other specified
S30.9   Unspecified

S31   **Other operations on flap of skin to other site**

S31.1   Delay of flap of skin NEC
S31.2   Transfer of flap of skin NEC
S31.3   Revision of flap of skin NEC
S31.4   Final inset of flap of skin NEC
S31.5   Thinning of flap of skin NEC
S31.6   Removal of flap of skin NEC
S31.8   Other specified
S31.9   Unspecified

S33   **Hair bearing graft of skin to scalp**

S33.1   Hair bearing punch graft to scalp for male pattern baldness
S33.2   Hair bearing strip graft to scalp for male pattern baldness
S33.3   Hair bearing graft to scalp for male pattern baldness NEC
S33.8   Other specified
S33.9   Unspecified

S34   **Hair bearing graft of skin to other site**
             Excludes: Hair bearing graft to eyebrow (C10.3)

S34.1   Hair bearing graft to nasolabial area
S34.2   Hair bearing graft to chin area
S34.8   Other specified
S34.9   Unspecified

S35   **Split autograft of skin**

S35.1   Meshed split autograft of skin to head or neck
S35.2   Meshed split autograft of skin NEC
S35.3   Split autograft of skin to head or neck NEC
S35.8   Other specified
S35.9   Unspecified

S36   **Other autograft of skin**

S36.1   Full thickness autograft of skin to head or neck
S36.2   Full thickness autograft of skin NEC
S36.3   Composite autograft of skin to head or neck
S36.4   Composite autograft of skin NEC
S36.5   Pinch graft of skin to head or neck
S36.6   Pinch graft of skin NEC
S36.8   Other specified
S36.9   Unspecified

S37   **Other graft of skin**

S37.1   Allograft of skin to head or neck
S37.2   Allograft of skin NEC
S37.3   Xenograft of skin to head or neck
S37.4   Xenograft of skin NEC
S37.8   Other specified
S37.9   Unspecified

S38   **Graft of mucosa**

S38.1   Graft of mucosa to head or neck
S38.8   Other specified
S38.9   Unspecified

S39   **Graft of other tissue to skin**
            Includes: Graft of tissue to subcutaneous tissue

S39.1   Allograft of amniotic membrane to head or neck
S39.2   Allograft of amniotic membrane NEC
S39.8   Other specified
S39.9   Unspecified

S40   **Other closure of skin**
            Includes: Wound

S40.1   Tape closure of skin NEC
S40.2   Tissue adhesive closure of skin NEC
            Includes: Glue closure of skin NEC
S40.3   Tape closure of skin of head or neck
S40.4   Tissue adhesive closure of skin of head or neck
            Includes: Glue closure of skin of head or neck
S40.8   Other specified
S40.9   Unspecified

S41   **Suture of skin of head or neck**
         Includes: *Insertion of clip into skin of head or neck*
                      Subcutaneous tissue of head or neck
                      Wound of head or neck

S41.1   Primary suture of skin of head or neck NEC
S41.2   Delayed primary suture of skin of head or neck
S41.3   Secondary suture of skin of head or neck
S41.4   Resuture of skin of head or neck
S41.8   Other specified
S41.9   Unspecified

S42   **Suture of skin of other site**
         Includes: *Insertion of clip into skin NEC*
                      Subcutaneous tissue NEC
                      Wound NEC

S42.1   Primary suture of skin NEC
S42.2   Delayed primary suture of skin NEC
S42.3   Secondary suture of skin NEC
S42.4   Resuture of skin NEC
S42.8   Other specified
S42.9   Unspecified

S43   **Removal of repair material from skin**
         Includes: *Subcutaneous tissue*
                      Wound

S43.1   Removal of clip from skin of head or neck
S43.2   Removal of clip from skin NEC
S43.3   Removal of suture from skin of head or neck
S43.4   Removal of suture from skin NEC
S43.8   Other specified
S43.9   Unspecified

S44   **Removal of other inorganic substance from skin**
         Includes: *Subcutaneous tissue*
                      Wound

S44.1   Removal of metal from skin of head or neck
S44.2   Removal of metal from skin NEC
S44.3   Removal of glass from skin of head or neck
S44.4   Removal of glass from skin NEC
S44.5   Removal of inorganic foreign body from skin of head or neck NEC
S44.6   Removal of inorganic foreign body from skin NEC
S44.8   Other specified
S44.9   Unspecified

S45   **Removal of other substance from skin**
          Includes: Subcutaneous tissue
          *   Wound*

S45.1   Removal of dirt from skin of head or neck
S45.2   Removal of dirt from skin NEC
S45.3   Removal of organic material from skin of head or neck NEC
S45.4   Removal of organic material from skin NEC
S45.5   Removal of foreign body from skin of head or neck NEC
S45.6   Removal of foreign body from skin NEC
S45.8   Other specified
S45.9   Unspecified

S47   **Opening of skin**
          Includes: Subcutaneous tissue

S47.1   Drainage of lesion of skin of head or neck
S47.2   Drainage of lesion of skin NEC
S47.3   Incision of lesion of skin of head or neck
S47.4   Incision of lesion of skin NEC
S47.5   Incision of skin of head or neck
S47.6   Incision of skin NEC
S47.8   Other specified
S47.9   Unspecified

S48   **Insertion of skin expander into subcutaneous tissue**

S48.1   Insertion of skin expander into subcutaneous tissue of head or neck
S48.2   Insertion of skin expander into subcutaneous tissue of breast
S48.8   Other specified
S48.9   Unspecified

S49   **Attention to skin expander in subcutaneous tissue**

S49.1   Adjustment to skin expander in subcutaneous tissue
          Includes: Inflation of skin expander in subcutaneous tissue
S49.2   Removal of skin expander from subcutaneous tissue of head or neck
S49.3   Removal of skin expander from subcutaneous tissue of breast
S49.4   Removal of skin expander from subcutaneous tissue NEC
S49.8   Other specified
S49.9   Unspecified

S50   **Introduction of other inert substance into subcutaneous tissue**

S50.1   Insertion of organic inert substance into subcutaneous tissue
S50.2   Injection of organic inert substance into subcutaneous tissue
S50.3   Insertion of inert substance into subcutaneous tissue NEC
S50.4   Injection of inert substance into subcutaneous tissue NEC
S50.8   Other specified
S50.9   Unspecified

S51   **Introduction of destructive substance into subcutaneous tissue**

S51.1   Injection of sclerosing substance into subcutaneous tissue
S51.8   Other specified
S51.9   Unspecified

S52   **Introduction of therapeutic substance into subcutaneous tissue**
               Excludes: Subcutaneous injections (X38)

S52.1   Insertion of steroid into subcutaneous tissue
S52.3   Insertion of therapeutic substance into subcutaneous tissue NEC
S52.5   Insertion of hormone into subcutaneous tissue
               Includes: Insertion of contraceptive substance into subcutaneous tissue
S52.6   Replacement of hormone in subcutaneous tissue
S52.8   Other specified
S52.9   Unspecified

S53   **Introduction of substance into skin**
               Includes: Introduction of substance into lesion of skin

S53.1   Insertion of therapeutic substance into skin
S53.2   Injection of therapeutic substance into skin
S53.3   Insertion of inert substance into skin
S53.4   Injection of inert substance into skin
S53.5   Insertion of diagnostic substance into skin
S53.6   Injection of diagnostic substance into skin
S53.8   Other specified
S53.9   Unspecified

S54   **Exploration of burnt skin of head or neck**
               Includes: Subcutaneous tissue of head or neck

S54.1   Debridement of burnt skin of head or neck
S54.2   Removal of slough from burnt skin of head or neck
               Includes: Escharotomy of burnt skin of head or neck
S54.3   Toilet to burnt skin of head or neck NEC
S54.4   Dressing of burnt skin of head or neck NEC
S54.5   Attention to dressing of burnt skin of head or neck
S54.6   Cleansing and sterilisation of burnt skin of head or neck
S54.7   Dressing of burnt skin of head or neck using vacuum assisted closure device
S54.8   Other specified
S54.9   Unspecified

S55   **Exploration of burnt skin of other site**
               Includes: Subcutaneous tissue NEC

S55.1   Debridement of burnt skin NEC
S55.2   Removal of slough from burnt skin NEC
               Includes: Escharotomy of burnt skin NEC
S55.3   Toilet to burnt skin NEC
S55.4   Dressing of burnt skin NEC
S55.5   Attention to dressing of burnt skin NEC
S55.6   Cleansing and sterilisation of burnt skin NEC
S55.7   Dressing of burnt skin using vacuum assisted closure device NEC
S55.8   Other specified
S55.9   Unspecified

S56   **Exploration of other skin of head or neck**
           Includes: *Subcutaneous tissue of head or neck NEC*
                      Wound of head or neck NEC

S56.1   Debridement of skin of head or neck NEC
           Includes: *Excision of devitalised skin of head or neck NEC*
S56.2   Removal of slough from skin of head or neck NEC
           Includes: *Escharotomy of skin of head or neck NEC*
S56.3   Toilet to skin of head or neck NEC
S56.4   Dressing of skin of head or neck NEC
S56.5   Attention to dressing of skin of head or neck NEC
S56.6   Cleansing and sterilisation of skin of head or neck NEC
S56.7   Dressing of skin of head or neck using vacuum assisted closure device NEC
S56.8   Other specified
S56.9   Unspecified

S57   **Exploration of other skin of other site**
           Includes: *Subcutaneous tissue NEC*
                      Wound NEC

S57.1   Debridement of skin NEC
           Includes: *Excision of devitalised skin NEC*
S57.2   Removal of slough from skin NEC
           Includes: *Escharotomy of skin NEC*
S57.3   Toilet of skin NEC
S57.4   Dressing of skin NEC
S57.5   Attention to dressing of skin NEC
S57.6   Cleansing and sterilisation of skin NEC
S57.7   Dressing of skin using vacuum assisted closure device NEC
S57.8   Other specified
S57.9   Unspecified

S58   **Larvae therapy of skin**
           Includes: *Subcutaneous tissue NEC*
                      Wound

S58.1   Larvae debridement therapy of skin of head or neck
S58.2   Larvae debridement therapy of skin NEC
S58.8   Other specified
S58.9   Unspecified

S59   **Leech therapy of skin**
           Includes: *Subcutaneous tissue NEC*
                      Wound

S59.1   Leech therapy of skin of head or neck
S59.2   Leech therapy of skin NEC
S59.8   Other specified
S59.9   Unspecified

S60 **Other operations on skin**
Includes: Wound

S60.1   Dermabrasion of skin of head or neck
S60.2   Dermabrasion of skin NEC
S60.3   Tattooing of skin
S60.4   Refashioning of scar NEC
S60.5   Diagnostic dermatoscopy of skin
S60.6   Electrolysis of hair
Includes: Electrolysis NEC
S60.7   Epilation NEC
S60.8   Other specified
S60.9   Unspecified

S62 **Other operations on subcutaneous tissue**
Note: Principal category, extended at S63

S62.1   Liposuction of subcutaneous tissue of head or neck
S62.2   Liposuction of subcutaneous tissue NEC
S62.3   Removal of inserted substance from subcutaneous tissue
S62.4   Removal of pack from subcutaneous tissue
S62.5   Removal of hormone implant from subcutaneous tissue
Includes: Removal of contraceptive from subcutaneous tissue
S62.6   Insertion of diagnostic substance into subcutaneous tissue
S62.7   Insertion of diagnostic device into subcutaneous tissue
S62.8   Other specified
S62.9   Unspecified

S63 **Operations on subcutaneous tissue**
Note: Principal S62

S63.1   Removal of diagnostic device from subcutaneous tissue
S63.2   Creation of subcutaneous storage pocket and placement of autologous tissue
Note: Use as a supplementary code when associated with decompressive craniectomy (V03.7)
S63.3   Removal of autologous tissue from subcutaneous storage pocket
Note: Use as a supplementary code when associated with replacement of stored cranial bone flap (V01.2)
S63.8   Other specified
S63.9   Unspecified

S64 **Extirpation of nail bed**
S64.1   Excision of nail bed
S64.2   Chemical destruction of nail bed
Includes: Phenolisation of nail bed
S64.3   Destruction of nail bed NEC
S64.8   Other specified
S64.9   Unspecified

S66 **Other operations on nail bed**

S66.1   Biopsy of lesion of nail bed
          Includes: Biopsy of nail bed
S66.2   Repair of nail bed
S66.3   Incision of nail bed
S66.8   Other specified
S66.9   Unspecified

S68 **Excision of nail**

S68.1   Total excision of nail
S68.2   Excision of wedge of nail
S68.3   Partial excision of nail NEC
S68.8   Other specified
S68.9   Unspecified

S70 **Other operations on nail**

S70.1   Avulsion of nail
          Includes: Removal of nail NEC
S70.2   Incision of nail
S70.3   Removal of foreign body from nail
S70.8   Other specified
S70.9   Unspecified

CHAPTER T
SOFT TISSUE
(CODES T01–T98)

Includes:	*CHEST WALL*
	ABDOMINAL WALL
	FASCIA
	TENDON
	MUSCLE
	LYMPHATIC TISSUE
	CONNECTIVE TISSUE

Excludes: MUSCLE OF EYE *(Chapter C)*

SOME OPERATIONS ON SOFT TISSUE FOR CORRECTION
OF CONGENITAL DEFORMITY OF LIMB *(Chapter X)*

Note: Use a subsidiary code for minimal access approach (Y74–Y76)

Use a subsidiary code to identify method of image control (Y53)

T01 **Partial excision of chest wall**

T01.1 Thoracoplasty
T01.2 Removal of plombage material from chest wall
T01.3 Excision of lesion of chest wall
T01.8 Other specified
T01.9 Unspecified

T02 **Reconstruction of chest wall**

T02.1 Correction of pectus deformity of chest wall
   Includes: Correction of pectus carinatum
   Correction of pectus excavatum
T02.2 Insertion of silicone implant for correction of pectus excavatum
T02.3 Insertion of prosthesis into chest wall NEC
T02.4 Removal of prosthesis from chest wall
T02.8 Other specified
T02.9 Unspecified

T03 **Opening of chest**
   Includes: Chest wall
   Pleura
   Pleural cavity
   Note: Do not use as approach code (Y49)

T03.1 Exploratory median sternotomy
T03.2 Reopening of chest and re-exploration of intrathoracic operation site and surgical arrest of postoperative bleeding
   Includes: Reopening of incision of chest and re-exploration of intrathoracic operation site and surgical arrest of bleeding
   Reopening of wound of chest and re-exploration of intrathoracic operation site and surgical arrest of bleeding
T03.3 Reopening of chest and re-exploration of intrathoracic operation site NEC
   Includes: Reopening of incision of chest and re-exploration of intrathoracic operation site NEC
   Reopening of wound of chest and re-exploration of intrathoracic operation site NEC
T03.4 Reopening of chest NEC
   Includes: Reopening of incision of chest NEC
   Reopening of wound of chest NEC
T03.8 Other specified
T03.9 Unspecified
   Includes: Exploratory thoracotomy NEC

T05   **Other operations on chest wall**

T05.1   Suture of chest wall
T05.2   Resuture of previous incision of chest wall
             Includes: Resuture of rupture of incision of chest wall
             *   Suture of dehiscence of wound of chest wall*
T05.3   Repair of chest wall NEC
T05.4   Removal of wire from chest wall
T05.8   Other specified
T05.9   Unspecified

T07   **Open excision of pleura**

T07.1   Decortication of pleura
T07.2   Open excision of lesion of pleura
T07.8   Other specified
T07.9   Unspecified
             Includes: Pleurectomy NEC

T08   **Open drainage of pleural cavity**

T08.1   Resection of rib and open drainage of pleural cavity
T08.2   Closure of open drainage of pleural cavity
T08.3   Fenestration of pleura
T08.4   Closure of fenestration of pleura
T08.8   Other specified
T08.9   Unspecified

T09   **Other open operations on pleura**

T09.1   Open destruction of lesion of pleura
T09.2   Open biopsy of lesion of pleura
             Includes: Open biopsy of pleura
T09.3   Mechanical open pleurodesis
T09.4   Chemical open pleurodesis
T09.5   Open pleurodesis NEC
T09.8   Other specified
T09.9   Unspecified

T10   **Therapeutic endoscopic operations on pleura**
             Note: It is not necessary to code additionally any mention of diagnostic endoscopic
             ***   examination of pleural cavity (T11.9)***
             ***   Therapeutic endoscopic operations specifically directed at individual***
             ***   intrathoracic organs are usually classified elsewhere***

T10.1   Endoscopic extirpation of lesion of pleura
T10.2   Endoscopic pleurodesis using talc
T10.3   Endoscopic pleurodesis NEC
T10.8   Other specified
T10.9   Unspecified

T11 **Diagnostic endoscopic examination of pleura**
Includes: Pleural cavity
Note: Diagnostic endoscopic examinations specifically directed at individual intrathoracic organs are usually classified elsewhere

T11.1 Diagnostic endoscopic examination of pleura and biopsy of lesion of pleura
*Includes: Diagnostic endoscopic examination of pleura and biopsy of pleura
Endoscopic biopsy of lesion of pleura
Endoscopic biopsy of pleura*

T11.2 Diagnostic endoscopic examination of pleura and biopsy of lesion of intrathoracic organ NEC
*Includes: Diagnostic endoscopic examination of pleura and biopsy of intrathoracic organ NEC
Thoracoscopic biopsy of lesion of intrathoracic organ NEC
Thoracoscopic biopsy of intrathoracic organ NEC*
Note: Use a subsidiary site code as necessary

T11.8 Other specified
T11.9 Unspecified
Includes: Thoracoscopy NEC

T12 **Puncture of pleura**

T12.1 Drainage of lesion of pleura NEC
Includes: Drainage of lesion of pleural cavity NEC

T12.2 Drainage of pleural cavity NEC
Includes: Paracentesis of chest
Excludes: Insertion of underwater drain into chest (T12.4)

T12.3 Aspiration of pleural cavity
Includes: Thoracocentesis

T12.4 Insertion of tube drain into pleural cavity
*Includes: Insertion of underwater drain into chest
Insertion of tunnelled catheter into pleural cavity*

T12.5 Attention to tube drain into pleural cavity
*Includes: Attention to underwater drain in chest
Attention to tunnelled catheter in pleural cavity*

T12.8 Other specified
T12.9 Unspecified

T13 **Introduction of substance into pleural cavity**

T13.1 Insufflation of talc into pleural cavity NEC
T13.2 Introduction of sclerosing substance into pleural cavity NEC
T13.3 Introduction of cytotoxic substance into pleural cavity
T13.4 Introduction of therapeutic substance into pleural cavity
T13.8 Other specified
T13.9 Unspecified

T14 **Other operations on pleura**
Includes: Pleural cavity

T14.1 Percutaneous biopsy of lesion of pleura
*Includes: Percutaneous biopsy of pleura
Biopsy of lesion of pleura NEC
Biopsy of pleura NEC*

T14.8 Other specified
T14.9 Unspecified

T15   **Repair of rupture of diaphragm**

T15.1   Repair of traumatic rupture of diaphragm
T15.2   Repair of postoperative rupture of diaphragm
T15.8   Other specified
T15.9   Unspecified

T16   **Other repair of diaphragm**
         Excludes: Repair of hiatus hernia (G23)

T16.1   Insertion of prosthesis for repair of diaphragm
T16.2   Plication of diaphragm
T16.3   Closure of fistula of diaphragm
T16.4   Repair of congenital diaphragmatic hernia
T16.5   Suture of diaphragm NEC
T16.8   Other specified
T16.9   Unspecified

T17   **Other operations on diaphragm**

T17.1   Excision of lesion of diaphragm
T17.2   Destruction of lesion of diaphragm
T17.8   Other specified
T17.9   Unspecified

T19   **Simple excision of inguinal hernial sac**
         Note: Use a supplementary code as necessary for tether of testis (N13.2)

T19.1   Bilateral herniotomy
T19.2   Unilateral herniotomy
T19.3   Ligation of patent processus vaginalis
         Includes: Correction of hydrocele of infancy
T19.8   Other specified
T19.9   Unspecified
         Includes: Herniotomy NEC

T20   **Primary repair of inguinal hernia**
         Includes: Repair of inguinal hernia NEC
         Note: Use a supplementary code as necessary for concurrent excision of bowel (e.g. G69.3, H11.1)
         Use a supplementary code as necessary for relief of strangulation of bowel (e.g. G76.2, H17.5)
         Use a subsidiary code to identify laterality (Z94)

T20.1   Primary repair of inguinal hernia using insert of natural material
T20.2   Primary repair of inguinal hernia using insert of prosthetic material
         Includes: Primary repair of inguinal hernia using insert NEC
T20.3   Primary repair of inguinal hernia using sutures
T20.4   Primary repair of inguinal hernia and reduction of sliding hernia
T20.8   Other specified
T20.9   Unspecified

T21   **Repair of recurrent inguinal hernia**
           Note: *Use a supplementary code as necessary for concurrent excision of bowel (e.g. G69.3, H11.1)*
                     Use a supplementary code as necessary for relief of strangulation of bowel (e.g. G76.2, H17.5)
                     Use a subsidiary code to identify laterality (Z94)

T21.1   Repair of recurrent inguinal hernia using insert of natural material
T21.2   Repair of recurrent inguinal hernia using insert of prosthetic material
           Includes: *Repair of recurrent inguinal hernia using insert NEC*
T21.3   Repair of recurrent inguinal hernia using sutures
T21.4   Removal of prosthetic material from previous repair of inguinal hernia
T21.8   Other specified
T21.9   Unspecified

T22   **Primary repair of femoral hernia**
           Includes: *Repair of femoral hernia NEC*
           Note: *Use a supplementary code as necessary for concurrent excision of bowel (e.g. G69.3, H11.1)*
                     Use a supplementary code as necessary for relief of strangulation of bowel (e.g. G76.2, H17.5)
                     Use a subsidiary code to identify laterality (Z94)

T22.1   Primary repair of femoral hernia using insert of natural material
T22.2   Primary repair of femoral hernia using insert of prosthetic material
           Includes: *Primary repair of femoral hernia using insert NEC*
T22.3   Primary repair of femoral hernia using sutures
T22.8   Other specified
T22.9   Unspecified

T23   **Repair of recurrent femoral hernia**
           Note: *Use a supplementary code as necessary for concurrent excision of bowel (e.g. G69.3, H11.1)*
                     Use a supplementary code as necessary for relief of strangulation of bowel (e.g. G76.2, H17.5)
                     Use a subsidiary code to identify laterality (Z94)

T23.1   Repair of recurrent femoral hernia using insert of natural material
T23.2   Repair of recurrent femoral hernia using insert of prosthetic material
           Includes: *Repair of recurrent femoral hernia using insert NEC*
T23.3   Repair of recurrent femoral hernia using sutures
T23.4   Removal of prosthetic material from previous repair of femoral hernia
T23.8   Other specified
T23.9   Unspecified

T24   **Primary repair of umbilical hernia**
           Includes: *Repair of umbilical hernia NEC*
           Excludes: *Repair of recurrent umbilical hernia (T97)*

T24.1   Repair of umbilical hernia using insert of natural material
T24.2   Repair of umbilical hernia using insert of prosthetic material
           Includes: *Repair of umbilical hernia using insert NEC*
T24.3   Repair of umbilical hernia using sutures
T24.4   Removal of prosthetic material from previous repair of umbilical hernia
T24.8   Other specified
T24.9   Unspecified

T25   **Primary repair of incisional hernia**
Includes: Repair of incisional hernia NEC
Primary repair of parastomal hernia
Repair of parastomal hernia NEC
Note: Use a supplementary code as necessary for concurrent excision of bowel (e.g. G69.3, H11.1)
Use a supplementary code as necessary for relief of strangulation of bowel (e.g. G76.2, H17.5)

T25.1   Primary repair of incisional hernia using insert of natural material
T25.2   Primary repair of incisional hernia using insert of prosthetic material
Includes: Primary repair of incisional hernia using insert NEC
T25.3   Primary repair of incisional hernia using sutures
T25.8   Other specified
T25.9   Unspecified

T26   **Repair of recurrent incisional hernia**
Includes: Repair of recurrent parastomal hernia
Note: Use a supplementary code as necessary for concurrent excision of bowel (e.g. G69.3, H11.1)
Use a supplementary code as necessary for relief of strangulation of bowel (e.g. G76.2, H17.5)

T26.1   Repair of recurrent incisional hernia using insert of natural material
T26.2   Repair of recurrent incisional hernia using insert of prosthetic material
Includes: Repair of recurrent incisional hernia using insert NEC
T26.3   Repair of recurrent incisional hernia using sutures
T26.4   Removal of prosthetic material from previous repair of incisional hernia
T26.8   Other specified
T26.9   Unspecified

T27   **Repair of other hernia of abdominal wall**
Excludes: Repair of recurrent other hernia of abdominal wall (T98)
Note: Use a supplementary code as necessary for concurrent excision of bowel (e.g. G69.3, H11.1)
Use a supplementary code as necessary for relief of strangulation of bowel (e.g. G76.2, H17.5)

T27.1   Repair of ventral hernia using insert of natural material
T27.2   Repair of ventral hernia using insert of prosthetic material
Includes: Repair of ventral hernia using insert NEC
T27.3   Repair of ventral hernia using sutures
T27.4   Removal of prosthetic material from previous repair of ventral hernia
T27.8   Other specified
T27.9   Unspecified

T28 **Other repair of anterior abdominal wall**
Includes: Abdominal wall NEC

T28.1   Closure of gastroschisis
Includes: Closure of exomphalos
T28.2   Suture of anterior abdominal wall
Includes: Suture of abdomen
Closure of anterior abdominal wall
Closure of abdomen
T28.3   Resuture of previous incision of anterior abdominal wall
Includes: Resuture of rupture of incision of anterior abdominal wall
Suture of dehiscence of wound of anterior abdominal wall
T28.8   Other specified
T28.9   Unspecified

T29 **Operations on umbilicus**
Includes: Skin of umbilicus
Excludes: Repair of umbilical hernia (T24)
   Note: Codes from Chapter S may be used to enhance these codes

T29.1   Excision of umbilicus
T29.2   Excision of urachus
Includes: Excision of lesion of urachus
T29.3   Extirpation of lesion of umbilicus
T29.4   Biopsy of lesion of umbilicus
Includes: Biopsy of umbilicus
T29.5   Excision of fistula of umbilicus
Includes: Excision of sinus of umbilicus
T29.6   Plastic operations on umbilicus
T29.8   Other specified
T29.9   Unspecified

T30 **Opening of abdomen**
Includes: Abdominal wall
Peritoneum
Peritoneal cavity
   Note: Do not use as approach code (Y50)

T30.1   Reopening of abdomen and re-exploration of intra-abdominal operation site and surgical arrest of postoperative bleeding
Includes: Reopening of incision of abdomen and re-exploration of intra-abdominal operation site and surgical arrest of bleeding
Reopening of wound of abdomen and re-exploration of intra-abdominal operation site and surgical arrest of bleeding
T30.2   Reopening of abdomen and re-exploration of intra-abdominal operation site NEC
Includes: Reopening of incision of abdomen and re-exploration of intra-abdominal operation site NEC
Reopening of wound of abdomen and re-exploration of intra-abdominal operation site NEC
T30.3   Reopening of abdomen NEC
Includes: Reopening of incision of abdomen NEC
Reopening of wound of abdomen NEC
T30.4   Opening of abdomen and exploration of groin
Excludes: Exploration of groin NEC (T31.7)
T30.8   Other specified
T30.9   Unspecified
Includes: Exploratory laparotomy NEC

T31   **Other operations on anterior abdominal wall**
            Includes: Abdominal wall NEC

T31.1   Biopsy of lesion of anterior abdominal wall
            Includes: Biopsy of anterior abdominal wall
T31.2   Excision of lesion of anterior abdominal wall and insert of prosthetic material into anterior abdominal wall
T31.3   Excision of lesion of anterior abdominal wall NEC
T31.4   Destruction of lesion of anterior abdominal wall
T31.5   Drainage of anterior abdominal wall
T31.6   Removal of foreign body from anterior abdominal wall
T31.7   Exploration of groin NEC
            Excludes: Opening of abdomen and exploration of groin (T30.4)
T31.8   Other specified
T31.9   Unspecified

T33   **Open extirpation of lesion of peritoneum**

T33.1   Open excision of lesion of peritoneum
T33.2   Open destruction of lesion of peritoneum
T33.8   Other specified
T33.9   Unspecified

T34   **Open drainage of peritoneum**
            Excludes: Operations to create drainage into peritoneum (A12.4, A53)
            *   Creation of peritoneovenous shunt (L81.1)*
            *   Peritoneal dialysis (X40.2)*

T34.1   Open drainage of subphrenic abscess
T34.2   Open drainage of pelvic abscess
T34.3   Open drainage of abdominal abscess NEC
T34.8   Other specified
T34.9   Unspecified

T36   **Operations on omentum**

T36.1   Omentectomy
T36.2   Excision of lesion of omentum
T36.3   Destruction of lesion of omentum
T36.4   Biopsy of lesion of omentum
            Includes: Biopsy of omentum
T36.5   Creation of omental flap
T36.8   Other specified
T36.9   Unspecified

T37   **Operations on mesentery of small intestine**

T37.1   Excision of lesion of mesentery of small intestine
T37.2   Destruction of lesion of mesentery of small intestine
T37.3   Biopsy of lesion of mesentery of small intestine
            Includes: Biopsy of mesentery of small intestine
            *   Biopsy of lesion of mesentery NEC*
            *   Biopsy of mesentery NEC*
T37.4   Repair of mesentery of small intestine
T37.8   Other specified
T37.9   Unspecified

T38 **Operations on mesentery of colon**

T38.1 Excision of lesion of mesentery of colon
T38.2 Destruction of lesion of mesentery of colon
T38.3 Biopsy of lesion of mesentery of colon
Includes: Biopsy of mesentery of colon
T38.4 Repair of mesentery of colon
T38.8 Other specified
T38.9 Unspecified

T39 **Operations on posterior peritoneum**
Includes: Posterior abdominal wall

T39.1 Excision of lesion of posterior peritoneum
T39.2 Destruction of lesion of posterior peritoneum
T39.3 Biopsy of lesion of posterior peritoneum
Includes: Biopsy of posterior peritoneum
T39.8 Other specified
T39.9 Unspecified

T41 **Other open operations on peritoneum**
Includes: Peritoneal cavity

T41.1 Open biopsy of lesion of peritoneum NEC
Includes: Open biopsy of peritoneum NEC
Biopsy of lesion of peritoneum NEC
Biopsy of peritoneum NEC
T41.2 Division of band of peritoneum
T41.3 Freeing of adhesions of peritoneum
Includes: Freeing of adhesions of mesentery
Freeing of adhesions of bowel
Division of adhesions of peritoneum NEC
Division of adhesions of mesentery NEC
Division of adhesions of bowel NEC
Division of limited adhesions of bowel
Excludes: Freeing of extensive adhesions of peritoneum (T41.5)
T41.4 Open removal of foreign body from peritoneum
Includes: Removal of foreign body from peritoneum NEC
T41.5 Freeing of extensive adhesions of peritoneum
Includes: Freeing of extensive adhesions of mesentery
Freeing of extensive adhesions of bowel
Division of extensive adhesions of peritoneum NEC
Division of extensive adhesions of mesentery NEC
Division of extensive adhesions of bowel
Excludes: Division of limited adhesions of bowel (T41.3)
T41.8 Other specified
T41.9 Unspecified

T42   **Therapeutic endoscopic operations on peritoneum**

       Includes: *Peritoneal cavity*

       Note: **It is not necessary to code additionally any mention of diagnostic endoscopic examination of peritoneum (T43.9)**
            Therapeutic endoscopic operations specifically directed at individual intra-abdominal organs are usually classified elsewhere

T42.1   Endoscopic resection of lesion of peritoneum

T42.2   Endoscopic destruction of lesion of peritoneum

T42.3   Endoscopic division of adhesions of peritoneum

       Includes: *Endoscopic division of adhesions of mesentery*
                 Endoscopic division of adhesions of bowel

T42.4   Endoscopic removal of foreign body from peritoneum

T42.8   Other specified

T42.9   Unspecified

T43   **Diagnostic endoscopic examination of peritoneum**

       Includes: *Peritoneal cavity*

       Note: **Diagnostic endoscopic examinations specifically directed at individual intra-abdominal organs are usually classified elsewhere**

T43.1   Diagnostic endoscopic examination of peritoneum and biopsy of lesion of peritoneum

       Includes: *Diagnostic endoscopic examination of peritoneum and biopsy of peritoneum*
                 Endoscopic biopsy of lesion of peritoneum
                 Endoscopic biopsy of peritoneum

T43.2   Diagnostic endoscopic examination of peritoneum and biopsy of lesion of intra-abdominal organ NEC

       Includes: *Diagnostic endoscopic examination of peritoneum and biopsy of intra-abdominal organ NEC*
                 Laparoscopic biopsy of lesion of intra-abdominal organ NEC
                 Laparoscopic biopsy of intra-abdominal organ NEC

       Note: **Use a subsidiary site code as necessary**

T43.3   Diagnostic endoscopic ultrasound examination of peritoneum

       Includes: *Laparoscopic ultrasound examination of peritoneum*

T43.4   Diagnostic endoscopic ultrasound examination of peritoneum and biopsy of intra-abdominal organ

       Includes: *Laparoscopic ultrasound examination of peritoneum and biopsy of intra-abdominal organ*

       Note: **Use a subsidiary site code as necessary**

T43.8   Other specified

T43.9   Unspecified

       Includes: *Gynaecological laparoscopy NEC*
                 Laparoscopy NEC
                 Peritoneoscopy NEC

T45   **Image controlled operations on abdominal cavity**

T45.1   Image controlled percutaneous drainage of subphrenic abscess

T45.2   Image controlled percutaneous drainage of pelvic abscess

T45.3   Image controlled percutaneous drainage of abdominal abscess NEC

T45.4   Image controlled percutaneous drainage of lesion of abdominal cavity NEC

T45.8   Other specified

T45.9   Unspecified

T46   **Other drainage of peritoneal cavity**
Excludes: Operations to create drainage into peritoneum (A12.4, A53)
Creation of peritoneovenous shunt (L81.1)
Peritoneal dialysis (X40.2)

T46.1   Paracentesis abdominis for ascites
T46.2   Drainage of ascites NEC
Includes: Tapping of ascites NEC
T46.3   Irrigation of peritoneal cavity
Includes: Lavage of peritoneal cavity
Washout of peritoneal cavity
T46.8   Other specified
T46.9   Unspecified

T48   **Other operations on peritoneum**
Includes: Peritoneal cavity

T48.1   Introduction of radioactive substance into peritoneal cavity
Note: Use an additional code to specify radiotherapy delivery (X65)
T48.2   Introduction of cytotoxic substance into peritoneal cavity
T48.3   Introduction of therapeutic substance into peritoneal cavity
T48.4   Introduction of substance into peritoneal cavity NEC
T48.8   Other specified
T48.9   Unspecified

T50   **Transplantation of fascia**
Excludes: With skin (S18, S25)

T50.1   Transfer of fascial tissue
T50.8   Other specified
T50.9   Unspecified

T51   **Excision of fascia of abdomen**
Includes: Release of fascia of abdomen

T51.1   Excision of fascia of posterior abdominal wall
T51.2   Excision of fascia of pelvis
T51.8   Other specified
T51.9   Unspecified

T52   **Excision of other fascia**
Note: Principal category, extended at T56

T52.1   Palmar fasciectomy
T52.2   Revision of palmar fasciectomy
T52.3   Plantar fasciectomy
T52.4   Revision of plantar fasciectomy
T52.5   Digital fasciectomy
T52.6   Revision of digital fasciectomy
T52.8   Other specified
T52.9   Unspecified
Includes: Fasciectomy NEC

T53   **Extirpation of lesion of fascia**

T53.1   Excision of lesion of fascia
T53.2   Destruction of lesion of fascia
T53.8   Other specified
T53.9   Unspecified

T54   **Division of fascia**

T54.1   Division of palmar fascia
T54.2   Division of plantar fascia
T54.8   Other specified
T54.9   Unspecified
         Includes: Fasciotomy NEC

T55   **Release of fascia**
         Excludes: Release of fascia of abdomen (T51)

T55.1   Release fasciotomy of upper arm
T55.2   Release fasciotomy of forearm
T55.3   Release fasciotomy of thigh
T55.4   Release fasciotomy of anterior compartment of lower leg
T55.5   Release fasciotomy of posterior compartment of lower leg
T55.6   Release fasciotomy of leg NEC
T55.8   Other specified
T55.9   Unspecified

T56   **Other excision of other fascia**
         Note: Principal T52

T56.1   Dermofasciectomy
T56.2   Revision of dermofasciectomy
T56.8   Other specified
T56.9   Unspecified

T57   **Other operations on fascia**

T57.1   Freeing of adhesions of fascia
T57.2   Biopsy of lesion of fascia
         Includes: Biopsy of fascia
T57.3   Repair of fascia
T57.4   Stripping of fascia
T57.8   Other specified
T57.9   Unspecified

T59   **Excision of ganglion**

T59.1   Excision of ganglion of wrist
T59.2   Excision of ganglion of hand NEC
T59.3   Excision of ganglion of knee
T59.4   Excision of ganglion of foot
         Includes: Excision of ganglion of ankle
T59.8   Other specified
T59.9   Unspecified

T60   **Re-excision of ganglion**

T60.1   Re-excision of ganglion of wrist
T60.2   Re-excision of ganglion of hand NEC
T60.3   Re-excision of ganglion of knee
T60.4   Re-excision of ganglion of foot
         Includes: Re-excision of ganglion of ankle
T60.8   Other specified
T60.9   Unspecified

T61   **Other operations on ganglion**

T61.1   Aspiration of ganglion
T61.2   Biopsy of ganglion
T61.3   Injection of ganglion
T61.8   Other specified
T61.9   Unspecified

T62   **Operations on bursa**

T62.1   Total excision of bursa
T62.2   Excision of bursa NEC
T62.3   Biopsy of lesion of bursa
         Includes: Biopsy of bursa
T62.4   Aspiration of bursa
T62.5   Injection into bursa
T62.6   Exploration of bursa
T62.8   Other specified
T62.9   Unspecified

T64   **Transposition of tendon**

T64.1   Multiple transfer of tendon to tendon
T64.2   Transfer of tendon to tendon NEC
T64.3   Multiple insertion of tendons into bone
T64.4   Insertion of tendon into bone NEC
         Excludes: For stabilisation of joint (W77)
T64.5   Tenodesis
T64.8   Other specified
T64.9   Unspecified

T65   **Excision of tendon**

T65.1   Sacrifice of tendon
T65.2   Excision of lesion of tendon
T65.8   Other specified
T65.9   Unspecified

T67   **Primary repair of tendon**
                   Includes: Repair of tendon NEC

T67.1	Primary repair of tendon using tendon transfer procedure
T67.2	Primary repair of tendon using lengthening procedure
T67.3	Primary repair of tendon using permanent prosthesis
T67.4	Primary repair of tendon using temporary prosthesis
T67.5	Primary repair of tendon using graft
T67.6	Primary simple repair of tendon

                   Includes: Primary end to end repair of tendon

T67.8	Other specified
T67.9	Unspecified

T68   **Secondary repair of tendon**

T68.1	Secondary repair of tendon using tendon transfer procedure
T68.2	Secondary repair of tendon using lengthening procedure
T68.3	Secondary repair of tendon using permanent prosthesis
T68.4	Secondary repair of tendon using temporary prosthesis
T68.5	Secondary repair of tendon using graft
T68.6	Secondary simple repair of tendon

                   Includes: Secondary end to end repair of tendon

T68.8	Other specified
T68.9	Unspecified

T69   **Freeing of tendon**
                   Excludes: For stabilisation of joint (W77)

T69.1	Primary tenolysis
T69.2	Revision of tenolysis
T69.8	Other specified
T69.9	Unspecified

T70   **Adjustment to length of tendon**

T70.1	Subcutaneous tenotomy
T70.2	Tenotomy NEC
T70.3	Adjustment to muscle origin of tendon
T70.4	Shortening of tendon NEC
T70.5	Lengthening of tendon

                   Includes: Lengthening of muscle

T70.8	Other specified
T70.9	Unspecified

T71   **Excision of sheath of tendon**

T71.1	Tenosynovectomy
T71.8	Other specified
T71.9	Unspecified

T72   **Other operations on sheath of tendon**

T72.1   Reconstruction of sheath of tendon
T72.2   Biopsy of lesion of sheath of tendon
               Includes: *Biopsy of sheath of tendon*
T72.3   Release of constriction of sheath of tendon
T72.4   Exploration of sheath of tendon
T72.8   Other specified
T72.9   Unspecified

T74   **Other operations on tendon**

T74.1   Biopsy of lesion of tendon NEC
               Includes: *Biopsy of tendon NEC*
T74.2   Removal of prosthesis from tendon
T74.3   Exploration of tendon NEC
T74.4   Injection of therapeutic substance into tendon NEC
T74.5   Extracorporeal shockwave lithotripsy of calculus of tendon
T74.6   Autologous blood injection into tendon
               Note: ***It is not necessary to code additionally any mention of venesection (X36.2)***
T74.8   Other specified
T74.9   Unspecified

T76   **Transplantation of muscle**
               Excludes: *With skin (S17, S24)*

T76.1   Microvascular free tissue transfer of flap of muscle
               Note: ***Use a supplementary code as necessary for concurrent vein graft (L93.5)***
T76.8   Other specified
T76.9   Unspecified

T77   **Excision of muscle**

T77.1   Excision of whole muscle group
T77.2   Wide excision of muscle
               Includes: *Wide excision of lesion of muscle*
T77.3   Partial excision of muscle NEC
               Includes: *Excision of lesion of muscle NEC*
                                Excision of Volkmann contracture of forearm
T77.4   Debridement of muscle NEC
T77.8   Other specified
T77.9   Unspecified

T79   **Repair of muscle**

T79.1   Plastic repair of rotator cuff of shoulder NEC
T79.2   Quadricepsplasty
T79.3   Revisional repair of rotator cuff NEC
T79.4   Plastic repair of multiple tears of rotator cuff of shoulder
T79.5   Revisional repair of multiple tears of rotator cuff of shoulder
T79.8   Other specified
T79.9   Unspecified

T80	**Release of contracture of muscle**
T80.1	Release of paralytic tether
T80.2	Release of cicatricial tether
T80.3	Release of webbing of neck
T80.4	Release of sternomastoid muscle
	Includes: Release of torticollis
T80.8	Other specified
T80.9	Unspecified

T81	**Biopsy of muscle**
T81.1	Percutaneous biopsy of muscle
	Includes: Percutaneous biopsy of lesion of muscle
T81.2	Biopsy of neuromuscular junction
	Includes: Biopsy of muscle for biochemical study
	Biopsy of muscle for physiological study
T81.3	Biopsy of lesion of muscle NEC
T81.8	Other specified
T81.9	Unspecified

T83	**Other operations on muscle**
T83.1	Destruction of lesion of muscle
T83.2	Division of muscle
	Excludes: Detrusor myotomy (M41.6)
T83.3	Stretching of muscle
T83.4	Exploration of muscle
T83.5	Catheter manometry of muscle compartment
T83.8	Other specified
T83.9	Unspecified

T85	**Block dissection of lymph nodes**
T85.1	Block dissection of cervical lymph nodes
T85.2	Block dissection of axillary lymph nodes
T85.3	Block dissection of mediastinal lymph nodes
T85.4	Block dissection of para-aortic lymph nodes
T85.5	Block dissection of inguinal lymph nodes
T85.6	Block dissection of pelvic lymph nodes
T85.8	Other specified
T85.9	Unspecified

T86	**Sampling of lymph nodes**
	Note: Use subsidiary code for sentinel lymph node (O14.2 (Z))
T86.1	Sampling of cervical lymph nodes
T86.2	Sampling of axillary lymph nodes
T86.3	Sampling of supraclavicular lymph nodes
T86.4	Sampling of internal mammary lymph nodes
T86.5	Sampling of mediastinal lymph nodes
T86.6	Sampling of para-aortic lymph nodes
T86.7	Sampling of inguinal lymph nodes
T86.8	Other specified
T86.9	Unspecified

T87   **Excision or biopsy of lymph node**
             Note: Use subsidiary code for sentinel lymph node (O14.2 (Z))

T87.1   Excision or biopsy of scalene lymph node
T87.2   Excision or biopsy of cervical lymph node NEC
T87.3   Excision or biopsy of axillary lymph node
           Includes: Excision or biopsy of supraclavicular lymph node NEC
T87.4   Excision or biopsy of mediastinal lymph node
T87.5   Excision or biopsy of para-aortic lymph node
T87.6   Excision or biopsy of porta hepatis lymph node
T87.7   Excision or biopsy of inguinal lymph node
T87.8   Other specified
T87.9   Unspecified

T88   **Drainage of lesion of lymph node**
             Note: Use subsidiary code for sentinel lymph node (O14.2 (Z))

T88.1   Drainage of lesion of cervical lymph node
T88.2   Drainage of lesion of axillary lymph node
T88.3   Drainage of lesion of inguinal lymph node
T88.8   Other specified
T88.9   Unspecified

T89   **Operations on lymphatic duct**

T89.1   Reconstruction of lymphatic duct
T89.2   Bypass of obstruction of lymphatic duct
T89.3   Ligation of lymphatic duct
T89.4   Cannulation of lymphatic duct
T89.8   Other specified
T89.9   Unspecified

T90   **Contrast radiology of lymphatic tissue**

T90.1   Lymphangiography of arm
T90.2   Lymphangiography of mediastinal lymph nodes
T90.3   Lymphangiography of para-aortic lymph nodes
T90.4   Lymphangiography of leg
T90.8   Other specified
T90.9   Unspecified
           Includes: Lymphangiography NEC

T91   **Operations on sentinel lymph node**

T91.1   Biopsy of sentinel lymph node NEC
T91.2   Scanning of sentinel lymph node
T91.8   Other specified
T91.9   Unspecified

T92   **Other operations on lymphatic tissue**

T92.1   Excision of lymphocele
T92.2   Excision of lymphoedematous tissue of arm
T92.3   Excision of lymphoedematous tissue of leg and buried flaps HFQ
T92.4   Excision of lymphoedematous tissue of leg NEC
T92.5   Excision of lymphoedematous tissue of scrotum
T92.6   Excision of lymphoedematous tissue NEC
T92.8   Other specified
T92.9   Unspecified

T94   **Operations on branchial cleft**

T94.1   Excision of branchial cyst
T94.2   Closure of branchial fistula
T94.8   Other specified
T94.9   Unspecified

T96   **Other operations on soft tissue**
                 Includes: Connective tissue

T96.1   Excision of cystic hygroma
T96.2   Excision of lesion of soft tissue NEC
T96.3   Debridement of soft tissue NEC
T96.4   Evacuation of seroma from soft tissue
T96.8   Other specified
T96.9   Unspecified

T97   **Repair of recurrent umbilical hernia**
                 Excludes: Removal of prosthetic material from previous repair of umbilical hernia (T24.4)

T97.1   Repair of recurrent umbilical hernia using insert of natural material
T97.2   Repair of recurrent umbilical hernia using insert of prosthetic material
                 Includes: Repair of recurrent umbilical hernia using insert NEC
T97.3   Repair of recurrent umbilical hernia using sutures
T97.8   Other specified
T97.9   Unspecified

T98   **Repair of recurrent other hernia of abdominal wall**
                 Note at T27 applies

T98.1   Repair of recurrent ventral hernia using insert of natural material
T98.2   Repair of recurrent ventral hernia using insert of prosthetic material
                 Includes: Repair of ventral hernia using insert NEC
T98.3   Repair of recurrent ventral hernia using sutures
T98.8   Other specified
T98.9   Unspecified

CHAPTER U
DIAGNOSTIC IMAGING, TESTING AND REHABILITATION (CODES U01–U54)

Note:	*Refer to anatomical chapter for diagnostic tests and image guided interventions on a specific organ or body part*

U01 **Diagnostic imaging of whole body**
Note: *Use subsidiary codes to identify radiology with contrast (Y97), radiology procedures (Y98)*

U01.1 Computed tomography of whole body
U01.2 Magnetic resonance imaging of whole body
U01.3 Thermography of whole body
U01.8 Other specified
U01.9 Unspecified

U04 **Diagnostic imaging of mouth**
Note: *Use subsidiary codes to identify radiology with contrast (Y97), radiology procedures (Y98)*

U04.1 Bitewing radiology
U04.2 Periapical radiology
U04.3 Occlusal radiology
U04.4 Lateral oblique jaw radiology
U04.8 Other specified
U04.9 Unspecified

U05 **Diagnostic imaging of central nervous system**
Note: *Use subsidiary codes to identify radiology with contrast (Y97), radiology procedures (Y98)*

U05.1 Computed tomography of head
U05.2 Magnetic resonance imaging of head
U05.3 Functional magnetic resonance imaging of head
U05.4 Computed tomography of spine
U05.5 Magnetic resonance imaging of spine
U05.8 Other specified
U05.9 Unspecified

U06 **Diagnostic imaging of face and neck**

U06.1 Computed tomography of sinuses
Note: *Use subsidiary codes to identify radiology with contrast (Y97), radiology procedures (Y98)*
U06.2 Dacryoscintigraphy
Note: *Use subsidiary codes to identify gallium-67 imaging (Y93), radiopharmaceutical imaging (Y94)*
U06.3 Ultrasound of thyroid gland
Note: *Use subsidiary codes to identify radiology with contrast (Y97), radiology procedures (Y98)*
U06.4 Plain x-ray of skull
Note: *Use subsidiary codes to identify radiology with contrast (Y97), radiology procedures (Y98)*
U06.5 Scanning of thyroid gland NEC
Note: *Use subsidiary codes to identify gallium-67 imaging (Y93), radiopharmaceutical imaging (Y94)*
U06.8 Other specified
U06.9 Unspecified

U07   **Diagnostic imaging of chest**
Excludes: Diagnostic imaging of breast (U18)
              Diagnostic imaging of respiratory system (U15)
Note: Use subsidiary codes to identify radiology with contrast (Y97), radiology procedures (Y98)

U07.1   Computed tomography of chest
U07.2   Magnetic resonance imaging of chest
U07.3   Plain x-ray of chest
U07.8   Other specified
U07.9   Unspecified

U08   **Diagnostic imaging of abdomen**
Excludes: Diagnostic imaging of digestive tract (U17)
Note: For laparoscopic ultrasound examination of organ – see body system chapter
          Use subsidiary codes to identify radiology with contrast (Y97), radiology procedures (Y98)

U08.1   Computed tomography of abdomen NEC
           Excludes: Computed tomography of colon (U17.5)
U08.2   Ultrasound of abdomen
U08.3   Plain x-ray of abdomen
U08.4   Upper gastrointestinal imaging series
U08.5   Magnetic resonance imaging of abdomen
U08.8   Other specified
U08.9   Unspecified

U09   **Diagnostic imaging of pelvis**
Note: Use subsidiary codes to identify radiology with contrast (Y97), radiology procedures (Y98)

U09.1   Computed tomography of pelvis
U09.2   Ultrasound of pelvis
           Includes: Hysterosonography
                       Transrectal ultrasound of pelvis
           Excludes: Transvaginal ultrasound (Q55.5)
U09.3   Magnetic resonance imaging of pelvis
U09.8   Other specified
U09.9   Unspecified

U10	**Diagnostic imaging of heart**
Excludes: Contrast radiology of heart (K63)

U10.1	Cardiac computed tomography for calcium scoring
	Note:	***Use subsidiary codes to identify radiology with contrast (Y97), radiology procedures (Y98)***

U10.2	Cardiac computed tomography angiography
	Note:	***Use subsidiary codes to identify radiology with contrast (Y97), radiology procedures (Y98)***

U10.3	Cardiac magnetic resonance imaging
	Note:	***Use subsidiary codes to identify radiology with contrast (Y97), radiology procedures (Y98)***

U10.4	Myocardial positron emission tomography
	Note:	***Use subsidiary codes to identify gallium-67 imaging (Y93), radiopharmaceutical imaging (Y94)***

U10.5	Radionuclide angiocardiography
	Includes: First pass cardiac angiogram
	Note:	***Use subsidiary codes to identify gallium-67 imaging (Y93), radiopharmaceutical imaging (Y94)***

U10.6	Myocardial perfusion scan
	Includes: Myocardial perfusion scan with combined rest and stress test
	Note:	***Use subsidiary codes to identify gallium-67 imaging (Y93), radiopharmaceutical imaging (Y94)***

U10.7	Cardiac multiple gated acquisition scan
	Note:	***Use subsidiary codes to identify gallium-67 imaging (Y93), radiopharmaceutical imaging (Y94)***

U10.8	Other specified
U10.9	Unspecified

U11	**Diagnostic imaging of vascular system**
Excludes: Diagnostic transluminal operations on arteries and veins (Chapter L)
	Note:	***Principal category, extended at U35***

U11.1	Ultrasound of carotid artery
	Note:	***Use subsidiary codes to identify radiology with contrast (Y97), radiology procedures (Y98)***

U11.2	Doppler ultrasound of vessels of extremities
	Note:	***Use subsidiary codes to identify radiology with contrast (Y97), radiology procedures (Y98)***

U11.3	Vascular ultrasound NEC
	Note:	***Use subsidiary codes to identify radiology with contrast (Y97), radiology procedures (Y98)***

U11.4	Computed tomography scan of cerebral vessels
	Note:	***Use subsidiary codes to identify radiology with contrast (Y97), radiology procedures (Y98)***

U11.5	Thallium stress test
	Includes: Myocardial perfusion scan stress test
	Note:	***Use subsidiary codes to identify gallium-67 imaging (Y93), radiopharmaceutical imaging (Y94)***

U11.6	D-dimer assay
	Note:	***Use subsidiary codes to identify radiology with contrast (Y97), radiology procedures (Y98)***

U11.7	Magnetic resonance angiography
	Includes: Magnetic resonance venography
	Note:	***Use subsidiary codes to identify radiology with contrast (Y97), radiology procedures (Y98)***

U11.8	Other specified
U11.9	Unspecified

U12	**Diagnostic imaging of genitourinary system**

Excludes: Diagnostic testing of genitourinary system (U26)
   Note: Principal category, extended at U37

U12.1   Voiding cystourethrogram
   Note: Use subsidiary codes to identify gallium-67 imaging (Y93), radiopharmaceutical imaging (Y94)

U12.2   Ultrasound of scrotum
   Includes: Ultrasound of testes
   Note: Use subsidiary codes to identify radiology with contrast (Y97), radiology procedures (Y98)

U12.3   Ultrasound of kidneys
   Note: Use subsidiary codes to identify radiology with contrast (Y97), radiology procedures (Y98)

U12.4   Ultrasound of bladder
   Note: Use subsidiary codes to identify radiology with contrast (Y97), radiology procedures (Y98)

U12.5   Static renogram
   Note: Use subsidiary codes to identify gallium-67 imaging (Y93), radiopharmaceutical imaging (Y94)

U12.6   Mercaptoacetyltriglycine renogram
   Note: Use subsidiary codes to identify gallium-67 imaging (Y93), radiopharmaceutical imaging (Y94)

U12.7   Nuclear cystography
   Note: Use subsidiary codes to identify gallium-67 imaging (Y93), radiopharmaceutical imaging (Y94)

U12.8   Other specified
U12.9   Unspecified

U13	**Diagnostic imaging of musculoskeletal system**

Excludes: Nuclear bone scan (U14)
   Note: Use a subsidiary site code as necessary
      Use subsidiary codes to identify radiology with contrast (Y97), radiology procedures (Y98)

U13.1   Bone densitometry
   Includes: Dual emission x-ray absorptiometry scan

U13.2   Ultrasound of bone
   Includes: Ultrasound of joint

U13.3   Magnetic resonance imaging of bone
   Includes: Magnetic resonance imaging of joint

U13.4   Plain x-ray of joint
U13.5   Plain x-ray of bone
U13.6   Computed tomography of bone
   Includes: Computed tomography of joint

U13.8   Other specified
U13.9   Unspecified

U14   **Nuclear bone scan**
Excludes: Diagnostic imaging of musculoskeletal system (U13)
> ***Note:*** *Use subsidiary codes to identify gallium-67 imaging (Y93), radiopharmaceutical imaging (Y94)*

U14.1   Nuclear bone scan of whole body
U14.2   Nuclear bone scan – special views
U14.3   Nuclear bone scan – three phase
U14.4   Nuclear bone scan – two phase
U14.8   Other specified
U14.9   Unspecified

U15   **Diagnostic imaging of respiratory system**
Excludes: Diagnostic imaging of chest (U07)
> ***Note:*** *Use subsidiary codes to identify gallium-67 imaging (Y93), radiopharmaceutical imaging (Y94)*

U15.1   Lung perfusion scanning NEC
U15.2   Lung ventilation scanning NEC
Includes: Ventilation scanning with krypton inhalation
U15.3   Ventilation perfusion quotient scan
U15.8   Other specified
U15.9   Unspecified

U16   **Diagnostic imaging of hepatobiliary system**

U16.1   Hepatobiliary nuclear scan
> ***Note:*** *Use subsidiary codes to identify gallium-67 imaging (Y93), radiopharmaceutical imaging (Y94)*
U16.2   Magnetic resonance cholangiopancreatography
> ***Note:*** *Use subsidiary codes to identify radiology with contrast (Y97), radiology procedures (Y98)*
U16.8   Other specified
U16.9   Unspecified

U17   **Diagnostic imaging of digestive tract**

U17.1   Meckel's scan
> ***Note:*** *Use subsidiary codes to identify gallium-67 imaging (Y93), radiopharmaceutical imaging (Y94)*
U17.2   Selenium 75 homocholic acid taurine study
> ***Note:*** *Use subsidiary codes to identify gallium-67 imaging (Y93), radiopharmaceutical imaging (Y94)*
U17.3   Barium swallow
> ***Note:*** *Use subsidiary codes to identify radiology with contrast (Y97), radiology procedures (Y98)*
U17.4   Barium enema
> ***Note:*** *Use subsidiary codes to identify radiology with contrast (Y97), radiology procedures (Y98)*
U17.5   Computed tomography of colon
> ***Note:*** *Use subsidiary codes to identify radiology with contrast (Y97), radiology procedures (Y98)*
U17.6   Patency capsule examination
U17.8   Other specified
U17.9   Unspecified

U18   **Diagnostic imaging of breast**

U18.1   Scintimammography
> *Note:*   *Use subsidiary codes to identify gallium-67 imaging (Y93), radiopharmaceutical imaging (Y94)*

U18.2   Thermography of breast
> *Note:*   *Use subsidiary codes to identify radiology with contrast (Y97), radiology procedures (Y98)*

U18.3   Mammography
> *Note:*   *Use subsidiary codes to identify radiology with contrast (Y97), radiology procedures (Y98)*

U18.8   Other specified

U18.9   Unspecified

U19   **Diagnostic electrocardiography**
> *Excludes:* *Diagnostic imaging of heart (U10)*
> > *Note:*   *Principal category, extended at U34*

U19.1   Implantation of electrocardiography loop recorder

U19.2   24 hour ambulatory electrocardiography
> *Includes:*   *24 hour event monitoring electrocardiography*

U19.3   48 hour ambulatory electrocardiography
> *Includes:*   *48 hour event monitoring electrocardiography*

U19.4   Exercise electrocardiography
> *Includes:* *Exercise stress test*

U19.5   Holter extended electrocardiographic recording

U19.6   Cardiomemo electrocardiographic monitoring

U19.7   Removal of electrocardiography loop recorder

U19.8   Other specified

U19.9   Unspecified

U20   **Diagnostic echocardiography**
> *Includes:* *Ultrasound of heart*

U20.1   Transthoracic echocardiography

U20.2   Transoesophageal echocardiography

U20.3   Intravascular echocardiography

U20.4   Epicardial echocardiography

U20.5   Stress echocardiography

U20.6   Fetal echocardiography

U20.8   Other specified

U20.9   Unspecified

U21   **Diagnostic imaging procedures**
             Note: Principal category, extended at U36

U21.1   Magnetic resonance imaging NEC
             Note: Use subsidiary codes to identify radiology with contrast (Y97), radiology
             *   procedures (Y98)*

U21.2   Computed tomography NEC
             Note: Use subsidiary codes to identify radiology with contrast (Y97), radiology
             *   procedures (Y98)*

U21.3   Positron emission tomography NEC
             Note: Use subsidiary codes to identify gallium-67 imaging (Y93), radiopharmaceutical
             *   imaging (Y94)*

U21.4   Single photon emission computed tomography NEC
             Note: Use subsidiary codes to identify gallium-67 imaging (Y93), radiopharmaceutical
             *   imaging (Y94)*

U21.5   Contrast fluoroscopy NEC
             Note: Use subsidiary codes to identify radiology with contrast (Y97), radiology
             *   procedures (Y98)*

U21.6   Ultrasound scan NEC
             Note: Use subsidiary codes to identify radiology with contrast (Y97), radiology
             *   procedures (Y98)*

U21.7   Plain x-ray NEC
             Note: Use subsidiary codes to identify radiology with contrast (Y97), radiology
             *   procedures (Y98)*

U21.8   Other specified
U21.9   Unspecified

U22   **Neuropsychology tests**

U22.1   Electroencephalograph telemetry
U22.2   Functional inactivation of single brain hemisphere test
U22.3   Neuropsychology test of intelligence
U22.4   Neuropsychology test of language
U22.5   Neuropsychology test of memory
U22.6   Neuropsychology test of perception
U22.7   Neuropsychology test of executive function
U22.8   Other specified
U22.9   Unspecified

U23   **Nuclear medicine haematological tests**
             Note: Use subsidiary codes to identify gallium-67 imaging (Y93), radiopharmaceutical
             *   imaging (Y94)*

U23.1   Red cell mass studies
U23.2   White cell scan using indium 111
U23.3   White cell scan using technetium 99
U23.4   Ferrokinetic studies
U23.8   Other specified
U23.9   Unspecified

U24   **Diagnostic audiology**

U24.1   Pure tone audiometry
U24.2   Balance assessment
U24.3   Hearing assessment
U24.8   Other specified
U24.9   Unspecified

U25   **Breath tests**

U25.1   C14 urea helicobacter pylori breath test
U25.2   C14 glycocholic acid breath test
U25.3   Hydrogen breath test
U25.4   Urea helicobacter pylori breath test NEC
U25.8   Other specified
U25.9   Unspecified

U26   **Diagnostic testing of genitourinary system**
          Excludes: Diagnostic imaging of genitourinary system (U12)

U26.1   Glomerular filtration rate testing
U26.2   Uroflowmetry NEC
U26.3   Test strip urinalysis
U26.4   Urodynamics NEC
          Excludes: Urodynamic studies using catheter (M47.4)
U26.5   Schilling test
U26.8   Other specified
U26.9   Unspecified

U27   **Diagnostic application tests on skin**

U27.1   Standard series patch testing of skin
U27.2   Extended series patch testing of skin
U27.3   Closed routine patch testing of skin
U27.4   Closed special patch testing of skin
U27.5   Open patch testing of skin
U27.6   Patch testing of skin with patient's own products
U27.7   Photopatch testing of skin
U27.8   Other specified
U27.9   Unspecified

U28   **Other diagnostic tests on skin**
          Note: Principal category, extended at U40

U28.1   Phototesting of skin using monochromator
U28.2   Phototesting of skin using solar simulator
U28.3   Provocation phototesting
U28.4   Passive transfer test for solar urticaria
U28.5   Reverse passive transfer test for solar urticaria
U28.6   Autologous serum skin test for urticaria
U28.7   Physical challenge tests for urticaria
          Includes: Dermographism
          Pressure tests
          Ice tests
          Sweat tests
          Water tests
          Exercise tests
          Vibration tests
U28.8   Other specified
U28.9   Unspecified

U29 **Diagnostic endocrinology**

U29.1   Insulin stress test of anterior pituitary function
U29.2   Insulin secretion glucagon test
U29.3   Glucose tolerance test
U29.4   Water deprivation test
U29.5   Adrenal suppression test
U29.6   Arginine vasopressin response to hypertonic saline test
U29.7   Short synacthen test
U29.8   Other specified
U29.9   Unspecified

U30 **Autonomic cardiovascular testing**

U30.1   Tilt table testing
U30.2   Carotid sinus massage test
U30.8   Other specified
U30.9   Unspecified

U31 **Pacemaker testing**

U31.1   Distant pacemaker test
U31.8   Other specified
U31.9   Unspecified

U32 **Diagnostic blood tests**

U32.1   Human Immunodeficiency Virus blood test
U32.8   Other specified
U32.9   Unspecified

U33 **Other diagnostic tests**

U33.1   Polysomnography
         Includes: Cardiopulmonary sleep studies
U33.2   Application of ambulatory blood pressure monitor
U33.3   Removal of ambulatory blood pressure monitor
U33.8   Other specified
U33.9   Unspecified

U34 **Other diagnostic electrocardiography**
         Excludes: Diagnostic imaging of heart (U10)
                  Note: Principal U19

U34.1   Cardiac provocation test
         Includes: Cardiac drug challenge test
U34.8   Other specified
U34.9   Unspecified

U35   **Other diagnostic imaging of vascular system**
> *Note:*   *Principal U11*
> *Use subsidiary codes to identify radiology with contrast (Y97), radiology procedures (Y98)*

U35.1   Thermography of blood flow
U35.2   Laser doppler ultrasound velocimetry
U35.3   Transcranial doppler ultrasound velocimetry
U35.4   Computed tomography of pulmonary arteries
U35.8   Other specified
U35.9   Unspecified

U36   **Other diagnostic imaging procedures**
> *Note:*   *Principal U21*

U36.1   Thermography NEC
> *Note:*   *Use subsidiary codes to identify radiology with contrast (Y97), radiology procedures (Y98)*

U36.2   Positron emission tomography with computed tomography NEC
> *Note:*   *Use subsidiary codes to identify gallium-67 imaging (Y93), radiopharmaceutical imaging (Y94)*

U36.3   Single photon emission computed tomography with computed tomography NEC
> *Note:*   *Use subsidiary codes to identify gallium-67 imaging (Y93), radiopharmaceutical imaging (Y94)*

U36.4   Ultrasound elastography
> *Note:*   *Use subsidiary codes to identify radiology with contrast (Y97), radiology procedures (Y98)*

U36.8   Other specified
U36.9   Unspecified

U37   **Other diagnostic imaging of genitourinary system**
> *Note:*   *Principal U12*
> *Use subsidiary codes to identify radiology with contrast (Y97), radiology procedures (Y98)*

U37.1   Magnetic resonance imaging of kidneys
U37.2   Computed tomography of kidneys
U37.8   Other specified
U37.9   Unspecified

U40   **Diagnostic tests on skin**
> *Excludes:*   *Diagnostic application tests on skin (U27)*
> *Note:*   *Principal U28*

U40.1   Diagnostic intradermal inoculation of skin
U40.2   Diagnostic ultraviolet skin test
U40.8   Other specified
U40.9   Unspecified

U50   **Rehabilitation for musculoskeletal disorders**

U50.1	Delivery of rehabilitation for amputation of limb
U50.2	Delivery of rehabilitation for hip fracture
	Excludes: When associated with joint replacement (U50.3)
U50.3	Delivery of rehabilitation for joint replacement
U50.4	Delivery of rehabilitation for rheumatoid arthritis
	Excludes: When associated with joint replacement (U50.3)
U50.5	Delivery of rehabilitation for osteoarthritis
	Excludes: When associated with joint replacement (U50.3)
U50.8	Other specified
U50.9	Unspecified

U51   **Rehabilitation for neurological disorders**

U51.1	Delivery of rehabilitation for brain injuries
U51.2	Delivery of rehabilitation for spinal cord injury
U51.3	Delivery of rehabilitation for pain syndromes
U51.8	Other specified
U51.9	Unspecified

U52   **Rehabilitation for psychiatric disorders**

U52.1	Delivery of rehabilitation for drug addiction
U52.2	Delivery of rehabilitation for alcohol addiction
U52.8	Other specified
U52.9	Unspecified

U53   **Rehabilitation for trauma and reconstructive surgery**

U53.1	Delivery of rehabilitation following plastic maxillofacial reconstructive surgery
U53.2	Delivery of rehabilitation following other plastic reconstructive surgery NEC
U53.3	Delivery of rehabilitation for burns
	Excludes: When associated with reconstructive surgery (U53.1, U53.2)
U53.4	Delivery of rehabilitation for trauma NEC
	Excludes: When associated with reconstructive surgery (U53.1,U53.2)
U53.8	Other specified
U53.9	Unspecified

U54   **Rehabilitation for other disorders**

U54.1	Delivery of rehabilitation for acute cardiac disorders
	Includes: Delivery of rehabilitation for acute myocardial infarction
U54.2	Delivery of rehabilitation for respiratory disorders
U54.3	Delivery of rehabilitation for stroke
U54.8	Other specified
U54.9	Unspecified

CHAPTER V
BONES AND JOINTS OF SKULL AND SPINE
(CODES V01–V68)

Excludes: *BONES AND JOINTS OF SACRUM AND COCCYX*   *(Chapter W)*

    Note: *Use a subsidiary code for minimal access approach (Y74–Y76)*

                Use a subsidiary code to identify method of image control (Y53)

V01   **Plastic repair of cranium**
                Note: *Principal category, extended at V02*
                          Use an additional code for application of distractors or springs (V18)

V01.1   Cranioplasty using prosthesis
V01.2   Cranioplasty using bone graft
                Note: *Use an additional code for associated removal of autologous bone flap from subcutaneous storage pocket (S63.3)*
V01.3   Opening of suture of cranium
V01.4   Removal of prosthesis from cranium
V01.5   Revision of cranioplasty NEC
V01.6   Strip craniectomy
V01.7   Strip craniectomy with remodelling of cranial bones HFQ
V01.8   Other specified
V01.9   Unspecified

V02   **Other plastic repair of cranium**
                Note: *Principal V01*
                          Use an additional code for application of distractors or springs (V18)

V02.1   Posterior calvarial release
V02.2   Remodelling of calvarium HFQ
V02.3   Reconstruction of cranium NEC
V02.8   Other specified
V02.9   Unspecified

V03   **Opening of cranium**
                Note: *Do not use as approach code (Y46, Y47)*

V03.1   Exploratory open craniotomy
                Includes: *Open craniotomy*
V03.2   Reopening of cranium and re-exploration of intracranial operation site and surgical arrest of postoperative bleeding
V03.3   Reopening of cranium and re-exploration of intracranial operation site NEC
V03.4   Reopening of cranium NEC
V03.5   Trephine of cranium
V03.6   Exploratory burrhole of cranium
V03.7   Decompressive craniectomy
                Includes: *Excision of cranial bone flap for relief of intracranial pressure*
                Note: *Use an additional code when associated with creation of subcutaneous storage pocket and placement of autologous bone flap (S63.2)*
V03.8   Other specified
V03.9   Unspecified
                Includes: *Exploratory craniotomy NEC*
                              Craniotomy NEC
                              Craniectomy NEC

V04   **Reshaping of cranium**

V04.1   Fitting dynamic cranioplasty bands
V04.8   Other specified
V04.9   Unspecified

V05   **Other operations on cranium**

V05.1   Extirpation of lesion of cranium
V05.2   Biopsy of lesion of cranium
        Includes: Biopsy of cranium
V05.3   Elevation of depressed fracture of cranium
V05.4   Repair of fracture of cranium NEC
V05.5   Graft of bone to cranium
V05.6   Transpetrous excision of lesion of jugular foramen
V05.7   Hemicraniotomy
V05.8   Other specified
V05.9   Unspecified

V06   **Excision of maxilla**

V06.1   Medial maxillectomy
V06.8   Other specified
V06.9   Unspecified
        Includes: Maxillectomy

V07   **Excision of bone of face**

V07.1   Extensive excision of bone of face
V07.2   Partial excision of bone of face NEC
V07.3   Excision of lesion of bone of face
        Excludes: Excision of dental lesion of maxilla (F18)
V07.4   Excision of lesion of infratemporal fossa
V07.8   Other specified
V07.9   Unspecified

V08   **Reduction of fracture of maxilla**

V08.1   Reduction of fracture of alveolus of maxilla
V08.2   Open reduction of fracture of maxilla NEC
V08.3   Closed reduction of fracture of maxilla NEC
V08.8   Other specified
V08.9   Unspecified

V09   **Reduction of fracture of other bone of face**
        Excludes: Fracture of orbit (C08)

V09.1   Reduction of fracture of nasoethmoid complex of bones
V09.2   Reduction of fracture of nasal bone NEC
        Includes: Reduction of fracture of nose
V09.3   Reduction of fracture of zygomatic complex of bones
V09.8   Other specified
V09.9   Unspecified

V10 **Division of bone of face**

    Note: ***Use an additional code for application of distractors or springs (V18)***

V10.1   Intracranial osteotomy of bone of face

V10.2   Transorbital subcranial osteotomy of bone of face

V10.3   Osteotomy of maxilla involving nasal complex

V10.4   Low level osteotomy of maxilla

    Includes: *Osteotomy of maxilla NEC*

V10.5   Osteotomy of alveolar segment of maxilla

    Includes: *Dentoalveolar level osteotomy of maxilla*

V10.6   Osteotomy of bones of face and translocation of orbit

V10.7   Subcranial U-osteotomy of bones of face and translocation of orbit

V10.8   Other specified

V10.9   Unspecified

V11 **Fixation of bone of face**

    Includes: *Fixator of bone of face*

V11.1   Intermaxillary fixation of maxilla

V11.2   Internal fixation of maxilla NEC

V11.3   Extraoral fixation of maxilla

V11.4   Fixation of maxilla NEC

V11.5   Removal of fixation from bone of face

V11.8   Other specified

V11.9   Unspecified

V12 **Operations on bones of skull**

V12.1   Advancement and remodelling of cranium and orbits HFQ

    Note: ***Use an additional code for application of distractors or springs (V18)***

V12.2   Advancement and remodelling of cranium and facial bones HFQ

    Note: ***Use an additional code for application of distractors or springs (V18)***

V12.3   Transcranial repair of craniofacial cleft and reconstruction of cranial and facial bones HFQ

    Excludes: *Correction of cleft lip (F03)*

                    Correction of cleft palate (F29)

V12.4   Subcranial repair of craniofacial cleft and reconstruction of cranial and facial bones HFQ

    Excludes: *Correction of cleft lip (F03)*

                    Correction of cleft palate (F29)

V12.5   Reconstruction of skull NEC

    Includes: *Skull base*

    Excludes: *Reconstruction of cranium NEC (V02.3)*

V12.8   Other specified

V12.9   Unspecified

V13 **Other operations on bone of face**

V13.1   Reconstruction of bone of face

V13.2   Alveolar bone graft to maxilla

V13.3   Biopsy of lesion of bone of face

    Includes: *Biopsy of bone of face*

V13.4   Bipartition of facial bones and maxilla

    Includes: *Bipartition and advancement of facial bones and maxilla*

    Note: ***Use an additional code for application of distractors or springs (V18)***

V13.8   Other specified

V13.9   Unspecified

V14   **Excision of mandible**
                 Includes: Jaw NEC

V14.1   Hemimandibulectomy
V14.2   Extensive excision of mandible NEC
V14.3   Partial excision of mandible NEC
                 Includes: Limited excision of mandible NEC
V14.4   Excision of lesion of mandible
                 Excludes: Excision of dental lesion of mandible (F18)
V14.8   Other specified
V14.9   Unspecified
                 Includes: Mandibulectomy NEC

V15   **Reduction of fracture of mandible**
                 Includes: Jaw NEC

V15.1   Reduction of fracture of alveolus of mandible
V15.2   Open reduction of fracture of mandible NEC
V15.3   Closed reduction of fracture of mandible NEC
V15.8   Other specified
V15.9   Unspecified

V16   **Division of mandible**
                 Includes: Jaw NEC

V16.1   Osteotomy of mandible and advancement of mandible
V16.2   Osteotomy of mandible and retrusion of mandible
V16.3   Osteotomy of alveolar segment of mandible
                 Includes: Dentoalveolar level osteotomy of mandible
V16.8   Other specified
V16.9   Unspecified

V17   **Fixation of mandible**
                 Includes: Fixator of mandible
                 *   Jaw NEC*

V17.1   Intermaxillary fixation of mandible
V17.2   Internal fixation of mandible NEC
V17.3   Extraoral fixation of mandible
V17.4   Removal of fixation from mandible
V17.8   Other specified
V17.9   Unspecified

V18   **Distraction osteogenesis of bones of skull**

V18.1   Application of external distractor to skull
V18.2   Insertion of internal distractor into skull
V18.3   Attention to external distractor of skull
V18.4   Attention to internal distractor of skull
V18.5   Removal of external distractor from skull
V18.6   Removal of internal distractor from skull
V18.8   Other specified
V18.9   Unspecified

V19   **Other operations on mandible**
            Includes: Jaw NEC

V19.1   Reconstruction of mandible
V19.2   Genioplasty of mandible
V19.3   Alveolar bone graft to mandible
V19.4   Biopsy of lesion of mandible
            Includes: Biopsy of mandible
V19.5   Manipulation of mandible NEC
V19.8   Other specified
V19.9   Unspecified

V20   **Reconstruction of temporomandibular joint**

V20.1   Total prosthetic replacement of temporomandibular joint
V20.2   Prosthetic replacement of temporomandibular joint NEC
V20.3   Intra-articular arthroplasty of temporomandibular joint
V20.8   Other specified
V20.9   Unspecified
            Includes: Arthroplasty of temporomandibular joint NEC

V21   **Other operations on temporomandibular joint**

V21.1   Meniscectomy of temporomandibular joint
V21.2   Reduction of dislocation of temporomandibular joint
V21.8   Other specified
V21.9   Unspecified

V22   **Primary decompression operations on cervical spine**
            Includes: Decompression operations on cervical spine NEC
            Note: Use an additional code to specify levels of spine (V55)

V22.1   Primary anterior decompression of cervical spinal cord and fusion of joint of cervical spine
V22.2   Primary anterior decompression of cervical spinal cord NEC
V22.3   Primary foraminotomy of cervical spine
V22.4   Primary anterior corpectomy of cervical spine with reconstruction HFQ
V22.5   Primary decompression of posterior fossa and upper cervical spinal cord and
            instrumentation
V22.6   Primary decompression of posterior fossa and upper cervical spinal cord NEC
V22.7   Primary laminoplasty of cervical spine
V22.8   Other specified
V22.9   Unspecified

V23   **Revisional decompression operations on cervical spine**
            Note: Use an additional code to specify levels of spine (V55)

V23.1   Revisional anterior decompression of cervical spinal cord and fusion of joint of cervical
            spine
V23.2   Revisional anterior decompression of cervical spinal cord NEC
V23.3   Revisional foraminotomy of cervical spine
V23.4   Revisional anterior corpectomy of cervical spine with reconstruction HFQ
V23.5   Revisional decompression of posterior fossa and upper cervical spinal cord and
            instrumentation
V23.6   Revisional decompression of posterior fossa and upper cervical spinal cord NEC
V23.7   Revisional laminoplasty of cervical spine
V23.8   Other specified
V23.9   Unspecified

V24 **Decompression operations on thoracic spine**
  Note: Use an additional code to specify levels of spine (V55)

V24.1 Primary decompression of thoracic spinal cord and fusion of joint of thoracic spine
  Includes: Decompression of thoracic spinal cord and fusion of joint of thoracic spine
V24.2 Primary decompression of thoracic spinal cord NEC
  Includes: Decompression of thoracic spinal cord NEC
V24.3 Revisional decompression of thoracic spinal cord NEC
V24.4 Primary anterior corpectomy of thoracic spine and reconstruction HFQ
  Includes: Anterior corpectomy of thoracic spine and reconstruction HFQ
V24.5 Revisional anterior corpectomy of thoracic spine and reconstruction HFQ
V24.8 Other specified
V24.9 Unspecified

V25 **Primary decompression operations on lumbar spine**
  Includes: Decompression operations on lumbar spine NEC
  Excludes: Primary insertion of lumbar interspinous process spacer (V28.1)
  Note: Principal category, extended at V67
  Use an additional code to specify levels of spine (V55)

V25.1 Primary extended decompression of lumbar spine and intertransverse fusion of joint of lumbar spine
V25.2 Primary extended decompression of lumbar spine NEC
V25.3 Primary posterior decompression of lumbar spine and intertransverse fusion of joint of lumbar spine
V25.4 Primary posterior laminectomy decompression of lumbar spine
V25.5 Primary posterior decompression of lumbar spine NEC
V25.6 Primary lateral foraminotomy of lumbar spine
V25.7 Primary anterior corpectomy of lumbar spine and reconstruction HFQ
V25.8 Other specified
V25.9 Unspecified

V26 **Revisional decompression operations on lumbar spine**
  Excludes: Revisional insertion of lumbar interspinous process spacer (V28.2)
  Note: Principal category, extended at V68
  Use an additional code to specify levels of spine (V55)

V26.1 Revisional extended decompression of lumbar spine and intertransverse fusion of joint of lumbar spine
V26.2 Revisional extended decompression of lumbar spine NEC
V26.3 Revisional posterior decompression of lumbar spine and intertransverse fusion of joint of lumbar spine
V26.4 Revisional posterior laminectomy decompression of lumbar spine
V26.5 Revisional posterior decompression of lumbar spine NEC
V26.6 Revisional lateral foraminotomy of lumbar spine
V26.7 Revisional anterior corpectomy of lumbar spine and reconstruction HFQ
V26.8 Other specified
V26.9 Unspecified

V27 **Decompression operations on unspecified spine**
Note: Use an additional code to specify levels of spine (V55)

V27.1   Primary decompression of spinal cord and fusion of joint of spine NEC
Includes: Decompression of spinal cord and fusion of joint of spine NEC
V27.2   Primary decompression of spinal cord NEC
Includes: Decompression of spinal cord NEC
V27.3   Revisional decompression of spinal cord NEC
V27.8   Other specified
V27.9   Unspecified

V28 **Insertion of lumbar interspinous process spacer**
Note: Use an additional code to specify levels of spine (V55)

V28.1   Primary insertion of lumbar interspinous process spacer
V28.2   Revisional insertion of lumbar interspinous process spacer
V28.8   Other specified
V28.9   Unspecified

V29 **Primary excision of cervical intervertebral disc**
Includes: Excision of cervical intervertebral disc NEC
Note: Use an additional code to specify level of spine (V55)

V29.1   Primary laminectomy excision of cervical intervertebral disc
V29.2   Primary hemilaminectomy excision of cervical intervertebral disc
V29.3   Primary fenestration excision of cervical intervertebral disc
V29.4   Primary anterior excision of cervical intervertebral disc and interbody fusion of joint of cervical spine
V29.5   Primary anterior excision of cervical intervertebral disc NEC
V29.6   Primary microdiscectomy of cervical intervertebral disc
V29.8   Other specified
V29.9   Unspecified

V30 **Revisional excision of cervical intervertebral disc**
Note: Use an additional code to specify levels of spine (V55)

V30.1   Revisional laminectomy excision of cervical intervertebral disc
V30.2   Revisional hemilaminectomy excision of cervical intervertebral disc
V30.3   Revisional fenestration excision of cervical intervertebral disc
V30.4   Revisional anterior excision of cervical intervertebral disc and interbody fusion of joint of cervical spine
V30.5   Revisional anterior excision of cervical intervertebral disc NEC
V30.6   Revisional microdiscectomy of cervical intervertebral disc
V30.8   Other specified
V30.9   Unspecified

V31 **Primary excision of thoracic intervertebral disc**
Includes: Excision of thoracic intervertebral disc NEC
Note: Use an additional code to specify levels of spine (V55)

V31.1   Primary anterolateral excision of thoracic intervertebral disc and graft HFQ
V31.2   Primary anterolateral excision of thoracic intervertebral disc NEC
V31.3   Primary costotransversectomy of thoracic intervertebral disc
V31.4   Primary percutaneous endoscopic excision of thoracic intervertebral disc
V31.8   Other specified
V31.9   Unspecified

V32 **Revisional excision of thoracic intervertebral disc**
        Note: Use an additional code to specify levels of spine (V55)

V32.1   Revisional anterolateral excision of thoracic intervertebral disc and graft HFQ
V32.2   Revisional anterolateral excision of thoracic intervertebral disc NEC
V32.3   Revisional costotransversectomy of thoracic intervertebral disc
V32.4   Revisional percutaneous endoscopic excision of thoracic intervertebral disc
V32.8   Other specified
V32.9   Unspecified

V33 **Primary excision of lumbar intervertebral disc**
        Includes: Excision of lumbar intervertebral disc NEC
        Note: Use an additional code to specify levels of spine (V55)

V33.1   Primary laminectomy excision of lumbar intervertebral disc
V33.2   Primary fenestration excision of lumbar intervertebral disc
V33.3   Primary anterior excision of lumbar intervertebral disc and interbody fusion of joint of lumbar spine
V33.4   Primary anterior excision of lumbar intervertebral disc NEC
V33.5   Primary anterior excision of lumbar intervertebral disc and posterior graft fusion of joint of lumbar spine
V33.6   Primary anterior excision of lumbar intervertebral disc and posterior instrumentation of lumbar spine
V33.7   Primary microdiscectomy of lumbar intervertebral disc
V33.8   Other specified
        Includes: Primary posterior excision of lumbar intervertebral disc
V33.9   Unspecified

V34 **Revisional excision of lumbar intervertebral disc**
        Note: Use an additional code to specify levels of spine (V55)

V34.1   Revisional laminectomy excision of lumbar intervertebral disc
V34.2   Revisional fenestration excision of lumbar intervertebral disc
V34.3   Revisional anterior excision of lumbar intervertebral disc and interbody fusion of joint of lumbar spine
V34.4   Revisional anterior excision of lumbar intervertebral disc NEC
V34.5   Revisional anterior excision of lumbar intervertebral disc and posterior graft fusion of joint of lumbar spine
V34.6   Revisional anterior excision of lumbar intervertebral disc and posterior instrumentation of lumbar spine
V34.7   Revisional microdiscectomy of lumbar intervertebral disc
V34.8   Other specified
        Includes: Revisional posterior excision of lumbar intervertebral disc
V34.9   Unspecified

V35 **Excision of unspecified intervertebral disc**
        Note: Use an additional code to specify levels of spine (V55)

V35.1   Primary excision of intervertebral disc NEC
        Includes: Excision of intervertebral disc NEC
V35.2   Revisional excision of intervertebral disc NEC
V35.8   Other specified
V35.9   Unspecified

V36 **Prosthetic replacement of intervertebral disc**
Note: *Use an additional code to specify levels of spine (V55)*

V36.1 Prosthetic replacement of cervical intervertebral disc
V36.2 Prosthetic replacement of thoracic intervertebral disc
V36.3 Prosthetic replacement of lumbar intervertebral disc
V36.8 Other specified
V36.9 Unspecified

V37 **Primary fusion of joint of cervical spine**
Includes: *Fusion of joint of cervical spine NEC*
Fusion of joint of cervical spine for stabilisation
Note: *Use an additional code to specify levels of spine (V55)*

V37.1 Posterior fusion of atlantoaxial joint NEC
V37.2 Posterior fusion of joint of cervical spine NEC
V37.3 Transoral fusion of atlantoaxial joint
V37.4 Fusion of atlanto-occipital joint
V37.5 Posterior fusion of atlantoaxial joint using transarticular screw
V37.6 Posterior fusion of atlantoaxial joint using pedicle screw
V37.7 Fusion of occipitocervical junction NEC
V37.8 Other specified
V37.9 Unspecified

V38 **Primary fusion of other joint of spine**
Includes: *Fusion of joint of spine NEC*
Unspecified spine
Fusion of joint of spine for stabilisation
Note: *Use an additional code to specify levels of spine (V55)*

V38.1 Primary fusion of joint of thoracic spine
V38.2 Primary posterior interlaminar fusion of joint of lumbar spine
V38.3 Primary posterior fusion of joint of lumbar spine NEC
Includes: *Primary posterior interspinous fusion of lumbar spine*
V38.4 Primary intertransverse fusion of joint of lumbar spine NEC
V38.5 Primary posterior interbody fusion of joint of lumbar spine
V38.6 Primary transforaminal interbody fusion of joint of lumbar spine
V38.8 Other specified
V38.9 Unspecified

V39 **Revisional fusion of joint of spine**
Includes: *Revisional fusion of joint of spine for stabilisation*
Note: *Principal category, extended at V66*
Use an additional code to specify levels of spine (V55)

V39.1 Revisional fusion of joint of cervical spine NEC
V39.2 Revisional fusion of joint of thoracic spine
V39.3 Revisional posterior interlaminar fusion of joint of lumbar spine
V39.4 Revisional posterior fusion of joint of lumbar spine NEC
Includes: *Revisional posterior interspinous fusion of lumbar spine*
V39.5 Revisional intertransverse fusion of joint of lumbar spine NEC
V39.6 Revisional posterior interbody fusion of joint of lumbar spine
V39.7 Revisional transforaminal interbody fusion of joint of lumbar spine
V39.8 Other specified
V39.9 Unspecified

V40   **Stabilisation of spine**
> *Note:*   *Use an additional code to specify levels of spine (V55)*

V40.1   Non-rigid stabilisation of spine
> *Excludes: Fusion of spine for stabilisation (V37–V39)*

V40.2   Posterior instrumented fusion of cervical spine NEC
V40.3   Posterior instrumented fusion of thoracic spine NEC
V40.4   Posterior instrumented fusion of lumbar spine NEC
V40.5   Removal of instrumentation from spine
> *Excludes: Removal of fixation device from spine (V46.5)*

V40.8   Other specified
V40.9   Unspecified

V41   **Instrumental correction of deformity of spine**
> *Excludes: Implantation of vertical expanding prosthetic titanium rib (O09.1 (W))*
> *Note:*   *Use an additional code to specify levels of spine (V55)*

V41.1   Posterior attachment of correctional instrument to spine
V41.2   Anterior attachment of correctional instrument to spine
V41.3   Removal of correctional instrument from spine
V41.4   Anterior and posterior attachment of correctional instrument to spine
V41.8   Other specified
V41.9   Unspecified

V42   **Other correction of deformity of spine**
> *Note:*   *Use an additional code to specify levels of spine (V55)*

V42.1   Excision of rib hump
V42.2   Epiphysiodesis of spinal apophyseal joint for correction of deformity
V42.3   Anterolateral release of spine for correction of deformity and graft HFQ
V42.4   Anterior and posterior epiphysiodesis of spine for correction of deformity
V42.5   Anterior epiphysiodesis of spine for correction of deformity NEC
V42.6   Posterior epiphysiodesis of spine for correction of deformity NEC
V42.8   Other specified
V42.9   Unspecified

V43   **Extirpation of lesion of spine**
> *Note:*   *Use an additional code to specify levels of spine (V55)*

V43.1   Excision of lesion of cervical vertebra
V43.2   Excision of lesion of thoracic vertebra
V43.3   Excision of lesion of lumbar vertebra
V43.8   Other specified
V43.9   Unspecified

V44   **Decompression of fracture of spine**
> *Note:*   *Use an additional code to specify levels of spine (V55)*

V44.1   Complex decompression of fracture of spine
V44.2   Anterior decompression of fracture of spine
V44.3   Posterior decompression of fracture of spine NEC
V44.4   Vertebroplasty of fracture of spine
V44.5   Balloon kyphoplasty of fracture of spine
V44.8   Other specified
V44.9   Unspecified

V45   **Other reduction of fracture of spine**
> *Note:*   *Use an additional code to specify levels of spine (V55)*

V45.1   Open reduction of fracture of spine and excision of facet of spine
V45.2   Open reduction of fracture of spine NEC
V45.3   Manipulative reduction of fracture of spine
V45.8   Other specified
V45.9   Unspecified

V46   **Fixation of fracture of spine**
> *Note:*   *Use an additional code to specify levels of spine (V55)*

V46.1   Fixation of fracture of spine using plate
V46.2   Fixation of fracture of spine using Harrington rod
V46.3   Fixation of fracture of spine using wire
V46.4   Fixation of fracture of spine and skull traction HFQ
V46.5   Removal of fixation device from spine
> *Excludes:*   *Removal of instrumentation from spine (V40.5)*

V46.8   Other specified
V46.9   Unspecified

V47   **Biopsy of spine**
> *Includes:*   *Biopsy of lesion of spine*
> *Note:*   *Use an additional code to specify levels of spine (V55)*

V47.1   Biopsy of cervical vertebra
V47.2   Biopsy of thoracic vertebra
V47.3   Biopsy of lumbar vertebra
V47.8   Other specified
V47.9   Unspecified

V48   **Denervation of spinal facet joint of vertebra**
> *Note:*   *Use an additional code to specify levels of spine (V55)*

V48.1   Radiofrequency controlled thermal denervation of spinal facet joint of cervical vertebra
V48.2   Denervation of spinal facet joint of cervical vertebra NEC
V48.3   Radiofrequency controlled thermal denervation of spinal facet joint of thoracic vertebra
V48.4   Denervation of spinal facet joint of thoracic vertebra NEC
V48.5   Radiofrequency controlled thermal denervation of spinal facet joint of lumbar vertebra
V48.6   Denervation of spinal facet joint of lumbar vertebra NEC
V48.7   Radiofrequency controlled thermal denervation of spinal facet joint of vertebra NEC
V48.8   Other specified
V48.9   Unspecified

V49   **Exploration of spine**
> *Note:*   *Do not use as approach code (Y48–Y50)*
>   *Use an additional code to specify levels of spine (V55)*

V49.1   Exploratory cervical laminectomy
V49.2   Exploratory thoracic laminectomy
V49.3   Exploratory lumbar laminectomy
V49.4   Exploratory laminectomy NEC
V49.5   Transthoracic exploration of spine
V49.6   Transperitoneal exploration of spine
V49.8   Other specified
V49.9   Unspecified

V50   **Manipulation of spine**
Note: *Use an additional code to specify levels of spine (V55)*

V50.1   Manipulation of spine using traction
V50.8   Other specified
V50.9   Unspecified

V52   **Other operations on intervertebral disc**
Note: *Use an additional code to specify levels of spine (V55)*

V52.1   Enzyme destruction of intervertebral disc
V52.2   Destruction of intervertebral disc NEC
Excludes: *Primary percutaneous intradiscal radiofrequency thermocoagulation to intervertebral disc (V62)*
Revisional percutaneous intradiscal radiofrequency thermocoagulation to intervertebral disc (V63)
V52.3   Discography of intervertebral disc
V52.4   Biopsy of lesion of intervertebral disc NEC
Includes: *Biopsy of intervertebral disc NEC*
V52.5   Aspiration of intervertebral disc NEC
V52.8   Other specified
V52.9   Unspecified

V54   **Other operations on spine**
Note: *Use an additional code to specify levels of spine (V55)*

V54.1   Transoral excision of odontoid process of axis
V54.2   Graft of bone to spine NEC
V54.3   Osteotomy of spine NEC
V54.4   Injection around spinal facet of spine
V54.8   Other specified
V54.9   Unspecified

V55   **Levels of spine**
Note: *Codes in this category are not intended as primary codes. They represent the number of levels operated upon not the anatomical region of the spine*

V55.1   One level of spine
V55.2   Two levels of spine
V55.3   Greater than two levels of spine
V55.8   Other specified
V55.9   Unspecified

V56   **Primary foraminoplasty of spine**
Includes: *Foraminoplasty of spine NEC*
Note: *Use an additional code to specify levels of spine (V55)*

V56.1   Primary laser foraminoplasty of cervical spine
V56.2   Primary laser foraminoplasty of thoracic spine
V56.3   Primary laser foraminoplasty of lumbar spine
V56.4   Primary laser foraminoplasty of spine NEC
V56.8   Other specified
V56.9   Unspecified

V57 **Revisional formaminoplasty of spine**
Note: *Use an additional code to specify levels of spine (V55)*

V57.1 Revisional laser foraminoplasty of cervical spine
V57.2 Revisional laser foraminoplasty of thoracic spine
V57.3 Revisional laser foraminoplasty of lumbar spine
V57.4 Revisional laser foraminoplasty of spine NEC
V57.8 Other specified
V57.9 Unspecified

V58 **Primary automated percutaneous mechanical excision of intervertebral disc**
Includes: *Automated percutaneous mechanical excision of intervertebral disc NEC*
Note: *Use an additional code to specify levels of spine (V55)*

V58.1 Primary automated percutaneous mechanical excision of cervical intervertebral disc
V58.2 Primary automated percutaneous mechanical excision of thoracic intervertebral disc
V58.3 Primary automated percutaneous mechanical excision of lumbar intervertebral disc
V58.8 Other specified
V58.9 Unspecified

V59 **Revisional automated percutaneous mechanical excision of intervertebral disc**
Note: *Use an additional code to specify levels of spine (V55)*

V59.1 Revisional automated percutaneous mechanical excision of cervical intervertebral disc
V59.2 Revisional automated percutaneous mechanical excision of thoracic intervertebral disc
V59.3 Revisional automated percutaneous mechanical excision of lumbar intervertebral disc
V59.8 Other specified
V59.9 Unspecified

V60 **Primary percutaneous decompression using coblation to intervertebral disc**
Includes: *Percutaneous decompression using coblation to intervertebral disc NEC*
Note: *Use an additional code to specify levels of spine (V55)*

V60.1 Primary percutaneous decompression using coblation to cervical intervertebral disc
V60.2 Primary percutaneous decompression using coblation to thoracic intervertebral disc
V60.3 Primary percutaneous decompression using coblation to lumbar intervertebral disc
V60.8 Other specified
V60.9 Unspecified

V61 **Revisional percutaneous decompression using coblation to intervertebral disc**
Note: *Use an additional code to specify levels of spine (V55)*

V61.1 Revisional percutaneous decompression using coblation to cervical intervertebral disc
V61.2 Revisional percutaneous decompression using coblation to thoracic intervertebral disc
V61.3 Revisional percutaneous decompression using coblation to lumbar intervertebral disc
V61.8 Other specified
V61.9 Unspecified

W14 **Diaphyseal division of bone**

W14.1   Angulation diaphyseal osteotomy and internal fixation HFQ
W14.2   Angulation diaphyseal osteotomy and external fixation HFQ
W14.3   Angulation diaphyseal osteotomy NEC
W14.4   Rotation diaphyseal osteotomy and internal fixation HFQ
W14.5   Rotation diaphyseal osteotomy and external fixation HFQ
W14.6   Rotation diaphyseal osteotomy NEC
W14.8   Other specified
W14.9   Unspecified

W15 **Division of bone of foot**

Excludes: For complex reconstruction of foot (W03, W04)
             Some similar operations for correction of congenital deformity (X19–X27)
   Note: Use as a secondary code when associated with soft tissue correction of hallux
             valgus (W79.1)

W15.1   Osteotomy of neck of first metatarsal bone
W15.2   Osteotomy of base of first metatarsal bone
W15.3   Osteotomy of first metatarsal bone NEC
W15.4   Osteotomy of head of metatarsal bone
W15.5   Osteotomy of midfoot tarsal bone
W15.6   Cuneiform osteotomy of proximal phalanx with resection of head of first metatarsal
W15.7   Osteotomy of bone of foot and fixation HFQ
W15.8   Other specified
W15.9   Unspecified

W16 **Other division of bone**

Excludes: Some similar operations for correction of congenital deformity (X19–X27)

W16.1   Multiple osteotomy and internal fixation HFQ
W16.2   Multiple osteotomy and external fixation HFQ
W16.3   Multiple osteotomy NEC
W16.4   Osteotomy and internal fixation NEC
W16.5   Osteotomy and external fixation NEC
W16.8   Other specified
W16.9   Unspecified
         Includes: Osteotomy NEC

W17 **Other reconstruction of bone**

Excludes: Some similar operations for correction of congenital deformity (X19–X27)

W17.1   Step cut lengthening of bone
W17.2   Traction lengthening of diaphysis of bone
W17.3   Traction lengthening of epiphyseal plate of bone
W17.4   Shortening of bone
W17.5   Revision of reconstruction of bone
W17.8   Other specified
W17.9   Unspecified

W18   **Drainage of bone**

W18.1   Fenestration of cortex of bone
W18.2   Saucerisation of bone
W18.3   Sequestrectomy of bone
W18.4   Decompression of fourage of bone
W18.5   Insertion of drainage system into bone
W18.6   Removal of drainage system from bone
W18.8   Other specified
W18.9   Unspecified

W19   **Primary open reduction of fracture of bone and intramedullary fixation**
        Includes: *Open reduction of fracture of bone and intramedullary fixation NEC*
        Excludes: *Fracture dislocation (W65)*

W19.1   Primary open reduction of fracture of neck of femur and open fixation using pin and plate
        Includes: *Primary open reduction of fracture of neck of femur and open fixation using dynamic hip screw*
W19.2   Primary open reduction of fracture of long bone and fixation using rigid nail NEC
W19.3   Primary open reduction of fracture of long bone and fixation using flexible nail
W19.4   Primary open reduction of fracture of small bone and fixation using screw
W19.5   Primary open reduction of fragment of bone and fixation using screw
W19.6   Primary open reduction of fragment of bone and fixation using wire system
W19.8   Other specified
W19.9   Unspecified

W20   **Primary open reduction of fracture of bone and extramedullary fixation**
        Includes: *Primary open reduction of fracture of bone and fixation NEC*
                 Open reduction of fracture of bone and extramedullary fixation NEC
                 Open reduction of fracture of bone and fixation NEC
        Excludes: *Fracture dislocation (W65)*

W20.1   Primary open reduction of fracture of long bone and extramedullary fixation using plate NEC
W20.2   Primary open reduction of fracture of long bone and extramedullary fixation using cerclage
        Includes: *Primary open reduction of fracture of long bone and extramedullary fixation using tension band wiring*
W20.3   Primary open reduction of fracture of long bone and extramedullary fixation using suture
W20.4   Primary open reduction of fracture of long bone and complex extramedullary fixation NEC
W20.5   Primary open reduction of fracture of ankle and extramedullary fixation NEC
W20.6   Wiring of sternum
W20.8   Other specified
W20.9   Unspecified

W21   **Primary open reduction of intra-articular fracture of bone**
        Includes: *Open reduction of intra-articular fracture of bone NEC*
        Excludes: *Fracture dislocation (W65)*

W21.1   Primary reduction of intra-articular fracture of bone using arthrotomy as approach
W21.2   Primary excision of intra-articular fragment of intra-articular fracture of bone
W21.3   Primary fixation of fragment of chondral cartilage of intra-articular fracture of bone
W21.4   Primary intra-articular fixation of intra-articular fracture of bone NEC
W21.5   Primary extra-articular reduction of intra-articular fracture of bone
W21.8   Other specified
W21.9   Unspecified

W32   **Other graft of bone**

W32.1   Prepared graft of bone
W32.2   Allograft of bone NEC
             Excludes: Allograft of bone marrow NEC (W34.2)
W32.3   Xenograft of bone
W32.4   Synthetic graft of bone
W32.5   Cancellous chip allograft of bone
             Includes: Morcellised allograft of bone
W32.6   Bulk allograft of bone
W32.8   Other specified
W32.9   Unspecified

W33   **Other open operations on bone**
             Excludes: Some similar operations for correction of congenital deformity (X19–X27)

W33.1   Open biopsy of lesion of bone
             Includes: Open biopsy of bone
W33.2   Debridement of open fracture of bone
             Includes: Debridement of fracture of bone
W33.3   Suture of periosteum
W33.4   Implantation of electromagnetic stimulator into bone
W33.5   Attention to electromagnetic stimulator in bone
W33.6   Debridement of bone NEC
W33.7   Lavage of bone
W33.8   Other specified
W33.9   Unspecified

W34   **Graft of bone marrow**
             Includes: Bone marrow transplant
             Excludes: Graft of cord blood stem cells to bone marrow (W99)

W34.1   Autograft of bone marrow
W34.2   Allograft of bone marrow NEC
W34.3   Allograft of bone marrow from sibling donor
W34.4   Allograft of bone marrow from matched unrelated donor
W34.5   Allograft of bone marrow from haploidentical donor
W34.6   Allograft of bone marrow from unmatched unrelated donor
W34.8   Other specified
W34.9   Unspecified

W35   **Therapeutic puncture of bone**

W35.1   Introduction of therapeutic substance into bone
W35.2   Introduction of destructive substance into bone
W35.3   Removal of implanted substance from bone
W35.4   Therapeutic drilling of bone NEC
W35.5   Therapeutic percutaneous puncture of bone
W35.6   Percutaneous radiofrequency ablation of lesion of bone
W35.8   Other specified
W35.9   Unspecified

W

W36 **Diagnostic puncture of bone**

W36.1 Percutaneous needle biopsy of lesion of bone
Includes: Percutaneous needle biopsy of bone
W36.2 Needle biopsy of lesion of bone NEC
Includes: Needle biopsy of bone NEC
Biopsy of lesion of bone NEC
Biopsy of bone NEC
W36.3 Diagnostic drilling of bone
W36.4 Diagnostic puncture of sternum
Includes: Aspiration of bone marrow of sternum
W36.5 Diagnostic extraction of bone marrow NEC
Includes: Aspiration of bone marrow NEC
Biopsy of bone marrow NEC
W36.8 Other specified
W36.9 Unspecified

W37 **Total prosthetic replacement of hip joint using cement**

W37.1 Primary total prosthetic replacement of hip joint using cement
W37.2 Conversion to total prosthetic replacement of hip joint using cement
Note: Use a subsidiary conversion from code as necessary
W37.3 Revision of total prosthetic replacement of hip joint using cement
W37.4 Revision of one component of total prosthetic replacement of hip joint using cement
W37.8 Other specified
W37.9 Unspecified
W37.0 Conversion from previous cemented total prosthetic replacement of hip joint

W38 **Total prosthetic replacement of hip joint not using cement**

W38.1 Primary total prosthetic replacement of hip joint not using cement
W38.2 Conversion to total prosthetic replacement of hip joint not using cement
Note: Use a subsidiary conversion from code as necessary
W38.3 Revision of total prosthetic replacement of hip joint not using cement
W38.4 Revision of one component of total prosthetic replacement of hip joint not using cement
W38.8 Other specified
W38.9 Unspecified
W38.0 Conversion from previous uncemented total prosthetic replacement of hip joint

W39 **Other total prosthetic replacement of hip joint**

W39.1 Primary total prosthetic replacement of hip joint NEC
W39.2 Conversion to total prosthetic replacement of hip joint NEC
Note: Use a subsidiary conversion from code as necessary
W39.3 Revision of total prosthetic replacement of hip joint NEC
W39.4 Attention to total prosthetic replacement of hip joint NEC
W39.5 Revision of one component of total prosthetic replacement of hip joint NEC
W39.6 Closed reduction of dislocated total prosthetic replacement of hip joint
W39.8 Other specified
W39.9 Unspecified
W39.0 Conversion from previous total prosthetic replacement of hip joint NEC

W40   **Total prosthetic replacement of knee joint using cement**

W40.1   Primary total prosthetic replacement of knee joint using cement
W40.2   Conversion to total prosthetic replacement of knee joint using cement
                Note: *Use a subsidiary conversion from code as necessary*
W40.3   Revision of total prosthetic replacement of knee joint using cement
W40.4   Revision of one component of total prosthetic replacement of knee joint using cement
W40.8   Other specified
W40.9   Unspecified
W40.0   Conversion from previous cemented total prosthetic replacement of knee joint

W41   **Total prosthetic replacement of knee joint not using cement**

W41.1   Primary total prosthetic replacement of knee joint not using cement
W41.2   Conversion to total prosthetic replacement of knee joint not using cement
                Note: *Use a subsidiary conversion from code as necessary*
W41.3   Revision of total prosthetic replacement of knee joint not using cement
W41.4   Revision of one component of total prosthetic replacement of knee joint not using cement
W41.8   Other specified
W41.9   Unspecified
W41.0   Conversion from previous uncemented total prosthetic replacement of knee joint

W42   **Other total prosthetic replacement of knee joint**

W42.1   Primary total prosthetic replacement of knee joint NEC
W42.2   Conversion to total prosthetic replacement of knee joint NEC
                Note: *Use a subsidiary conversion from code as necessary*
W42.3   Revision of total prosthetic replacement of knee joint NEC
W42.4   Attention to total prosthetic replacement of knee joint NEC
W42.5   Revision of one component of total prosthetic replacement of knee joint NEC
W42.6   Arthrolysis of total prosthetic replacement of knee joint
W42.8   Other specified
W42.9   Unspecified
W42.0   Conversion from previous total prosthetic replacement of knee joint NEC

W43   **Total prosthetic replacement of other joint using cement**

W43.1   Primary total prosthetic replacement of joint using cement NEC
W43.2   Conversion to total prosthetic replacement of joint using cement NEC
                Note: *Use a subsidiary conversion from code as necessary*
W43.3   Revision of total prosthetic replacement of joint using cement NEC
W43.4   Revision of one component of total prosthetic replacement of joint using cement NEC
W43.8   Other specified
W43.9   Unspecified
W43.0   Conversion from previous cemented total prosthetic replacement of joint NEC

W44   **Total prosthetic replacement of other joint not using cement**

W44.1   Primary total prosthetic replacement of joint not using cement NEC
W44.2   Conversion to total prosthetic replacement of joint not using cement NEC
                Note: *Use a subsidiary conversion from code as necessary*
W44.3   Revision of total prosthetic replacement of joint not using cement NEC
W44.4   Revision of one component of total prosthetic replacement of joint not using cement NEC
W44.8   Other specified
W44.9   Unspecified
W44.0   Conversion from previous uncemented total prosthetic replacement of joint NEC

W45   **Other total prosthetic replacement of other joint**

W45.1   Primary total prosthetic replacement of joint NEC
W45.2   Conversion to total prosthetic replacement of joint NEC
          Note: Use a subsidiary conversion from code as necessary
W45.3   Revision of total prosthetic replacement of joint NEC
W45.4   Attention to total prosthetic replacement of joint NEC
W45.5   Revision of one component of total prosthetic replacement of joint NEC
W45.8   Other specified
W45.9   Unspecified
W45.0   Conversion from previous total prosthetic replacement of joint NEC

W46   **Prosthetic replacement of head of femur using cement**
          Includes: Prosthetic hemiarthroplasty of head of femur using cement

W46.1   Primary prosthetic replacement of head of femur using cement
W46.2   Conversion to prosthetic replacement of head of femur using cement
          Note: Use a subsidiary conversion from code as necessary
W46.3   Revision of prosthetic replacement of head of femur using cement
W46.8   Other specified
W46.9   Unspecified
W46.0   Conversion from previous cemented prosthetic replacement of head of femur

W47   **Prosthetic replacement of head of femur not using cement**
          Includes: Prosthetic hemiarthroplasty of head of femur not using cement

W47.1   Primary prosthetic replacement of head of femur not using cement
W47.2   Conversion to prosthetic replacement of head of femur not using cement
          Note: Use a subsidiary conversion from code as necessary
W47.3   Revision of prosthetic replacement of head of femur not using cement
W47.8   Other specified
W47.9   Unspecified
W47.0   Conversion from previous uncemented prosthetic replacement of head of femur

W48   **Other prosthetic replacement of head of femur**
          Includes: Prosthetic hemiarthroplasty of head of femur NEC

W48.1   Primary prosthetic replacement of head of femur NEC
W48.2   Conversion to prosthetic replacement of head of femur NEC
          Note: Use a subsidiary conversion from code as necessary
W48.3   Revision of prosthetic replacement of head of femur NEC
W48.4   Attention to prosthetic replacement of head of femur NEC
W48.5   Closed reduction of dislocated prosthetic replacement of head of femur
W48.8   Other specified
W48.9   Unspecified
W48.0   Conversion from previous prosthetic replacement of head of femur NEC

W49   **Prosthetic replacement of head of humerus using cement**
            Includes: Prosthetic hemiarthroplasty of head of humerus using cement

W49.1   Primary prosthetic replacement of head of humerus using cement
W49.2   Conversion to prosthetic replacement of head of humerus using cement
            Note: Use a subsidiary conversion from code as necessary
W49.3   Revision of prosthetic replacement of head of humerus using cement
W49.4   Resurfacing hemiarthroplasty of head of humerus using cement
W49.8   Other specified
W49.9   Unspecified
W49.0   Conversion from previous cemented prosthetic replacement of head of humerus

W50   **Prosthetic replacement of head of humerus not using cement**
            Includes: Prosthetic hemiarthroplasty of head of humerus not using cement

W50.1   Primary prosthetic replacement of head of humerus not using cement
W50.2   Conversion to prosthetic replacement of head of humerus not using cement
            Note: Use a subsidiary conversion from code as necessary
W50.3   Revision of prosthetic replacement of head of humerus not using cement
W50.4   Resurfacing hemiarthroplasty of head of humerus not using cement
W50.8   Other specified
W50.9   Unspecified
W50.0   Conversion from previous uncemented prosthetic replacement of head of humerus

W51   **Other prosthetic replacement of head of humerus**
            Includes: Prosthetic hemiarthroplasty of head of humerus NEC

W51.1   Primary prosthetic replacement of head of humerus NEC
W51.2   Conversion to prosthetic replacement of head of humerus NEC
            Note: Use a subsidiary conversion from code as necessary
W51.3   Revision of prosthetic replacement of head of humerus NEC
W51.4   Attention to prosthetic replacement of head of humerus NEC
W51.5   Resurfacing hemiarthroplasty of head of humerus NEC
W51.8   Other specified
W51.9   Unspecified
W51.0   Conversion from previous prosthetic replacement of head of humerus NEC

W52   **Prosthetic replacement of articulation of other bone using cement**
            Includes: Prosthetic hemiarthroplasty of articulation of bone using cement NEC

W52.1   Primary prosthetic replacement of articulation of bone using cement NEC
W52.2   Conversion to prosthetic replacement of articulation of bone using cement NEC
            Note: Use a subsidiary conversion from code as necessary
W52.3   Revision of prosthetic replacement of articulation of bone using cement NEC
W52.8   Other specified
W52.9   Unspecified
W52.0   Conversion from previous cemented prosthetic replacement of articulation of bone NEC

W53   **Prosthetic replacement of articulation of other bone not using cement**
Includes: Prosthetic hemiarthroplasty of articulation of bone not using cement NEC

W53.1   Primary prosthetic replacement of articulation of bone not using cement NEC
W53.2   Conversion to prosthetic replacement of articulation of bone not using cement NEC
           Note: Use a subsidiary conversion from code as necessary
W53.3   Revision of prosthetic replacement of articulation of bone not using cement NEC
W53.8   Other specified
W53.9   Unspecified
W53.0   Conversion from previous uncemented prosthetic replacement of articulation of bone NEC

W54   **Other prosthetic replacement of articulation of other bone**
Includes: Prosthetic hemiarthroplasty of articulation of bone NEC

W54.1   Primary prosthetic replacement of articulation of bone NEC
W54.2   Conversion to prosthetic replacement of articulation of bone NEC
           Note: Use a subsidiary conversion from code as necessary
W54.3   Revision of prosthetic replacement of articulation of bone NEC
W54.4   Attention to prosthetic replacement of articulation of bone NEC
W54.8   Other specified
W54.9   Unspecified
W54.0   Conversion from previous prosthetic replacement of articulation of bone NEC

W55   **Prosthetic interposition reconstruction of joint**
Excludes: Some similar operations for correction of congenital deformity (X19–X27)

W55.1   Primary prosthetic interposition arthroplasty of joint
           Includes: Prosthetic interposition arthroplasty of joint
W55.2   Revision of prosthetic interposition arthroplasty of joint
W55.3   Conversion to prosthetic interposition arthroplasty of joint
           Note: Use a subsidiary conversion from code as necessary
W55.4   Attention to prosthetic interposition arthroplasty of joint NEC
W55.8   Other specified
W55.9   Unspecified
W55.0   Conversion from previous prosthetic interposition arthroplasty of joint

W56   **Other interposition reconstruction of joint**
Includes: Interposition reconstruction of joint using natural tissue
Excludes: Some similar operations for correction of congenital deformity (X19–X27)

W56.1   Primary interposition arthroplasty of metatarsophalangeal joint NEC
           Includes: Interposition arthroplasty of metatarsophalangeal joint NEC
W56.2   Primary interposition arthroplasty of joint NEC
           Includes: Interposition arthroplasty of joint NEC
W56.3   Revision of interposition arthroplasty of joint NEC
W56.4   Conversion to interposition arthroplasty of joint NEC
           Note: Use a subsidiary conversion from code as necessary
W56.8   Other specified
W56.9   Unspecified
W56.0   Conversion from previous interposition arthroplasty of joint NEC

W57 **Excision reconstruction of joint**
Excludes: Some similar operations for correction of congenital deformity (X19–X27)

W57.1   Primary excision arthroplasty of first metatarsophalangeal joint
Includes: Excision arthroplasty of first metatarsophalangeal joint

W57.2   Primary excision arthroplasty of joint NEC
Includes: Excision arthroplasty of joint NEC

W57.3   Revision of excision arthroplasty of joint

W57.4   Conversion to excision arthroplasty of joint
> ***Note: Use a subsidiary conversion from code as necessary***

W57.8   Other specified

W57.9   Unspecified

W57.0   Conversion from previous excision arthroplasty of joint

W58 **Other reconstruction of joint**
Excludes: Some similar operations for correction of congenital deformity (X19–X27)

W58.1   Primary resurfacing arthroplasty of joint

W58.2   Revision of resurfacing arthroplasty of joint

W58.8   Other specified

W58.9   Unspecified

W58.0   Conversion from previous resurfacing arthroplasty of joint

W59 **Fusion of joint of toe**
Excludes: For complex reconstruction of foot (W03, W04)
> ***Note: Use as a secondary code when associated with soft tissue correction of hallux valgus (W79.1)***

W59.1   Fusion of first metatarsophalangeal joint and replacement of lesser metatarsophalangeal joint

W59.2   Fusion of first metatarsophalangeal joint and excision of lesser metatarsophalangeal joint

W59.3   Fusion of first metatarsophalangeal joint NEC

W59.4   Fusion of interphalangeal joint of great toe

W59.5   Fusion of interphalangeal joint of toe NEC

W59.6   Revision of fusion of joint of toe

W59.8   Other specified

W59.9   Unspecified

W60 **Fusion of other joint and extra-articular bone graft**
Includes: Fusion of joint and bone graft NEC

W60.1   Primary arthrodesis and extra-articular bone graft NEC
Includes: Arthrodesis and extra-articular bone graft NEC

W60.2   Revision of arthrodesis and extra-articular bone graft NEC

W60.3   Conversion to arthrodesis and extra-articular bone graft NEC
> ***Note: Use a subsidiary conversion from code as necessary***

W60.8   Other specified

W60.9   Unspecified

W60.0   Conversion from previous arthrodesis and extra-articular bone graft NEC

W61   **Fusion of other joint and other articular bone graft**

W61.1   Primary arthrodesis and articular bone graft NEC
Includes: Arthrodesis and articular bone graft NEC
W61.2   Revision of arthrodesis and articular bone graft NEC
W61.3   Conversion to arthrodesis and articular bone graft NEC
Note: Use a subsidiary conversion from code as necessary
W61.8   Other specified
W61.9   Unspecified
W61.0   Conversion from previous arthrodesis and articular bone graft NEC

W62   **Other primary fusion of other joint**
Includes: Fusion of joint NEC

W62.1   Primary arthrodesis and internal fixation of joint NEC
W62.2   Primary arthrodesis and external fixation of joint NEC
W62.8   Other specified
W62.9   Unspecified
Includes: Primary arthrodesis NEC
Simple arthrodesis NEC
Arthrodesis NEC

W63   **Revisional fusion of other joint**

W63.1   Revision of arthrodesis and internal fixation NEC
W63.2   Revision of arthrodesis and external fixation NEC
W63.8   Other specified
W63.9   Unspecified
Includes: Revision of simple arthrodesis NEC
Revision of arthrodesis NEC

W64   **Conversion to fusion of other joint**

W64.1   Conversion to arthrodesis and internal fixation NEC
W64.2   Conversion to arthrodesis and external fixation NEC
W64.8   Other specified
W64.9   Unspecified
Includes: Conversion to simple arthrodesis NEC
Conversion to arthrodesis NEC
W64.0   Conversion from previous arthrodesis NEC

W65 **Primary open reduction of traumatic dislocation of joint**
Excludes: Some similar operations for correction of congenital deformity (X19–X27)

W65.1   Primary open reduction of fracture dislocation of joint and skeletal traction HFQ
Includes: Open reduction of fracture dislocation of joint and skeletal traction HFQ

W65.2   Primary open reduction of traumatic dislocation of joint and skeletal traction NEC
Includes: Open reduction of traumatic dislocation of joint and skeletal traction NEC

W65.3   Primary open reduction of fracture dislocation of joint NEC
Includes: Open reduction of fracture dislocation of joint NEC

W65.4   Primary open reduction of fracture dislocation of joint and internal fixation NEC
Includes: Open reduction of fracture dislocation of joint and internal fixation NEC

W65.5   Primary open reduction of fracture dislocation of joint and combined internal and external fixation
Includes: Open reduction of fracture dislocation of joint and combined internal and external fixation NEC

W65.8   Other specified

W65.9   Unspecified
Includes: Open reduction of traumatic dislocation of joint NEC
Open reduction of dislocation of joint NEC

W66 **Primary closed reduction of traumatic dislocation of joint**
Excludes: Some similar operations for correction of congenital deformity (X19–X27)

W66.1   Primary closed reduction of fracture dislocation of joint and skeletal traction HFQ
Includes: Closed reduction of fracture dislocation of joint and skeletal traction HFQ

W66.2   Primary closed reduction of traumatic dislocation of joint and skeletal traction NEC
Includes: Closed reduction of traumatic dislocation of joint and skeletal traction NEC
Reduction of traumatic dislocation of joint and skeletal traction NEC
Reduction of dislocation of joint and skeletal traction NEC

W66.3   Primary manipulative closed reduction of fracture dislocation of joint NEC
Includes: Closed reduction of fracture dislocation of joint NEC
Manipulative reduction of fracture dislocation of joint NEC

W66.4   Primary closed reduction of fracture dislocation of joint and internal fixation
Includes: Closed reduction of fracture dislocation of joint and internal fixation

W66.8   Other specified

W66.9   Unspecified
Includes: Manipulative reduction of traumatic dislocation of joint NEC
Manipulative reduction of dislocation of joint NEC
Reduction of traumatic dislocation of joint NEC
Reduction of dislocation of joint NEC

W67 **Secondary reduction of traumatic dislocation of joint**
Excludes: Some similar operations for correction of congenital deformity (X19–X27)

W67.1   Secondary open reduction of fracture dislocation of joint and skeletal traction HFQ

W67.2   Secondary open reduction of traumatic dislocation of joint and skeletal traction NEC
Includes: Secondary open reduction of dislocation of joint and skeletal traction NEC

W67.3   Secondary open reduction of fracture dislocation of joint NEC

W67.4   Secondary open reduction of traumatic dislocation of joint NEC
Includes: Secondary open reduction of dislocation of joint NEC

W67.5   Remanipulation of fracture dislocation of joint

W67.6   Remanipulation of traumatic dislocation of joint
Includes: Remanipulation of dislocation of joint NEC

W67.7   Secondary open reduction of fracture dislocation of joint and internal fixation NEC

W67.8   Other specified

W67.9   Unspecified

W68   **Primary reduction of injury to growth plate**

W68.1   Open reduction of injury to growth plate and internal fixation HFQ
W68.2   Open reduction of injury to growth plate and traction HFQ
W68.3   Open reduction of injury to growth plate NEC
W68.4   Closed reduction of injury to growth plate and internal fixation HFQ
W68.5   Closed reduction of injury to growth plate and traction HFQ
W68.6   Closed reduction of injury to growth plate NEC
W68.8   Other specified
W68.9   Unspecified

W69   **Open operations on synovial membrane of joint**

W69.1   Total synovectomy
W69.2   Subtotal synovectomy
W69.3   Partial synovectomy
         Includes: *Synovectomy NEC*
W69.4   Open biopsy of synovial membrane of joint
         Includes: *Open biopsy of lesion of synovial membrane of joint*
                       Biopsy of synovial membrane of joint NEC
                       Biopsy of lesion of synovial membrane of joint NEC
W69.5   Open division of synovial plica
W69.8   Other specified
W69.9   Unspecified

W70   **Open operations on semilunar cartilage**
         Includes: *Operations on semilunar cartilage NEC*

W70.1   Open total excision of semilunar cartilage
W70.2   Open excision of semilunar cartilage NEC
         Includes: *Open excision of lesion of semilunar cartilage*
W70.3   Open repair of semilunar cartilage
W70.8   Other specified
W70.9   Unspecified

W71   **Other open operations on intra-articular structure**
         Includes: *Operations on intra-articular structure NEC*

W71.1   Open drilling of articular cartilage
W71.2   Open excision of intra-articular osteophyte
W71.3   Forage of joint
W71.4   Open autologous chondrocyte implantation into articular structure
W71.8   Other specified
W71.9   Unspecified

W72   **Prosthetic replacement of ligament**
         Note: **Use as a secondary code when associated with transposition of ligament for stabilisation of joint (W77.7)**

W72.1   Primary prosthetic replacement of multiple ligaments
W72.2   Prosthetic replacement of multiple ligaments NEC
W72.3   Primary prosthetic replacement of intra-articular ligament
W72.4   Prosthetic replacement of intra-articular ligament NEC
W72.5   Primary prosthetic replacement of extra-articular ligament
W72.6   Prosthetic replacement of extra-articular ligament NEC
W72.8   Other specified
W72.9   Unspecified

W73   **Prosthetic reinforcement of ligament**

W73.1   Primary extra-articular prosthetic augmentation of intra-articular ligament NEC
W73.2   Extra-articular prosthetic augmentation of intra-articular ligament NEC
W73.3   Primary prosthetic reinforcement of intra-articular ligament NEC
W73.4   Prosthetic reinforcement of intra-articular ligament NEC
W73.8   Other specified
W73.9   Unspecified

W74   **Other reconstruction of ligament**

W74.1   Reconstruction of multiple ligaments NEC
W74.2   Reconstruction of intra-articular ligament NEC
W74.3   Reconstruction of extra-articular ligament NEC
               Excludes: Reconstruction of extra-articular ligament for stabilisation of joint (O27.1)
W74.8   Other specified
W74.9   Unspecified

W75   **Other open repair of ligament**
               Includes: Repair of ligament NEC

W75.1   Open repair of multiple ligaments NEC
W75.2   Open repair of intra-articular ligament NEC
W75.3   Open repair of extra-articular ligament NEC
W75.8   Other specified
W75.9   Unspecified

W76   **Other operations on ligament**

W76.1   Excision of ligament
W76.2   Excision of lesion of ligament
W76.3   Biopsy of lesion of ligament
               Includes: Biopsy of ligament
W76.8   Other specified
W76.9   Unspecified

W77   **Stabilising operations on joint**
               Excludes: Some similar operations for correction of congenital deformity (X19–X27)
                   *Note: **Principal category, extended at O27***

W77.1   Repair of capsule of joint for stabilisation of joint NEC
W77.2   Transposition of muscle for stabilisation of joint
W77.3   Blocking operations on joint using prosthesis for stabilisation of joint
W77.4   Blocking operations on joint using bone for stabilisation of joint
W77.5   Periarticular osteotomy for stabilisation of joint
W77.6   Annular ligament reconstruction for stabilisation of joint
W77.7   Transposition of ligament for stabilisation of joint
                   *Note: **Use a supplementary code for concurrent prosthetic replacement of ligament (W72)***
W77.8   Other specified
W77.9   Unspecified

W78   **Release of contracture of joint**
            Excludes: Some similar operations for correction of congenital deformity (X19–X27)

W78.1   Release of contracture of shoulder joint
W78.2   Release of contracture of hip joint
W78.3   Release of contracture of knee joint
W78.4   Limited release of contracture of capsule of joint
            Includes: Release of contracture of capsule of joint NEC
W78.5   Release of contracture of elbow joint
            Includes: Arthrolysis of elbow joint NEC
W78.8   Other specified
W78.9   Unspecified

W79   **Soft tissue operations on joint of toe**
            Excludes: Some similar operations for correction of congenital deformity (X19–X27)

W79.1   Soft tissue correction of hallux valgus
            Includes: Soft tissue correction of hallux valgus and excision of bunion
                **Note: Use a supplementary code for concurrent osteotomy of first metatarsal
                bone (W15)
                Use a supplementary code for concurrent arthrodesis (W59)**
W79.2   Excision of bunion NEC
            *Includes: Bunionectomy
                        Simple excision of bunion
                        Excision of bunionette*
W79.3   Syndactylisation of lesser toes
W79.8   Other specified
W79.9   Unspecified

W80   **Debridement and irrigation of joint**

W80.1   Open debridement and irrigation of joint
W80.2   Open debridement of joint NEC
W80.3   Open irrigation of joint NEC
W80.8   Other specified
W80.9   Unspecified

W81   **Other open operations on joint**
            Excludes: Some similar operations for correction of congenital deformity (X19–X27)

W81.1   Excision of lesion of joint NEC
W81.2   Open removal of loose body from joint
W81.3   Drainage of joint
W81.4   Incision of joint NEC
            Includes: Arthrotomy NEC
W81.5   Exploration of joint NEC
W81.6   Capsulorrhaphy of joint
            Includes: Plication of capsule of joint
W81.7   Insertion of therapeutic spacer into joint
W81.8   Other specified
W81.9   Unspecified

W82   **Therapeutic endoscopic operations on semilunar cartilage**
Note: It is not necessary to code additionally any mention of diagnostic endoscopic examination of knee joint (W87.9)

W82.1   Endoscopic total excision of semilunar cartilage
W82.2   Endoscopic resection of semilunar cartilage NEC
W82.3   Endoscopic repair of semilunar cartilage
W82.8   Other specified
W82.9   Unspecified

W83   **Therapeutic endoscopic operations on other articular cartilage**
Note: Principal category, extended at W89
It is not necessary to code additionally any mention of diagnostic endoscopic examination of same joint (W87.9, W88.9)

W83.1   Endoscopic drilling of lesion of articular cartilage
W83.2   Endoscopic fixation of lesion of articular cartilage
W83.3   Endoscopic shaving of articular cartilage
W83.4   Endoscopic articular abrasion chondroplasty
W83.5   Endoscopic articular thermal chondroplasty
W83.6   Endoscopic excision of articular cartilage NEC
W83.7   Endoscopic osteochondral autograft
Includes: Endoscopic osteoarticular transfer system
Endoscopic mosaicplasty
W83.8   Other specified
W83.9   Unspecified

W84   **Therapeutic endoscopic operations on other joint structure**
Note: Principal category, extended at O19
It is not necessary to code additionally any mention of diagnostic endoscopic examination of same joint (W87.9, W88.9)

W84.1   Endoscopic repair of intra-articular ligament
W84.2   Endoscopic reattachment of intra-articular ligament
W84.3   Endoscopic division of synovial plica
W84.4   Endoscopic decompression of joint
W84.5   Endoscopic drilling of epiphysis for repair of articular cartilage
Includes: Microfracture of bone for repair of articular cartilage
W84.6   Endoscopic excision of synovial plica
W84.7   Endoscopic repair of superior labrum anterior to posterior tear
W84.8   Other specified
W84.9   Unspecified

W85   **Therapeutic endoscopic operations on cavity of knee joint**
Note: It is not necessary to code additionally any mention of diagnostic endoscopic examination of knee joint (W87.9)

W85.1   Endoscopic removal of loose body from knee joint
W85.2   Endoscopic irrigation of knee joint
Includes: Endoscopic lavage of knee joint
Endoscopic washout of knee joint
W85.3   Endoscopic autologous chondrocyte implantation of knee joint
W85.8   Other specified
W85.9   Unspecified

W86　　**Therapeutic endoscopic operations on cavity of other joint**
　　　　　　Note:　It is not necessary to code additionally any mention of diagnostic endoscopic
　　　　　　　　　　examination of same joint (W88.9)

W86.1　Endoscopic removal of loose body from joint NEC
W86.8　Other specified
W86.9　Unspecified

W87　　**Diagnostic endoscopic examination of knee joint**
　　　　　　Note:　Do not use as approach code (Y76.7)

W87.1　Diagnostic endoscopic examination of knee joint and biopsy of lesion of knee joint
　　　　　Includes:　Diagnostic endoscopic examination of knee joint and biopsy of knee joint
　　　　　　　　　　　Endoscopic biopsy of lesion of knee joint
　　　　　　　　　　　Endoscopic biopsy of knee joint
W87.8　Other specified
W87.9　Unspecified
　　　　　Includes:　Arthroscopy of knee joint NEC

W88　　**Diagnostic endoscopic examination of other joint**

W88.1　Diagnostic endoscopic examination of joint and biopsy of lesion of joint NEC
　　　　　Includes:　Diagnostic endoscopic examination of joint and biopsy of joint NEC
　　　　　　　　　　　Endoscopic biopsy of lesion of joint NEC
　　　　　　　　　　　Endoscopic biopsy of joint NEC
W88.8　Other specified
W88.9　Unspecified
　　　　　Includes:　Arthroscopy NEC

W89　　**Other therapeutic endoscopic operations on other articular cartilage**
　　　　　　Note:　Principal W83

W89.1　Endoscopic chondroplasty NEC
W89.2　Endoscopic harvest of autologous chondrocytes
W89.8　Other specified
W89.9　Unspecified

W90　　**Puncture of joint**

W90.1　Aspiration of joint
W90.2　Arthrography
W90.3　Injection of therapeutic substance into joint
W90.4　Injection into joint NEC
W90.8　Other specified
W90.9　Unspecified

W91　　**Other manipulation of joint**

W91.1　Manipulation of joint using traction NEC
W91.2　Ponsetti manipulation
　　　　　Includes:　Ponsetti treatment
W91.3　Manipulation of prosthetic joint NEC
W91.8　Other specified
W91.9　Unspecified

W92   **Other operations on joint**
Excludes: *Some similar operations for correction of congenital deformity (X19–X27)*

W92.1   Biopsy of lesion of joint NEC
         Includes: Biopsy of joint NEC
W92.2   Distension of joint
W92.3   Examination of joint under image intensifier
W92.4   Examination of joint under anaesthetic
W92.5   Examination of joint NEC
W92.8   Other specified
W92.9   Unspecified

W93   **Hybrid prosthetic replacement of hip joint using cemented acetabular component**

W93.1   Primary hybrid prosthetic replacement of hip joint using cemented acetabular component
W93.2   Conversion to hybrid prosthetic replacement of hip joint using cemented acetabular component
         Note: Use a subsidiary conversion from code as necessary
W93.3   Revision of hybrid prosthetic replacement of hip joint using cemented acetabular component
W93.8   Other specified
W93.9   Unspecified
W93.0   Conversion from previous hybrid prosthetic replacement of hip joint using cemented acetabular component

W94   **Hybrid prosthetic replacement of hip joint using cemented femoral component**

W94.1   Primary hybrid prosthetic replacement of hip joint using cemented femoral component
W94.2   Conversion to hybrid prosthetic replacement of hip joint using cemented femoral component
         Note: Use a subsidiary conversion from code as necessary
W94.3   Revision of hybrid prosthetic replacement of hip joint using cemented femoral component
W94.8   Other specified
W94.9   Unspecified
W94.0   Conversion from previous hybrid prosthetic replacement of hip joint using cemented femoral component

W95   **Hybrid prosthetic replacement of hip joint using cement**
Includes: *Hybrid prosthetic replacement of hip joint NEC*

W95.1   Primary hybrid prosthetic replacement of hip joint using cement NEC
W95.2   Conversion to hybrid prosthetic replacement of hip joint using cement NEC
         Note: Use a subsidiary conversion from code as necessary
W95.3   Revision of hybrid prosthetic replacement of hip joint using cement NEC
W95.4   Attention to hybrid prosthetic replacement of hip joint using cement NEC
W95.8   Other specified
W95.9   Unspecified
W95.0   Conversion from previous hybrid prosthetic replacement of hip joint using cement NEC

W96 **Total prosthetic replacement of shoulder joint using cement**

W96.1 Primary total prosthetic replacement of shoulder joint using cement
W96.2 Conversion to total prosthetic replacement of shoulder joint using cement
Note: Use a subsidiary conversion from code as necessary
W96.3 Revision of total prosthetic replacement of shoulder joint using cement
W96.4 Revision of one component of total prosthetic replacement of shoulder joint using cement
W96.5 Primary reverse polarity total prosthetic replacement of shoulder joint using cement
W96.6 Revision of reverse polarity total prosthetic replacement of shoulder joint using cement
W96.8 Other specified
W96.9 Unspecified
W96.0 Conversion from total prosthetic replacement of shoulder joint using cement

W97 **Total prosthetic replacement of shoulder joint not using cement**

W97.1 Primary total prosthetic replacement of shoulder joint not using cement
W97.2 Conversion to total prosthetic replacement of shoulder joint not using cement
Note: Use a subsidiary conversion from code as necessary
W97.3 Revision of total prosthetic replacement of shoulder joint not using cement
W97.4 Revision of one component of total prosthetic replacement of shoulder joint not using cement
W97.5 Primary reverse polarity total prosthetic replacement of shoulder joint not using cement
W97.6 Revision of reverse polarity total prosthetic replacement of shoulder joint not using cement
W97.8 Other specified
W97.9 Unspecified
W97.0 Conversion from total prosthetic replacement of shoulder joint not using cement

W98 **Total prosthetic replacement of shoulder joint**

Includes: Total prosthetic replacement of shoulder joint NEC

W98.1 Primary total prosthetic replacement of shoulder joint NEC
W98.2 Conversion to total prosthetic replacement of shoulder joint NEC
Note: Use a subsidiary conversion from code as necessary
W98.3 Revision of total prosthetic replacement of shoulder joint NEC
W98.4 Attention to total prosthetic replacement of shoulder joint NEC
W98.5 Revision of one component of total prosthetic replacement of shoulder joint NEC
W98.6 Primary reverse polarity total prosthetic replacement of shoulder joint NEC
W98.7 Revision of reverse polarity total prosthetic replacement of shoulder joint NEC
W98.8 Other specified
W98.9 Unspecified
W98.0 Conversion from total prosthetic replacement of shoulder joint NEC

W99 **Graft of cord blood stem cells to bone marrow**

W99.1 Allograft of cord blood stem cells to bone marrow
W99.8 Other specified
W99.9 Unspecified

O06 **Hybrid prosthetic replacement of shoulder joint using cemented humeral component**

O06.1 Primary hybrid prosthetic replacement of shoulder joint using cemented humeral component

O06.2 Conversion to hybrid prosthetic replacement of shoulder joint using cemented humeral component
Note: Use a subsidiary conversion from code as necessary

O06.3 Revision of hybrid prosthetic replacement of shoulder joint using cemented humeral component

O06.8 Other specified

O06.9 Unspecified

O06.0 Conversion from previous hybrid prosthetic replacement of shoulder joint using cemented humeral component

O07 **Hybrid prosthetic replacement of shoulder joint using cemented glenoid component**

O07.1 Primary hybrid prosthetic replacement of shoulder joint using cemented glenoid component

O07.2 Conversion to hybrid prosthetic replacement of shoulder joint using cemented glenoid component
Note: Use a subsidiary conversion from code as necessary

O07.3 Revision of hybrid prosthetic replacement of shoulder joint using cemented glenoid component

O07.8 Other specified

O07.9 Unspecified

O07.0 Conversion from previous hybrid prosthetic replacement of shoulder joint using cemented glenoid component

O08 **Hybrid prosthetic replacement of shoulder joint using cement**
Includes: Hybrid prosthetic replacement of shoulder joint NEC

O08.1 Primary hybrid prosthetic replacement of shoulder joint using cement NEC

O08.2 Conversion to hybrid prosthetic replacement of shoulder joint using cement NEC
Note: Use a subsidiary conversion from code as necessary

O08.3 Revision of hybrid prosthetic replacement of shoulder joint using cement NEC

O08.4 Attention to hybrid prosthetic replacement of shoulder joint using cement NEC

O08.8 Other specified

O08.9 Unspecified

O08.0 Conversion from previous hybrid prosthetic replacement of shoulder joint using cement NEC

O09 **Placement of bone prosthesis**
Excludes: Prosthetic replacement of bone (W05)

O09.1 Implantation of vertical expanding prosthetic titanium rib

O09.8 Other specified

O09.9 Unspecified

O10 **Complex reconstruction of shoulder**

O10.1 Extra-articular scapular resection with reconstruction of shoulder

O10.8 Other specified

O10.9 Unspecified

O17 **Secondary closed reduction of fracture of bone and internal fixation**
Includes: Secondary internal fixation of fracture of bone without mention of reduction
Remanipulation of fracture of bone and internal fixation
Excludes: Fracture dislocation (W66)

O17.1 Remanipulation of intracapsular fracture of neck of femur and fixation using nail or screw
O17.2 Remanipulation of fracture of long bone and rigid internal fixation NEC
O17.3 Remanipulation of fracture of long bone and flexible internal fixation HFQ
O17.4 Remanipulation of fracture of small bone and fixation using screw
O17.5 Remanipulation of fragment of bone and fixation using screw
O17.8 Other specified
O17.9 Unspecified

O18 **Hybrid prosthetic replacement of knee joint using cement**
Includes: Hybrid prosthetic replacement of knee joint NEC

O18.1 Primary hybrid prosthetic replacement of knee joint using cement
O18.2 Conversion to hybrid prosthetic replacement of knee joint using cement
Note: Use a subsidiary conversion from code as necessary
O18.3 Revision of hybrid prosthetic replacement of knee joint using cement
O18.4 Attention to hybrid prosthetic replacement of knee joint using cement
O18.8 Other specified
O18.9 Unspecified
O18.0 Conversion from previous hybrid prosthetic replacement of knee joint using cement

O19 **Other therapeutic endoscopic operations on other joint structure**
Note: Principal W84
It is not necessary to code additionally any mention of diagnostic endoscopic examination of same joint (W87.9, W88.9)

O19.1 Endoscopic autologous matrix induced chondrogenesis of joint
O19.2 Endoscopic excision of infrapatellar fat pad
O19.8 Other specified
O19.9 Unspecified

O21 **Total prosthetic replacement of elbow joint using cement**

O21.1 Primary total prosthetic replacement of elbow joint using cement
O21.2 Conversion to total prosthetic replacement of elbow joint using cement
Note: Use a subsidiary conversion from code as necessary
O21.3 Revision of total prosthetic replacement of elbow joint using cement
O21.4 Revision of one component of total prosthetic replacement of elbow joint using cement
O21.8 Other specified
O21.9 Unspecified
O21.0 Conversion from total prosthetic replacement of elbow joint using cement

O22 **Total prosthetic replacement of elbow joint not using cement**

O22.1 Primary total prosthetic replacement of elbow joint not using cement
O22.2 Conversion to total prosthetic replacement of elbow joint not using cement
Note: Use a subsidiary conversion from code as necessary
O22.3 Revision of total prosthetic replacement of elbow joint not using cement
O22.4 Revision of one component of total prosthetic replacement of elbow joint not using cement
O22.8 Other specified
O22.9 Unspecified
O22.0 Conversion from total prosthetic replacement of elbow joint not using cement

O23   **Total prosthetic replacement of elbow joint**
         Includes: *Total prosthetic replacement of elbow joint NEC*

O23.1   Primary total prosthetic replacement of elbow joint NEC
O23.2   Conversion to total prosthetic replacement of elbow joint NEC
         Note: ***Use a subsidiary conversion from code as necessary***
O23.3   Revision of total prosthetic replacement of elbow joint NEC
O23.4   Attention to total prosthetic replacement of elbow joint NEC
O23.5   Revision of one component of total prosthetic replacement of elbow joint NEC
O23.8   Other specified
O23.9   Unspecified
O23.0   Conversion from total prosthetic replacement of elbow joint NEC

O24   **Prosthetic replacement of head of radius using cement**
         Includes: *Prosthetic hemiarthroplasty of head of radius using cement*

O24.1   Primary prosthetic replacement of head of radius using cement
O24.2   Conversion to prosthetic replacement of head of radius using cement
         Note: ***Use a subsidiary conversion from code as necessary***
O24.3   Revision of prosthetic replacement of head of radius using cement
O24.8   Other specified
O24.9   Unspecified
O24.0   Conversion from previous cemented prosthetic replacement of head of radius

O25   **Prosthetic replacement of head of radius not using cement**
         Includes: *Prosthetic hemiarthroplasty of head of radius not using cement*

O25.1   Primary prosthetic replacement of head of radius not using cement
O25.2   Conversion to prosthetic replacement of head of radius not using cement
         Note: ***Use a subsidiary conversion from code as necessary***
O25.3   Revision of prosthetic replacement of head of radius not using cement
O25.8   Other specified
O25.9   Unspecified
O25.0   Conversion from previous uncemented prosthetic replacement of head of radius

O26   **Other prosthetic replacement of head of radius**
         Includes: *Prosthetic hemiarthroplasty of head of radius NEC*

O26.1   Primary prosthetic replacement of head of radius NEC
O26.2   Conversion to prosthetic replacement of head of radius NEC
         Note: ***Use a subsidiary conversion from code as necessary***
O26.3   Revision of prosthetic replacement of head of radius NEC
O26.4   Attention to prosthetic replacement of head of radius NEC
O26.8   Other specified
O26.9   Unspecified
O26.0   Conversion from previous prosthetic replacement of head of radius NEC

O27   **Other stabilising operations on joint**
         Note: ***Principal W77***

O27.1   Extra-articular ligament reconstruction for stabilisation of joint
O27.2   Repair of capsule and anterior and posterior labrum for stabilisation of glenohumeral joint
O27.3   Repair of capsule and anterior labrum for stabilisation of glenohumeral joint
O27.4   Repair of capsule and posterior labrum for stabilisation of glenohumeral joint
O27.8   Other specified
O27.9   Unspecified

O29   **Excision of bone**
            Note: Principal W08

O29.1   Subacromial decompression
            Includes: Acromioplasty NEC
O29.8   Other specified
O29.9   Unspecified

O32   **Total prosthetic replacement of ankle joint**

O32.1   Primary total prosthetic replacement of ankle joint NEC
O32.2   Conversion to total prosthetic replacement of ankle joint NEC
            Note: Use a subsidiary conversion from code as necessary
O32.3   Revision of total prosthetic replacement of ankle joint NEC
O32.4   Attention to total prosthetic replacement of ankle joint NEC
O32.5   Revision of one component of total prosthetic replacement of ankle joint NEC
O32.8   Other specified
O32.9   Unspecified
O32.0   Conversion from total prosthetic replacement of ankle joint NEC

CHAPTER X
MISCELLANEOUS OPERATIONS
(CODES X01-X98)

Includes: *OPERATIONS COVERING MULTIPLE SYSTEMS*
Note: *This chapter contains certain codes designed to precede codes in Chapter Y when more precise preceding codes cannot be determined or are not applicable*
Use a subsidiary code for minimal access approach (Y74-Y76)
Use a subsidiary code to identify method of image control (Y53)

X01   **Replantation of upper limb**

X01.1   Replantation of whole arm
X01.2   Replantation of forearm
X01.3   Replantation of hand
X01.4   Replantation of thumb
X01.5   Replantation of finger NEC
X01.8   Other specified
X01.9   Unspecified
         Includes: *Replantation of arm NEC*

X02   **Replantation of lower limb**

X02.1   Replantation of whole leg
X02.2   Replantation of foot
X02.3   Replantation of toe
X02.8   Other specified
X02.9   Unspecified
         Includes: *Replantation of leg NEC*

X03   **Replantation of other organ**

X03.1   Replantation of ear
X03.2   Replantation of nose
X03.8   Other specified
X03.9   Unspecified

X04   **Transplantation between systems**

X04.1   Autotransplantation of adrenal medulla to caudate nucleus of brain
X04.8   Other specified
X04.9   Unspecified

X05   **Implantation of prosthesis for limb**

X05.1   Implantation of bioelectrical prosthesis for limb
X05.2   Implantation of kineplastic prosthesis for limb
X05.3   Attention to prosthesis for limb
X05.8   Other specified
X05.9   Unspecified

X07   **Amputation of arm**

X07.1   Forequarter amputation
X07.2   Disarticulation of shoulder
X07.3   Amputation of arm above elbow
X07.4   Amputation of arm through elbow
X07.5   Amputation of arm through forearm
X07.8   Other specified
X07.9   Unspecified

X08   **Amputation of hand**

X08.1   Amputation of hand at wrist
X08.2   Amputation of thumb
          Excludes: Amputation of duplicate thumb (X21.5)
X08.3   Amputation of phalanx of finger
X08.4   Amputation of finger NEC
          Excludes: Amputation of supernumerary finger (X21.6)
X08.8   Other specified
X08.9   Unspecified

X09   **Amputation of leg**

X09.1   Hindquarter amputation
X09.2   Disarticulation of hip
X09.3   Amputation of leg above knee
X09.4   Amputation of leg through knee
X09.5   Amputation of leg below knee
X09.8   Other specified
X09.9   Unspecified

X10   **Amputation of foot**

X10.1   Amputation of foot through ankle
X10.2   Disarticulation of tarsal bones
X10.3   Disarticulation of metatarsal bones
X10.4   Amputation through metatarsal bones
X10.8   Other specified
X10.9   Unspecified

X11   **Amputation of toe**
          Excludes: Amputation of supernumerary toe (X27.3)

X11.1   Amputation of great toe
X11.2   Amputation of phalanx of toe
X11.8   Other specified
X11.9   Unspecified
          Includes: Disarticulation of toe

X12 Operations on amputation stump

X12.1 Reamputation at higher level
X12.2 Excision of lesion of amputation stump
X12.3 Shortening of length of amputation stump
X12.4 Revision of coverage of amputation stump
X12.5 Drainage of amputation stump
X12.8 Other specified
X12.9 Unspecified

X14 Clearance of pelvis

X14.1 Total exenteration of pelvis
   Includes: Exenteration of pelvis NEC
X14.2 Anterior exenteration of pelvis
X14.3 Posterior exenteration of pelvis
X14.8 Other specified
X14.9 Unspecified

X15 Operations for sexual transformation
Excludes: Operations for disorders of sex development (X16)

X15.1 Combined operations for transformation from male to female
X15.2 Combined operations for transformation from female to male
X15.3 Code retired - refer to introduction
X15.4 Construction of scrotum
X15.8 Other specified
X15.9 Unspecified

X16 Operations for disorders of sex development
Excludes: Operations for sexual transformation (X15)

X16.1 Excision of Mullerian duct remnant
   Includes: Excision of uterine horn
             Excision of rudimentary uterus
   Excludes: Excision of accessory uterus (Q07.6)
X16.2 Excision of lesion of Mullerian duct remnant
X16.3 Excision of gonad from abdomen
   Note: Use a supplementary code for concurrent excision of fallopian tube (Q22-Q24)
X16.4 Excision of gonad from pelvis
   Note: Use a supplementary code for concurrent excision of fallopian tube (Q22-Q24)
X16.5 Excision of gonad from inguinal canal
   Note: Use a supplementary code for concurrent excision of fallopian tube (Q22-Q24)
X16.6 Excision of gonad NEC
   Note: Use a supplementary code for concurrent excision of fallopian tube (Q22-Q24)
X16.8 Other specified
X16.9 Unspecified

X17 Separation of conjoined twins

X17.1 Combined operations to separate conjoined twins
X17.8 Other specified
X17.9 Unspecified

X19   **Correction of congenital deformity of shoulder or upper arm**

X19.1   Reduction of Sprengel deformity
X19.2   Correction of obstetric palsy
X19.8   Other specified
X19.9   Unspecified

X20   **Correction of congenital deformity of forearm**

X20.1   Excision of anlage of radius
X20.2   Excision of anlage of ulna
X20.3   Centralisation of carpus for correction of congenital deformity of forearm
X20.4   Revision of release of radius for correction of congenital deformity of forearm
X20.5   Revision of release of ulna for correction of congenital deformity of forearm
X20.8   Other specified
X20.9   Unspecified

X21   **Correction of congenital deformity of hand**

X21.1   Reduction of gigantism of hand
X21.2   Correction of mirror hand
X21.3   Correction of syndactyly of fingers using skin graft
X21.4   Correction of syndactyly of fingers using skin expander
X21.5   Amputation of duplicate thumb
X21.6   Amputation of supernumerary finger NEC
X21.7   Reconstruction of radial club hand
X21.8   Other specified
X21.9   Unspecified

X22   **Correction of congenital deformity of hip**

X22.1   Open reduction of congenital deformity of hip
X22.2   Primary osteotomy of pelvis for correction of congenital deformity of hip
            Includes: Osteotomy of pelvis for correction of congenital deformity of hip
X22.3   Secondary arthroplasty of hip for correction of congenital deformity of hip
X22.4   Intra-articular soft tissue procedures for correction of congenital deformity of hip
X22.5   Extra-articular procedures for correction of congenital deformity of hip
X22.8   Other specified
X22.9   Unspecified

X23   **Correction of congenital deformity of leg**

X23.1   Operative reduction of congenital dislocation of knee
X23.2   Correction of pseudoarthrosis of tibia
X23.3   Excision of anlage of fibula
X23.4   Excision of anlage of tibia
X23.5   Centralisation of tarsus for correction of congenital deformity of leg
X23.6   Reversal of rotation plasty of ankle for correction of congenital deformity of leg
X23.8   Other specified
X23.9   Unspecified

X24   **Primary correction of congenital deformity of foot**

X24.1   Release of pantalar joints for correction of congenital deformity of foot
X24.2   Posterior release of joints of foot for correction of congenital deformity of foot
X24.3   Medial release of joints of foot for correction of congenital deformity of foot
X24.4   Anterior release of joints of foot for correction of congenital deformity of foot
X24.8   Other specified
X24.9   Unspecified

X25   **Other correction of congenital deformity of foot**
        Includes: Late correction of congenital deformity of foot

X25.1   Osteotomy of body of os calcis
X25.2   Wedge tarsectomy for correction of congenital deformity of foot
X25.3   Reduction of gigantism of foot
X25.4   Separation of tarsal coalition
X25.8   Other specified
X25.9   Unspecified

X27   **Correction of minor congenital deformity of foot**

X27.1   Release of Streeter band
X27.2   Release of syndactyly of toes
X27.3   Amputation of supernumerary toe
X27.4   Correction of curly fifth toe
X27.5   Correction of congenital crossed toes
X27.8   Other specified
X27.9   Unspecified

X28   **Intermittent infusion of therapeutic substance**
        Excludes: Continuous infusion of therapeutic substance (X29)

X28.1   Intermittent intravenous infusion of therapeutic substance
X28.2   Intermittent subcutaneous infusion of therapeutic substance
X28.8   Other specified
X28.9   Unspecified

X29   **Continuous Infusion of therapeutic substance**
        Excludes: Intermittent infusion of therapeutic substance (X28)

X29.1   Continuous subcutaneous infusion of insulin
        Includes: Subcutaneous infusion with insulin pump
X29.2   Continuous intravenous infusion of therapeutic substance NEC
X29.3   Continuous subcutaneous infusion of therapeutic substance NEC
        Includes: Subcutaneous infusion of fluids NEC
X29.8   Other specified
X29.9   Unspecified

X30   **Injection of therapeutic substance**
              Includes: Injection of prophylactic substance

X30.1   Injection of Rh immune globulin
X30.2   Injection of gamma globulin
              Includes: Intravenous immunoglobulin NEC
X30.3   Injection of immune serum NEC
X30.4   Injection of thrombin NEC
X30.5   Injection of sclerosing substance NEC
X30.6   Injection of anaesthetic agent NEC
X30.8   Other specified
X30.9   Unspecified

X31   **Injection of radiocontrast material**

X31.1   Intravenous cholecystography
X31.2   Intravenous pyelography
              Includes: Intravenous urogram
X31.3   Intravenous injection of radiocontrast material NEC
X31.8   Other specified
X31.9   Unspecified

X32   **Exchange blood transfusion**
              Includes: Therapeutic apheresis
                   Note: Principal category, extended at X47

X32.1   Neonatal exchange blood transfusion
X32.2   Exchange of plasma (single)
              Includes: Plasmapheresis (single)
              Plasma separation (single)
X32.3   Exchange of plasma (2-9)
              Includes: Plasmapheresis (2-9)
              Plasma separation (2-9)
X32.4   Exchange of plasma (10-19)
              Includes: Plasmapheresis (10-19)
              Plasma separation (10-19)
X32.5   Exchange of plasma (>19)
              Includes: Plasmapheresis (>19)
              Plasma separation (>19)
X32.6   Red cell exchange
              Includes: Erythrocytopheresis
              Excludes: Autologous transfusion of red blood cells (X33.7)
X32.7   Leucopheresis
X32.8   Other specified
X32.9   Unspecified

X33   **Other blood transfusion**

X33.1   Intra-arterial blood transfusion
X33.2   Intravenous blood transfusion of packed cells
X33.3   Intravenous blood transfusion of platelets
X33.4   Autologous peripheral blood stem cell transplant
X33.5   Syngeneic peripheral blood stem cell transplant
X33.6   Allogeneic peripheral blood stem cell transplant
X33.7   Autologous transfusion of red blood cells
         Excludes: Exchange blood transfusion (X32)
X33.8   Other specified
X33.9   Unspecified
         Includes: Intravenous blood transfusion NEC

X34   **Other intravenous transfusion**

X34.1   Transfusion of coagulation factor
X34.2   Transfusion of plasma NEC
X34.3   Transfusion of serum NEC
X34.4   Transfusion of blood expander
X34.8   Other specified
X34.9   Unspecified

X35   **Other intravenous injection**
         Includes: Intravenous bolus injection
                   Intravenous bolus NEC

X35.1   Intravenous induction of labour
X35.2   Intravenous chemotherapy
X35.3   Intravenous immunotherapy
         Excludes: Intravenous injection of vaccine (X44.1)
X35.4   Intravenous injection of non radioactive diagnostic substance
X35.5   Intravenous injection of antimicrobial therapy
X35.8   Other specified
X35.9   Unspecified

X36   **Blood withdrawal**

X36.1   Blood donation
X36.2   Venesection
X36.3   Venous sampling
X36.4   Autologous blood salvage
X36.8   Other specified
X36.9   Unspecified

X37   **Intramuscular injection**

X37.1   Intramuscular calcitonin therapy
X37.2   Intramuscular gold therapy
X37.3   Intramuscular chemotherapy
X37.4   Intramuscular immunotherapy
         Excludes: Intramuscular injection of vaccine (X44.2)
X37.5   Intramuscular injection for local action
X37.6   Intramuscular hormone therapy
X37.8   Other specified
X37.9   Unspecified

X38   **Subcutaneous injection**

X38.1   Injection of triamcinolone for local action
Includes: Injection of triamcinolone
X38.2   Injection of steroid for local action NEC
Includes: Injection of steroid NEC
X38.3   Injection of hormone for local action NEC
Includes: Injection of hormone NEC
X38.4   Subcutaneous chemotherapy
X38.5   Subcutaneous immunotherapy
Excludes: Subcutaneous injection of vaccine (X44.3)
X38.6   Subcutaneous injection for local action NEC
Includes: Subcutaneous injection NEC
X38.7   Subcutaneous injection of haematological growth factor
X38.8   Other specified
X38.9   Unspecified

X39   **Other route of administration of therapeutic substance**

X39.1   Oral administration of therapeutic substance
Excludes: Oral administration of vaccine (X44.4)
X39.2   Sublingual administration of therapeutic substance
X39.3   Intranasal administration of therapeutic substance
X39.4   Inhalation administration of therapeutic substance
X39.5   Transdermal administration of therapeutic substance
X39.6   Intraocular administration of therapeutic substance
X39.8   Other specified
X39.9   Unspecified

X40   **Compensation for renal failure**

X40.1   Renal dialysis
X40.2   Peritoneal dialysis NEC
X40.3   Haemodialysis NEC
X40.4   Haemofiltration
X40.5   Automated peritoneal dialysis
X40.6   Continuous ambulatory peritoneal dialysis
X40.7   Haemoperfusion
X40.8   Other specified
X40.9   Unspecified

X41   **Placement of ambulatory apparatus for compensation for renal failure**

X41.1   Insertion of ambulatory peritoneal dialysis catheter
X41.2   Removal of ambulatory peritoneal dialysis catheter
X41.8   Other specified
X41.9   Unspecified

X42   **Placement of other apparatus for compensation for renal failure**

X42.1   Insertion of temporary peritoneal dialysis catheter
X42.8   Other specified
X42.9   Unspecified

X43   **Compensation for liver failure**

X43.1   Extracorporeal albumin haemodialysis
X43.8   Other specified
X43.9   Unspecified

X44   **Administration of vaccine**
Excludes: Administration of Bacillus Calmette-Guerin vaccine (E95.2)

X44.1   Intravenous injection of vaccine
X44.2   Intramuscular injection of vaccine
X44.3   Subcutaneous injection of vaccine
X44.4   Oral administration of vaccine
X44.8   Other specified
X44.9   Unspecified

X45   **Donation of organ**

X45.1   Donation of kidney
X45.2   Donation of heart
X45.3   Donation of lobe of lung
X45.8   Other specified
X45.9   Unspecified

X46   **Donation of other tissue**

X46.1   Donation of bone marrow
X46.2   Donation of skin
X46.8   Other specified
X46.9   Unspecified

X47   **Other exchange blood transfusion**
Includes: Therapeutic apheresis
        Note: Principal X32

X47.1   Low-density lipoprotein apheresis
X47.8   Other specified
X47.9   Unspecified

X48   **Immobilisation using plaster cast**

X48.1   Application of plaster cast
        Note: This code is not normally used when associated with another operation for treatment of fracture or disease of bone (Chapter V-W)
X48.2   Change of plaster cast
X48.3   Removal of plaster cast
X48.8   Other specified
X48.9   Unspecified

X49   **Other external support of limb**

                 Note: *These codes are not normally used when associated with another operation for treatment of fracture or disease of bone (Chapter V-W)*

X49.1   Application of splint NEC
X49.2   Change of splint NEC
X49.3   Removal of splint NEC
X49.4   Skin traction
X49.5   Application of sling NEC
           Includes: *Collar and cuff*
X49.6   Application of elastic support bandage NEC
X49.7   Application of gauze support bandage NEC
X49.8   Other specified
X49.9   Unspecified

X50   **External resuscitation**

X50.1   Direct current cardioversion
X50.2   External cardioversion NEC
X50.3   Advanced cardiac pulmonary resuscitation
X50.4   External ventricular defibrillation
           Includes: *Cardiac defibrillation NEC*
X50.5   Evaluation of cardioverter defibrillator
           Includes: *Evaluation of transvenous cardioverter defibrillator by induction of ventricular fibrillation*
                           Evaluation of subcutaneous cardioverter defibrillator by induction of ventricular fibrillation

X50.8   Other specified
X50.9   Unspecified

X51   **Change of body temperature**

X51.1   Hypothermia therapy
X51.2   Active cooling
X51.8   Other specified
X51.9   Unspecified

X52   **Oxygen therapy**

           Excludes: *Extracorporeal membrane oxygenation (X58.1)*
                      Oxygen therapy support (E87)

X52.1   Hyperbaric therapy
X52.8   Other specified
X52.9   Unspecified

X53   **Extirpation of unspecified organ**

X53.1   Excision of unspecified organ
X53.2   Excision of lesion of unspecified organ
X53.3   Destruction of lesion of unspecified organ
           Includes: *Photodynamic therapy of lesion of unspecified organ*
X53.8   Other specified
X53.9   Unspecified

X55   **Other operations on unspecified organ**

X55.1   Biopsy of lesion of unspecified organ
           Includes: Biopsy of unspecified organ
              Note: Use a subsidiary code to identify biopsy of abdominal mass (Z31.9)
X55.2   Incision of unspecified organ
X55.3   Fenestration of unspecified organ
X55.8   Other specified
X55.9   Unspecified

X56   **Intubation of trachea**

X56.1   Nasotracheal intubation
X56.2   Endotracheal intubation
              Note: Use Y80.2 for endotracheal intubation as part of general anaesthetic
X56.3   Tracheal intubation using laryngeal mask airway
           Includes: Intubation using laryngeal mask airway
X56.8   Other specified
X56.9   Unspecified
           Includes: Intubation trachea NEC

X58   **Artificial support for body system**

X58.1   Extracorporeal membrane oxygenation
X58.8   Other specified
X58.9   Unspecified

X59   **Anaesthetic without surgery**

X59.1   Preoperative anaesthetic death
X59.8   Other specified
X59.9   Unspecified

X60   **Rehabilitation assessment**
           Excludes: Assessment (X62)

X60.1   Rehabilitation assessment by multidisciplinary non-specialised team
X60.2   Rehabilitation assessment by multidisciplinary specialised team
X60.3   Rehabilitation assessment by unidisciplinary non-specialised team
X60.4   Rehabilitation assessment by unidisciplinary specialised team
X60.8   Other specified
X60.9   Unspecified

X61   **Complementary therapy**

X61.1   Functional therapy session
X61.2   Relaxation therapy session
X61.3   Body massage
           Includes: Acupressure
X61.4   Movement therapy NEC
           Includes: Yoga
                  Tai chi
X61.8   Other specified
X61.9   Unspecified

X62   **Assessment**
    Excludes: Rehabilitation assessment (X60)

X62.1   Assessment by uniprofessional team NEC
X62.2   Assessment by multiprofessional team NEC
X62.3   Assessment by multidisciplinary team NEC
X62.8   Other specified
X62.9   Unspecified

X63   **Category retired – refer to introduction**

X64   **Category retired – refer to introduction**

X65   **Radiotherapy delivery**

X65.1   Delivery of a fraction of total body irradiation
    Note: Use a subsidiary code to identify external beam radiotherapy (Y91)
X65.2   Delivery of a fraction of intracavitary radiotherapy
    Note: Use a subsidiary code to identify introduction of radioactive material (Y35, Y36)
    Use a subsidiary code to identify brachytherapy (Y89)
X65.3   Delivery of a fraction of interstitial radiotherapy
    Note: Use a subsidiary code to identify introduction of radioactive material (Y35, Y36)
    Use a subsidiary code to identify brachytherapy (Y89)
X65.4   Delivery of a fraction of external beam radiotherapy NEC
    Note: Use a subsidiary code to identify external beam radiotherapy (Y91)
X65.5   Oral delivery of radiotherapy for thyroid ablation
    Includes: Oral radioactive iodine therapy
    Excludes: Delivery of radionuclide therapy NEC (X65.7)
X65.6   Delivery of a fraction of intraluminal brachytherapy
    Note: Use a subsidiary code to identify introduction of radioactive material (Y35, Y36)
    Use a subsidiary code to identify brachytherapy (Y89)
X65.7   Delivery of radionuclide therapy NEC
    Excludes: Oral delivery of radiotherapy for thyroid ablation (X65.5)
X65.8   Other specified
X65.9   Unspecified

X66   **Cognitive behavioural therapy**

X66.1   Cognitive behavioural therapy by unidisciplinary team
X66.2   Cognitive behavioural therapy by multidisciplinary team
X66.8   Other specified
X66.9   Unspecified

X67   **Preparation for external beam radiotherapy**
    Note: Use a subsidiary code to identify the use of technical support (Y92)

X67.1   Preparation for intensity modulated radiation therapy
    Includes: Imaging and dosimetry
X67.2   Preparation for total body irradiation
X67.3   Preparation for hemi body irradiation
X67.4   Preparation for simple radiotherapy with imaging and dosimetry
X67.5   Preparation for simple radiotherapy with imaging and simple calculation
X67.6   Preparation for superficial radiotherapy with simple calculation
X67.7   Preparation for complex conformal radiotherapy
X67.8   Other specified
X67.9   Unspecified

X68 **Preparation for brachytherapy**
        Note: *Use a subsidiary code to identify the use of technical support (Y92)*

X68.1   Preparation for intraluminal brachytherapy
X68.2   Preparation for intracavitary brachytherapy
X68.3   Preparation for interstitial brachytherapy
X68.8   Other specified
X68.9   Unspecified

X70 **Procurement of drugs for chemotherapy for neoplasm in Bands 1-5**
        Excludes: *Other chemotherapy drugs (X74)*

X70.1   Procurement of drugs for chemotherapy for neoplasm for regimens in Band 1
X70.2   Procurement of drugs for chemotherapy for neoplasm for regimens in Band 2
X70.3   Procurement of drugs for chemotherapy for neoplasm for regimens in Band 3
X70.4   Procurement of drugs for chemotherapy for neoplasm for regimens in Band 4
X70.5   Procurement of drugs for chemotherapy for neoplasm for regimens in Band 5
X70.8   Other specified
X70.9   Unspecified

X71 **Procurement of drugs for chemotherapy for neoplasm in Bands 6-10**
        Excludes: *Other chemotherapy drugs (X74)*

X71.1   Procurement of drugs for chemotherapy for neoplasm for regimens in Band 6
X71.2   Procurement of drugs for chemotherapy for neoplasm for regimens in Band 7
X71.3   Procurement of drugs for chemotherapy for neoplasm for regimens in Band 8
X71.4   Procurement of drugs for chemotherapy for neoplasm for regimens in Band 9
X71.5   Procurement of drugs for chemotherapy for neoplasm for regimens in Band 10
X71.8   Other specified
X71.9   Unspecified

X72 **Delivery of chemotherapy for neoplasm**
        Excludes: *Exclusive delivery of oral chemotherapy (X73)*
                         Other chemotherapy drugs (X74)

X72.1   Delivery of complex chemotherapy for neoplasm including prolonged infusional treatment at first attendance
X72.2   Delivery of complex parenteral chemotherapy for neoplasm at first attendance
X72.3   Delivery of simple parenteral chemotherapy for neoplasm at first attendance
X72.4   Delivery of subsequent element of cycle of chemotherapy for neoplasm
X72.8   Other specified
X72.9   Unspecified

X73 **Delivery of oral chemotherapy for neoplasm**
        Excludes: *Other chemotherapy drugs (X74)*

X73.1   Delivery of exclusively oral chemotherapy for neoplasm
X73.8   Other specified
X73.9   Unspecified

X74   **Other chemotherapy drugs**
Excludes: Procurement of drugs for chemotherapy for neoplasm (X70-X71)
Delivery of chemotherapy for neoplasm (X72-X73)
High cost drugs (X81-X98)

X74.1   Cancer hormonal treatment drugs Band 1
X74.2   Cancer supportive drugs Band 1
X74.8   Other specified
X74.9   Unspecified

X81   **High cost gastrointestinal drugs**
Excludes: Other chemotherapy drugs (X74)

X81.8   Other specified
X81.9   Unspecified

X82   **High cost hypertension drugs**
Excludes: Other chemotherapy drugs (X74)

X82.1   Pulmonary arterial hypertension drugs Band 1
X82.2   Pulmonary arterial hypertension drugs Band 2
X82.3   Pulmonary arterial hypertension drugs Band 3
X82.4   Pulmonary arterial hypertension drugs Band 4
X82.8   Other specified
X82.9   Unspecified

X83   **High cost other cardiovascular drugs**
Excludes: Other chemotherapy drugs (X74)

X83.1   Blood products Band 1
X83.2   Blood products Band 2
X83.3   Fibrinolytic drugs Band 1
X83.8   Other specified
X83.9   Unspecified

X84   **High cost respiratory drugs**
Excludes: Other chemotherapy drugs (X74)

X84.1   Medical gases Band 1
X84.2   Pulmonary surfactant drugs Band 1
X84.3   Mucolytic drugs Band 1
X84.8   Other specified
X84.9   Unspecified

X85   **High cost neurology drugs**
Excludes: Other chemotherapy drugs (X74)

X85.1   Torsion dystonias and other involuntary movements drugs Band 1
X85.2   Amyotrophic lateral sclerosis drugs Band 1
X85.3   Hypnotic drugs Band 1
X85.4   Analgesic drugs Band 1
X85.5   Neurodegenerative condition drugs Band 1
X85.6   Neuromuscular disorder drugs Band 1
X85.8   Other specified
X85.9   Unspecified

X86 **High cost anti-infective drugs**
    SEE ALSO X98
    Excludes: *Other chemotherapy drugs (X74)*

X86.1 Antifungal drugs Band 1
X86.2 Antifungal drugs Band 2
X86.3 Hepatitis B treatment drugs Band 1
X86.4 Respiratory syncytial virus treatment and Hepatitis C treatment drugs Band 1
X86.5 Respiratory syncytial virus prevention drugs Band 1
X86.6 Antiretroviral drugs Band 1
X86.7 Cytomegalovirus drugs Band 1
X86.8 Other specified
X86.9 Unspecified

X87 **High cost endocrinology drugs**
    Excludes: *Other chemotherapy drugs (X74)*

X87.1 Growth hormone receptor antagonist drugs Band 1
X87.2 Growth hormone analogue drugs Band 1
X87.3 Bone metabolism drugs Band 1
X87.4 Vasopressin antagonist drugs Band 1
X87.8 Other specified
X87.9 Unspecified

X88 **High cost reproductive and urinary tract drugs**
    Excludes: *Other chemotherapy drugs (X74)*

X88.8 Other specified
X88.9 Unspecified

X89 **High cost immunosuppressant drugs**
    Excludes: *Other chemotherapy drugs (X74)*

X89.1 Monoclonal antibodies Band 1
X89.2 Monoclonal antibodies Band 2
X89.3 Immunomodulating drugs Band 1
X89.4 Somatostatin analogues Band 1
X89.5 Allergic emergency drugs Band 1
X89.8 Other specified
X89.9 Unspecified

X90 **High cost haematology and nutrition drugs**
    Excludes: *Other chemotherapy drugs (X74)*

X90.1 Hypoplastic haemolytic and renal anaemia drugs Band 1
X90.2 Hypoplastic haemolytic and renal anaemia drugs Band 2
X90.3 Neutropenia drugs Band 1
X90.4 Intravenous nutrition Band 1
X90.5 Platelet disorder drugs Band 1
X90.6 Protein tyrosine kinase inhibitors Band 1
X90.7 Myelodysplastic syndrome drugs Band 1
X90.8 Other specified
X90.9 Unspecified

X91   **High cost metabolic drugs**
          Excludes: Other chemotherapy drugs (X74)

X91.1   Metabolic disorder drugs Band 1
X91.2   Metabolic disorder drugs Band 2
X91.3   Metabolic disorder drugs Band 3
X91.4   Metabolic disorder drugs Band 4
X91.8   Other specified
X91.9   Unspecified

X92   **High cost musculoskeletal drugs**
          Excludes: Other chemotherapy drugs (X74)

X92.1   Cytokine inhibitor drugs Band 1
X92.2   Hyperuricaemia drugs Band 1
X92.3   Bone morphogenetic proteins Band 1
X92.4   Soft tissue disorder drugs Band 1
X92.8   Other specified
X92.9   Unspecified

X93   **High cost ophthalmology drugs**
          Excludes: Other chemotherapy drugs (X74)

X93.1   Subfoveal choroidal neovascularisation drugs Band 1
X93.2   Macular oedema drugs Band 1
X93.3   Retinal disorder drugs Band 1
X93.8   Other specified
X93.9   Unspecified

X94   **High cost ear, nose and throat drugs**
          Excludes: Other chemotherapy drugs (X74)

X94.8   Other specified
X94.9   Unspecified

X95   **High cost dermatology drugs**
          Excludes: Other chemotherapy drugs (X74)

X95.1   Immune response drugs Band 1
X95.2   Skin condition drugs Band 1
X95.8   Other specified
X95.9   Unspecified

X96   **High cost immunology drugs**
          Excludes: Other chemotherapy drugs (X74)

X96.1   Immunoglobulins Band 1
X96.2   Allergen immunotherapy drugs Band 1
X96.3   Poison management drugs Band 1
X96.8   Other specified
X96.9   Unspecified

X97   **High cost anaesthesia drugs**
          Excludes: Other chemotherapy drugs (X74)

X97.8   Other specified
X97.9   Unspecified

X98   **Other high cost drugs**
            SEE ALSO X86

            Excludes: Other chemotherapy drugs (X74)

X98.1   Antibacterial drugs Band 1
X98.8   Other specified
X98.9   Unspecified

Y05	**Excision of organ NOC**
Y05.1	Total excision of organ NOC
Y05.2	Partial excision of organ NOC
Y05.3	Excision of sinus track from organ NOC
	Includes: *Excision of fistula from organ NOC*
	Note: ***Site specific chapter related code can be used only when precise identification of organ from which sinus track or fistula originates is given***
	This does not include skin of site of original operation otherwise X55.8 should be used
Y05.4	Ex vivo resection of organ NOC
	Includes: *Ante situm hypothermic resection of organ NOC*
Y05.5	Debridement of organ NOC
Y05.8	Other specified
Y05.9	Unspecified

Y06	**Excision of lesion of organ NOC**
Y06.1	Marsupialisation of organ NOC
Y06.2	Deroofing of cyst of organ NOC
Y06.3	Enucleation of lesion of organ NOC
Y06.4	Excision of scar tissue NOC
Y06.5	Gamma wave excision of lesion of organ NOC
Y06.6	Vacuum excision of lesion of organ NOC
	Includes: *Vacuum assisted excision of lesion of organ NOC*
Y06.7	Radiofrequency excision of lesion of organ NOC
Y06.8	Other specified
Y06.9	Unspecified

Y07	**Obliteration of cavity of organ NOC**
Y07.1	Ligation of organ NOC
Y07.2	Clipping of organ NOC
Y07.3	Obliteration of sinus track from organ NOC
	Includes: *Obliteration of fistula from organ NOC*
	Closure of sinus track from organ NOC
	Closure of fistula from organ NOC
	Note: ***Site specific chapter related code can be used only when precise identification of organ from which sinus track or fistula originates is given***
	This does not include skin of site of original operation otherwise X55.8 should be used
Y07.4	Obliteration of diverticulum of organ NOC
Y07.5	Occlusion of organ NOC
Y07.8	Other specified
Y07.9	Unspecified

Y08	**Laser therapy to organ NOC**
Y08.1	Laser excision of organ NOC
Y08.2	Laser excision of lesion of organ NOC
Y08.3	Laser destruction of organ NOC
Y08.4	Laser destruction of lesion of organ NOC
Y08.5	Laser modification of organ NOC
Y08.6	Laser incision of organ NOC
Y08.8	Other specified
Y08.9	Unspecified

Y09   **Chemical destruction of organ NOC**

Y09.1   Injection of sclerosing substance into organ NOC
     Includes: Sclerotherapy to organ NOC
Y09.2   Injection of other destructive substance into organ NOC
Y09.8   Other specified
Y09.9   Unspecified

Y10   **Destruction of organ NOC**
     Includes: Destruction of tissue of organ
         Note: Principal Y11

Y10.1   Coblation of organ NOC
Y10.2   Electrocauterisation of organ NOC
Y10.8   Other specified
Y10.9   Unspecified

Y11   **Other destruction of organ NOC**
     Includes: Other destruction of tissue of organ
         Note: Principal category, extended at Y10

Y11.1   Cauterisation of organ NOC
Y11.2   Cryotherapy to organ NOC
Y11.3   Curettage of organ NOC
Y11.4   Radiofrequency controlled thermal destruction of organ NOC
     Includes: Radiofrequency ablation of organ NOC
Y11.5   Ultrasonic destruction of organ NOC
Y11.6   Microwave destruction of organ NOC
Y11.7   Gamma wave destruction of organ NOC
Y11.8   Other specified
Y11.9   Unspecified

Y12   **Chemical destruction of lesion of organ NOC**

Y12.1   Injection of sclerosing substance into lesion of organ NOC
     Includes: Sclerotherapy to lesion of organ NOC
Y12.2   Injection of other destructive substance into lesion of organ NOC
Y12.3   Electrochemotherapy to lesion of organ NOC
     Includes: Electroporation to lesion of organ NOC
Y12.8   Other specified
Y12.9   Unspecified

Y13   **Other destruction of lesion of organ NOC**
         Note: Principal category, extended at Y17

Y13.1   Cauterisation of lesion of organ NOC
Y13.2   Cryotherapy to lesion of organ NOC
Y13.3   Curettage of lesion of organ NOC
Y13.4   Radiofrequency controlled thermal destruction of lesion of organ NOC
     Includes: Radiofrequency ablation of lesion of organ NOC
Y13.5   Ultrasonic destruction of lesion of organ NOC
Y13.6   Photodynamic therapy of lesion of organ NOC
Y13.7   Microwave destruction of lesion of organ NOC
Y13.8   Other specified
Y13.9   Unspecified

Y29   **Removal of foreign body from organ NOC**

Y29.1   Surgical removal of foreign body from organ NOC
Y29.2   Manipulative removal of foreign body from organ NOC
Y29.8   Other specified
Y29.9   Unspecified

Y30   **Incision of organ NOC**

Y30.1   Incision of lesion of organ NOC
Y30.8   Other specified
Y30.9   Unspecified

Y31   **Exploration of organ NOC**

Y31.1   Exploration of sinus track from organ NOC
          Includes: Exploration of fistula from organ NOC
             Note: Site specific chapter related code can be used only when precise identification of organ from which sinus track or fistula originates is given
                   This does not include skin of site of original operation otherwise X55.8 should be used
Y31.8   Other specified
Y31.9   Unspecified

Y32   **Re-exploration of organ NOC**

Y32.1   Re-exploration of organ and surgical arrest of postoperative bleeding NOC
Y32.2   Re-exploration of organ and other repair of organ NOC
          Includes: Re-exploration of organ and resuture of organ NOC
Y32.3   Re-exploration of organ and packing of organ NOC
Y32.8   Other specified
Y32.9   Unspecified

Y33   **Puncture of organ NOC**

Y33.1   Acupuncture of organ NOC
Y33.2   Drilling of organ NOC
Y33.8   Other specified
Y33.9   Unspecified

Y35   **Introduction of removable radioactive material into organ NOC**

Y35.1   Introduction of radioactive caesium into organ NOC
Y35.2   Introduction of iridium wire into organ NOC
Y35.3   Introduction of radium into organ NOC
Y35.4   Introduction of radioactive substance into organ for brachytherapy NOC
Y35.8   Other specified
Y35.9   Unspecified

Y36   **Introduction of non-removable material into organ NOC**

Y36.1   Introduction of gold seeds into organ NOC
Y36.2   Introduction of therapeutic implant into organ NOC
Y36.3   Radioactive seed implantation NOC
Y36.4   Introduction of non-removable radioactive substance into organ for brachytherapy NOC
Y36.8   Other specified
Y36.9   Unspecified

Y37 **Introduction of other substance into organ NOC**

Y37.1 Introduction of photodynamic substance into organ NOC
Includes: Instillation of photodynamic substance into organ NOC
Y37.8 Other specified
Y37.9 Unspecified

Y38 **Injection of therapeutic substance into organ NOC**

Y38.1 Continuous injection of therapeutic substance into organ NOC
Y38.8 Other specified
Y38.9 Unspecified

Y39 **Injection of other substance into organ NOC**

Y39.1 Injection of radiocontrast substance into sinus track from organ NOC
Includes: Injection of radiocontrast substance into fistula from organ NOC
Fistulogram NOC
Sinogram NOC
Note: Site specific chapter related code can be used only when precise identification
of organ from which sinus track or fistula originates is given
This does not include skin of site of original operation otherwise X55.8 should
be used
Y39.2 Other injection of radiocontrast substance into organ NOC
Y39.3 Injection of inert substance into organ NOC
Y39.4 Lipofilling injection into organ NOC
Y39.5 Tattooing of organ NOC
Includes: Tattooing of lesion of organ
Y39.8 Other specified
Y39.9 Unspecified

Y40 **Dilation of organ NOC**

Y40.1 Dilation of stricture of organ NOC
Y40.2 Stretching of organ NOC
Y40.3 Balloon dilation of organ NOC
Y40.8 Other specified
Y40.9 Unspecified

Y41 **Examination of organ NOC**

Y41.1 Examination of organ under anaesthetic NOC
Y41.2 Endoscopic ultrasound staging examination of organ NOC
Y41.3 Endoscopic ultrasound examination of organ NOC
Y41.8 Other specified
Y41.9 Unspecified

Y42 **Manipulation of organ NOC**

Y42.1 External manipulation of organ NOC
Y42.8 Other specified
Y42.9 Unspecified

Y67   **Harvest of other multiple tissue**

Y67.1   Harvest of composite of skin and cartilage from ear
         Excludes: Harvest of cartilage from ear (Y69.2)
Y67.2   Harvest of composite of skin and fat
         Includes: Harvest of dermis fat NEC
Y67.8   Other specified
Y67.9   Unspecified

Y69   **Harvest of other tissue**

Y69.1   Harvest of omentum
Y69.2   Harvest of cartilage from ear
Y69.3   Harvest of vein
Y69.4   Harvest of cartilage NEC
Y69.8   Other specified
Y69.9   Unspecified

Y70   **Early operations NOC**

Y70.1   Emergency operations NOC
Y70.2   Immediate operations NOC
Y70.3   First stage of staged operations NOC
Y70.4   Primary operations NOC
Y70.5   Temporary operations
Y70.8   Other specified
Y70.9   Unspecified

Y71   **Late operations NOC**

Y71.1   Subsequent stage of staged operations NOC
Y71.2   Secondary operations NOC
Y71.3   Revisional operations NOC
Y71.4   Failed minimal access approach converted to open
Y71.5   Failed percutaneous transluminal approach converted to open
Y71.6   Second revisional operation NOC
Y71.7   Third or greater revisional operation NOC
Y71.8   Other specified
Y71.9   Unspecified

Y73   **Facilitating operations NOC**

Y73.1   Cardiopulmonary bypass
Y73.2   Extracorporeal circulation NEC
Y73.3   Ventilatory support
Y73.4   Modified ultrafiltration adjunct to cardiopulmonary bypass
Y73.5   Circulatory arrest
Y73.6   Intraoperative fluid monitoring
Y73.8   Other specified
Y73.9   Unspecified

Y74	Minimal access to thoracic cavity
Y74.1	Thoracoscopically assisted approach to thoracic cavity
Y74.2	Thoracoscopic approach to thoracic cavity NEC
Y74.3	Robotic minimal access approach to thoracic cavity
	Includes: Robotic assisted minimal access approach to thoracic cavity
Y74.4	Thoracoscopic video-assisted approach to thoracic cavity
	Excludes: Approach to organ under video control NEC (Y53.6)
Y74.5	Mediastinoscopic approach to mediastinal cavity
Y74.8	Other specified
Y74.9	Unspecified

Y75	Minimal access to abdominal cavity
Y75.1	Laparoscopically assisted approach to abdominal cavity
Y75.2	Laparoscopic approach to abdominal cavity NEC
Y75.3	Robotic minimal access approach to abdominal cavity
	Includes: Robotic assisted minimal access approach to abdominal cavity
Y75.4	Hand assisted minimal access approach to abdominal cavity
Y75.5	Laparoscopic ultrasonic approach to abdominal cavity
	Excludes: Approach to organ under ultrasonic control NEC (Y53.2)
Y75.8	Other specified
Y75.9	Unspecified

Y76	Minimal access to other body cavity
	Includes: Minimal access to other body area
Y76.1	Functional endoscopic sinus surgery
Y76.2	Functional endoscopic nasal surgery
Y76.3	Endoscopic approach to other body cavity
Y76.4	Endoscopic ultrasonic approach to other body cavity
	Excludes: Approach to organ under ultrasonic control (Y53.2)
Y76.5	Robotic assisted minimal access approach to other body cavity
	Includes: Robotic minimal access approach to other body cavity
Y76.6	Endonasal endoscopic approach to other body cavity
	Excludes: Functional endoscopic nasal surgery (Y76.2)
Y76.7	Arthroscopic approach to joint
Y76.8	Other specified
Y76.9	Unspecified

Y78	Arteriotomy approach to organ under image control
Y78.1	Arteriotomy approach to organ using image guidance with fluoroscopy
Y78.2	Arteriotomy approach to organ using image guidance with computed tomography
Y78.3	Arteriotomy approach to organ using image guidance with ultrasound
Y78.4	Arteriotomy approach to organ using image guidance with image intensifier
Y78.5	Arteriotomy approach to organ using image guidance with video control
Y78.6	Arteriotomy approach to organ using image guidance with magnetic resonance imaging control
Y78.8	Other specified
Y78.9	Unspecified

Y79   **Approach to organ through artery**

Y79.1   Transluminal approach to organ through subclavian artery
          Includes: Transluminal approach to organ through axillary artery
Y79.2   Transluminal approach to organ through brachial artery
Y79.3   Transluminal approach to organ through femoral artery
Y79.4   Transluminal approach to organ through aortic artery
Y79.8   Other specified
Y79.9   Unspecified

ANAESTHETICS

Y80   **General anaesthetic**

Y80.1   Inhalation anaesthetic using muscle relaxant
Y80.2   Inhalation anaesthetic using endotracheal intubation NEC
Y80.3   Inhalation anaesthetic NEC
Y80.4   Intravenous anaesthetic NEC
Y80.5   Rapid sequence induction of anaesthetic
Y80.8   Other specified
Y80.9   Unspecified

Y81   **Spinal anaesthetic**

Y81.1   Epidural anaesthetic using lumbar approach
          Includes: Epidural anaesthetic NEC
Y81.2   Epidural anaesthetic using sacral approach
Y81.8   Other specified
Y81.9   Unspecified

Y82   **Local anaesthetic**
          Excludes: Local anaesthetics for ophthalmology procedures (C90)

Y82.1   Local anaesthetic nerve block
          Excludes: Destructive nerve block (Chapter A)
Y82.2   Injection of local anaesthetic NEC
Y82.3   Application of local anaesthetic NEC
Y82.8   Other specified
Y82.9   Unspecified

Y84   **Other anaesthetic**

Y84.1   Gas and air analgesia in labour
Y84.2   Sedation NEC
Y84.8   Other specified
Y84.9   Unspecified

Y89   **Brachytherapy**

Y89.1   High dose rate brachytherapy treatment
Y89.2   Pulsed dose rate brachytherapy treatment
Y89.8   Other specified
Y89.9   Unspecified

Y91 **External beam radiotherapy**

Y91.1 Megavoltage treatment for complex radiotherapy
Y91.2 Megavoltage treatment for simple radiotherapy
Y91.3 Superficial or orthovoltage treatment for radiotherapy
Y91.4 Megavoltage treatment for adaptive radiotherapy
Y91.5 Megavoltage treatment for hypofractionated stereotactic radiotherapy
Y91.8 Other specified
Y91.9 Unspecified

Y92 **Support for preparation for radiotherapy**

Y92.1 Technical support for preparation for radiotherapy
Y92.8 Other specified
Y92.9 Unspecified

Y93 **Gallium-67 imaging**

Y93.1 Gallium-67 imaging scan
Y93.8 Other specified
Y93.9 Unspecified

Y94 **Radiopharmaceutical imaging**
Excludes: Gallium-67 imaging (Y93)

Y94.1 Dopamine transporter scan
Y94.2 Octreotide imaging
Y94.3 Metaiodobenzylguanidine imaging
Y94.4 Diethylenetriamine pentacetic acid imaging
Y94.8 Other specified
Y94.9 Unspecified

Y95 **Gestational age**

Y95.1 Over 20 weeks gestational age
Y95.2 From 14 weeks to 20 weeks gestational age
Y95.3 From 9 weeks to < 14 weeks gestational age
Y95.4 Under 9 weeks gestational age
Y95.8 Other specified
Y95.9 Unspecified

Y96 **In vitro fertilisation**

Y96.1 In vitro fertilisation with donor sperm
Y96.2 In vitro fertilisation with donor eggs
Y96.3 In vitro fertilisation with intracytoplasmic sperm injection
Y96.4 In vitro fertilisation with intracytoplasmic sperm injection and donor egg
Y96.5 In vitro fertilisation with pre-implantation for genetic diagnosis
Y96.6 In vitro fertilisation with surrogacy
Y96.8 Other specified
Y96.9 Unspecified

Z59   **Muscle of foot**
           Includes: Tendon of muscle of foot

Z59.1   Flexor hallucis longus
Z59.2   Flexor digitorum muscle of foot
Z59.3   Short hallux muscle
Z59.4   Short sole muscle
Z59.5   Interosseous muscle of foot
Z59.6   Lumbrical muscle of foot
Z59.8   Specified muscle of foot NEC
Z59.9   Muscle of foot NEC

Z60   **Other muscle**
           Includes: Tendon of muscle NEC

Z60.1   Muscle of face
Z60.2   Muscle of neck
Z60.3   Muscle of anterior abdominal wall
Z60.4   Muscle of back
Z60.5   Muscle of chest
           Includes: Muscle of thorax
Z60.8   Specified muscle NEC
Z60.9   Muscle NEC

Z61   **Lymph node**
           Note: Principal category, extended at O14

Z61.1   Cervical lymph node
Z61.2   Scalene lymph node
Z61.3   Axillary lymph node
Z61.4   Mediastinal lymph node
Z61.5   Para-aortic lymph node
Z61.6   Inguinal lymph node
Z61.7   Retroperitoneal lymph node
Z61.8   Specified lymph node NEC
Z61.9   Lymph node NEC

Z62   **Other soft tissue**

Z62.1   Fascia
Z62.2   Lymphatic duct
Z62.3   Lymphatic tissue
Z62.4   Connective tissue
Z62.8   Specified soft tissue NEC
Z62.9   Soft tissue NEC

Z63   **Bone of cranium**
           Excludes: Mastoid (Z20.3)

Z63.1   Frontal bone
Z63.2   Parietal bone
Z63.3   Temporal bone
Z63.4   Occipital bone
Z63.8   Specified bone of cranium NEC
Z63.9   Bone of cranium NEC

Z64   **Bone of face**

Z64.1   Nasoethmoid complex of bones
Z64.2   Nasal bone
Z64.3   Zygomatic complex of bones
Z64.4   Maxilla
Z64.8   Specified bone of face NEC
Z64.9   Bone of face NEC

Z65   **Jaw**

Z65.1   Mandible
Z65.2   Temporomandibular joint
Z65.8   Specified jaw NEC
Z65.9   Jaw NEC

Z66   **Vertebra**

Z66.1   Atlas
Z66.2   Axis bone
Z66.3   Cervical vertebra
Z66.4   Thoracic vertebra
Z66.5   Lumbar vertebra
Z66.8   Specified vertebra NEC
Z66.9   Vertebra NEC

Z67   **Intervertebral joint**

Z67.1   Atlanto-occipital joint
Z67.2   Atlantoaxial joint
Z67.3   Cervical intervertebral joint
Z67.4   Thoracic intervertebral joint
Z67.5   Lumbar intervertebral joint
Z67.6   Lumbosacral joint
Z67.7   Sacrococcygeal joint
Z67.8   Specified intervertebral joint NEC
Z67.9   Intervertebral joint NEC

Z68   **Bone of shoulder girdle**

Z68.1   Clavicle
Z68.2   Acromion process of scapula
Z68.3   Coracoid process of scapula
Z68.4   Glenoid cavity of scapula
Z68.5   Scapula NEC
Z68.8   Specified bone of shoulder girdle NEC
Z68.9   Bone of shoulder girdle NEC

Z78   **Other bone of lower leg**

Z78.1   Shafts of tibia and fibula in combination
Z78.2   Head of fibula
Z78.3   Shaft of fibula NEC
Z78.4   Lateral malleolus
Z78.5   Lower end of fibula NEC
        Includes: Articular surface of fibula at ankle
Z78.6   Fibula NEC
Z78.7   Patella
Z78.8   Specified bone of lower leg NEC
Z78.9   Bone of lower leg NEC

Z79   **Bone of tarsus**

Z79.1   Talus
        Includes: Articular surface of talus at ankle
Z79.2   Os calcis
Z79.3   Navicular bone of foot
Z79.4   Cuboid bone
Z79.5   Cuneiform bone
Z79.8   Specified bone of tarsus NEC
Z79.9   Bone of tarsus NEC

Z80   **Other bone of foot**

Z80.1   First metatarsal
Z80.2   Metatarsal NEC
Z80.3   Phalanx of great toe
Z80.4   Phalanx of toe NEC
Z80.8   Specified bone of foot NEC
Z80.9   Bone of foot NEC

Z81   **Joint of shoulder girdle or arm**
        Note: For operations on one bone of joint use site code for bone in preference to site code for joint (Z68-Z80)

Z81.1   Sternoclavicular joint
Z81.2   Acromioclavicular joint
Z81.3   Glenohumeral joint
Z81.4   Shoulder joint
Z81.5   Elbow joint
Z81.6   Superior radioulnar joint
Z81.7   Inferior radioulnar joint
Z81.8   Specified joint of shoulder girdle or arm NEC
Z81.9   Joint of shoulder girdle or arm NEC

Z82   **Joint of wrist or hand**
        Note at Z81 applies

Z82.1   Radiocarpal joint
Z82.2   Intercarpal joint
Z82.3   Carpometacarpal joint of thumb
Z82.4   Carpometacarpal joint of finger
Z82.8   Specified joint of wrist or hand NEC
Z82.9   Joint of wrist or hand NEC

Z83   **Joint of finger**
            Note at Z81 applies

Z83.1   Metacarpophalangeal joint of thumb
Z83.2   Metacarpophalangeal joint of finger
Z83.3   Interphalangeal joint of thumb
Z83.4   Proximal interphalangeal joint of finger
Z83.5   Distal interphalangeal joint of finger
Z83.6   Interphalangeal joint of finger NEC
Z83.8   Specified joint of finger NEC
Z83.9   Joint of finger NEC

Z84   **Joint of pelvis or upper leg**
            Note at Z81 applies

Z84.1   Sacroiliac joint
Z84.2   Pubic symphysis
Z84.3   Hip joint
Z84.4   Patellofemoral joint
Z84.5   Tibiofemoral joint
Z84.6   Knee joint
Z84.8   Specified joint of pelvis or upper leg NEC
Z84.9   Joint of pelvis or upper leg NEC

Z85   **Joint of lower leg or tarsus**
            Note at Z81 applies

Z85.1   Upper tibiofibular joint
Z85.2   Lower tibiofibular joint
Z85.3   Talocalcaneal joint
Z85.4   Talonavicular joint
Z85.5   Calcaneocuboid joint
Z85.6   Ankle joint
Z85.8   Specified joint of lower leg or tarsus NEC
Z85.9   Joint of lower leg or tarsus NEC

Z86   **Other joint of foot**
            Note at Z81 applies

Z86.1   Midtarsal joint
Z86.2   Intertarsal joint
Z86.3   Tarsometatarsal joint
Z86.4   Metatarsophalangeal joint of great toe
Z86.5   Metatarsophalangeal joint of toe NEC
Z86.6   Interphalangeal joint of toe
Z86.8   Specified joint of foot NEC
Z86.9   Joint of foot NEC

Z87   **Other part of musculoskeletal system**

Z87.1   Bone NEC
Z87.2   Ligament of joint
Z87.3   Capsule of joint
Z87.4   Joint NEC
Z87.8   Specified part of musculoskeletal system NEC
Z87.9   Musculoskeletal system NEC

Z89   **Arm region**
> *Note:*   *Principal category, extended at O31*
> *These codes should not normally be used when more specific site codes may be identified (Z01-Z87)*

Z89.1   Shoulder NEC
Z89.2   Upper arm NEC
Z89.3   Forearm NEC
Z89.4   Hand NEC
Z89.5   Thumb NEC
Z89.6   Finger NEC
Z89.7   Multiple digits of hand NEC
Z89.8   Specified arm region NEC
Z89.9   Arm NEC

Z90   **Leg region**
> *Note at Z89 applies*
> *Note:*   *Principal category, extended at O13*

Z90.1   Buttock NEC
Z90.2   Hip NEC
Z90.3   Upper leg NEC
Z90.4   Lower leg NEC
Z90.5   Foot NEC
Z90.6   Great toe NEC
Z90.7   Toe NEC
Z90.8   Specified leg region NEC
Z90.9   Leg region NEC

Z91   **Other vein of upper body**
> *SEE ALSO Z39*

Z91.1   Cephalic vein
Z91.2   Brachiocephalic vein
Z91.3   Brachial vein
Z91.4   Subclavian vein
Z91.5   Axillary vein
Z91.8   Specified vein of upper body NEC
Z91.9   Vein of upper body NEC

Z92   **Other region of body**
> *Note at Z89 applies*
> *Note:*   *Principal category, extended at O16*

Z92.1   Head NEC
Z92.2   Face NEC
Z92.3   Neck NEC
Z92.4   Chest NEC
Z92.5   Back NEC
Z92.6   Abdomen NEC
Z92.7   Trunk NEC
Z92.8   Specified region of body NEC
Z92.9   Region of body NEC

Z93   **Other veins of pelvis**
            SEE ALSO Z39

Z93.1   Iliac vein
Z93.2   Ovarian vein
Z93.3   Testicular vein
Z93.4   Vulval vein
Z93.5   Uterine vein
Z93.8   Specified vein of pelvis NEC
Z93.9   Vein of pelvis NEC

Z94   **Laterality of operation**

Z94.1   Bilateral operation
Z94.2   Right sided operation
Z94.3   Left sided operation
Z94.4   Unilateral operation
Z94.8   Specified laterality NEC
Z94.9   Laterality NEC

Z95   **Other branch of thoracic aorta**
            Note: Principal Z36
Z95.1   Intercostal artery
Z95.2   Bronchial artery
Z95.3   Ulnar artery
Z95.4   Radial artery
Z95.5   External carotid artery
Z95.6   Common carotid artery
Z95.7   Internal carotid artery
Z95.8   Specified other branch of thoracic aorta NEC
Z95.9   Other branch of thoracic aorta NEC

Z96   **Other lateral branch of abdominal aorta**
            Note: Principal Z37

Z96.1   Gastroduodenal artery
Z96.2   Pancreaticoduodenal artery
Z96.3   Lumbar artery
Z96.4   Ovarian artery
Z96.5   Pudendal artery
Z96.6   Uterine artery
Z96.7   Testicular artery
Z96.8   Specified other lateral branch of abdominal aorta NEC
Z96.9   Other lateral branch of abdominal aorta NEC

Z97   **Other terminal branch of aorta**
            Note: Principal Z38

Z97.1   Anterior tibial artery
Z97.2   Posterior tibial artery
Z97.3   Peroneal artery
Z97.4   Dorsalis pedis artery
Z97.5   External iliac artery
Z97.6   Iliac artery NEC
Z97.7   Tibial artery NEC
Z97.8   Specified other terminal branch of aorta NEC
Z97.9   Other terminal branch of aorta NEC

Z98   **Other veins of lower limb**
           SEE ALSO Z39
           Excludes: Saphenous vein unspecified (Z39.5)

Z98.1   Common femoral vein
Z98.2   Deep femoral vein
Z98.3   Superficial femoral vein
Z98.4   Popliteal vein
Z98.5   Long saphenous vein
Z98.6   Short saphenous vein
Z98.7   Tibial vein
Z98.8   Specified vein of lower limb NEC
Z98.9   Vein of lower limb NEC

Z99   **Intervertebral disc**

Z99.1   Intervertebral disc of cervical spine
Z99.2   Intervertebral disc of thoracic spine
Z99.3   Intervertebral disc of lumbar spine
Z99.8   Specified intervertebral disc NEC
Z99.9   Intervertebral disc NEC

O11 **Other upper digestive tract**
Note: Principal Z27

O11.1   Gastro-oesophageal junction
O11.8   Specified other upper digestive tract NEC
O11.9   Other upper digestive tract NEC

O12 **Branch of external carotid artery**
Excludes: External carotid artery (Z95.5)

O12.1   Superficial temporal artery
O12.2   Maxillary artery
O12.8   Specified branch of external carotid artery
O12.9   Branch of external carotid artery NEC

O13 **Other leg region**
Note at Z89 applies
Note: Principal Z90

O13.1   Multiple digits of foot NEC
O13.2   Knee NEC
O13.8   Specified other leg region NEC
O13.9   Other leg region NEC

O14 **Other lymph node**
Note: Principal Z61

O14.1   Pelvic lymph node
O14.2   Sentinel lymph node
O14.8   Specified other lymph node NEC
O14.9   Other lymph node NEC

O16 **Body region**
Note at Z89 applies
Note: Principal Z92

O16.1   Pelvis NEC
O16.2   Spine NEC
O16.8   Specified body region NEC
O16.9   Body region NEC

O28 **Other cerebral artery**
Note: Principal Z35

O28.1   Basilar artery
O28.8   Specified other cerebral artery NEC
O28.9   Other cerebral artery NEC

O30 **Other large intestine**
Note: Principal Z28

O30.1   Hepatic flexure
O30.2   Splenic flexure
O30.8   Specified other large intestine NEC
O30.9   Other large intestine NEC

O31 **Other arm region**
Note at Z89 applies
Note: Principal Z89

O31.1 Wrist NEC
O31.8 Specified other arm region NEC
O31.9 Other arm region NEC

O33 **Bone of skull**
Excludes: Bone of cranium (Z63)
Bone of face (Z64)
Jaw (Z65)

O33.1 Skull base
O33.8 Specified bone of skull NEC
O33.9 Bone of skull NEC